Gaining Knowledge and Skills with Dyslexia and other SpLDs

'Great! This is a book for dyslexic/SpLD people about strategies for gaining knowledge (input, storage), and about accessing and demonstrating knowledge (recall, output). The book allows you to navigate the content in your own way and be rewarded with personally relevant information. It encourages you to develop your "tool bag for living confidently". Exploring the useful preface and glossary guides you around the content of this book and links you to others in the series. I have been using techniques Ginny taught me for many years.'
– **Dr Mary Eld, former SpLD student of Ginny Stacey, UK**

Gaining Knowledge and Skills with Dyslexia and other SpLDs lays the foundation for skilling dyslexic/ SpLD people so that they can be autonomous, confident people, who can use their full potential with minimal disruption from the dyslexia/ SpLD. It is a comprehensive manual for helping dyslexic/ SpLD people, whether the help is given by specialist teachers, subject teachers, professionals of all kinds, family and friends, or the general public such as shop keepers. There are lists of the most important ideas for policy-makers and general readers so that they can support best practice for helping dyslexic/ SpLD people. The book advocates changes of attitude that will be good for everyone but which are VITAL for dyslexic/ SpLD people. It is not proposing expensive solutions, though it does recognise that there will be times when accommodation is needed for some effects of dyslexia/ SpLD that an individual cannot work round.

The book recognises that dyslexia/ SpLDs are variable syndromes that need constant monitoring. Given a range of skills and knowledge to draw on, a dyslexic/ SpLD person needs to be able to select the most suitable ones for any particular situation.

Confidence grows when dyslexia/ SpLD can be managed well;
dyslexic/ SpLD people can then function at their best.

The book is addressed to someone alongside a dyslexic/ SpLD person, who may also be dyslexic/ SpLD, so the style of the book is suitable for dyslexic/ SpLD people. It uses a special layout to emphasise stories, insights, examples, exercises, tips, key points and summaries.

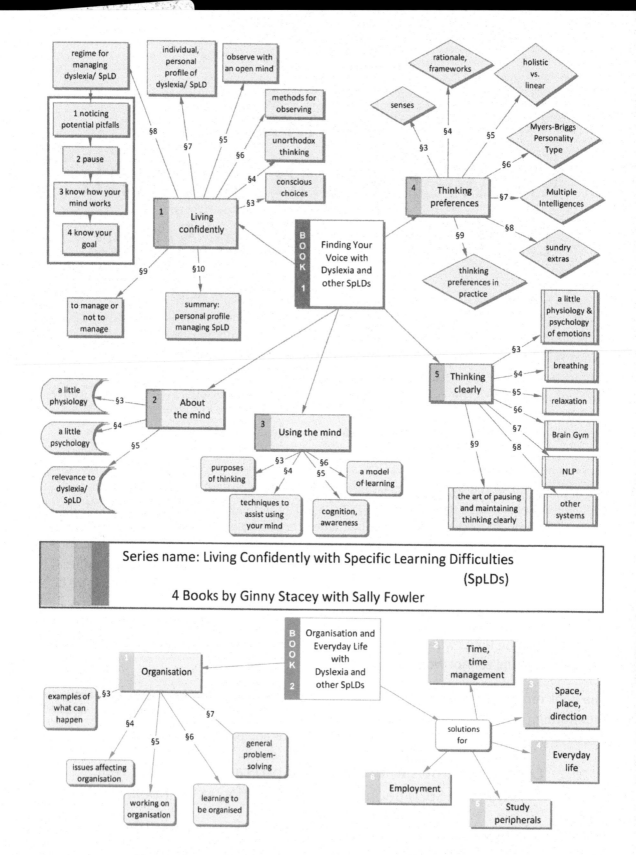

Series name: Living Confidently with Specific Learning Difficulties (SpLDs)

4 Books by Ginny Stacey with Sally Fowler

Different, larger maps of each book: Book 1: p 33; Book 2: p 35

Contents p xvi   Where to start p viii

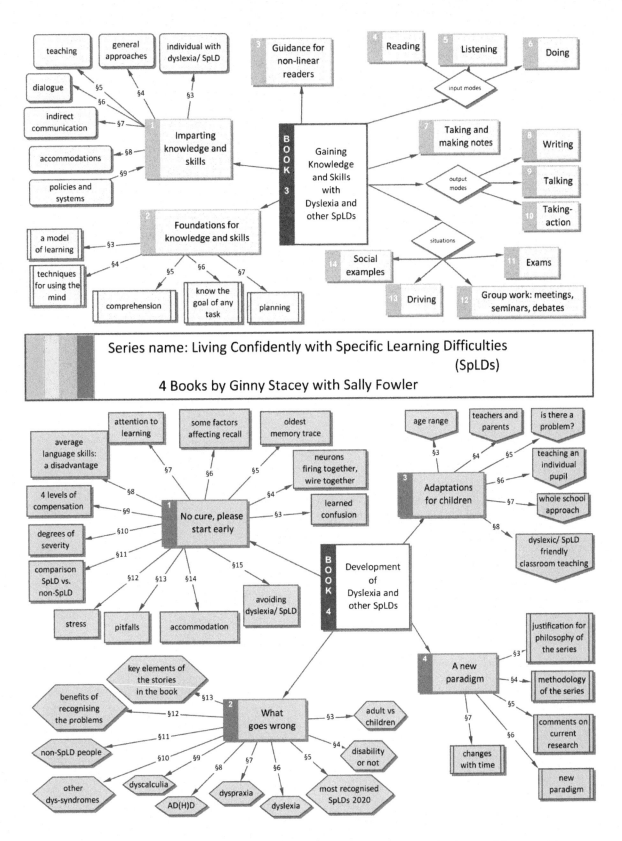

Book 3: Gaining Knowledge and Skills with Dyslexia and other SpLDs

1 Imparting knowledge and skills
- §5 teaching
- §6 dialogue
- §7 indirect communication
- §8 accommodations
- §9 policies and systems
- §4 general approaches
- §3 individual with dyslexia/ SpLD

2 Foundations for knowledge and skills
- §3 a model of learning
- §4 techniques for using the mind
- §5 comprehension
- §6 know the goal of any task
- §7 planning

3 Guidance for non-linear readers

input modes
- 4 Reading
- 5 Listening
- 6 Doing

output modes
- 7 Taking and making notes
- 8 Writing
- 9 Talking
- 10 Taking-action

situations
- 11 Exams
- 12 Group work: meetings, seminars, debates
- 13 Driving
- 14 Social examples

Series name: Living Confidently with Specific Learning Difficulties (SpLDs)

4 Books by Ginny Stacey with Sally Fowler

Book 4: Development of Dyslexia and other SpLDs

1 No cure, please start early
- §3 learned confusion
- §4 neurons firing together, wire together
- §5 oldest memory trace
- §6 some factors affecting recall
- §7 attention to learning
- §8 average language skills: a disadvantage
- §9 4 levels of compensation
- §10 degrees of severity
- §11 comparison SpLD vs. non-SpLD
- §12 stress
- §13 pitfalls
- §14 accommodation
- §15 avoiding dyslexia/ SpLD

2 What goes wrong
- §3 adult vs children
- §4 disability or not
- §5 most recognised SpLDs 2020
- §6 dyslexia
- §7 dyspraxia
- §8 AD(H)D
- §9 dyscalculia
- §10 other dys-syndromes
- §11 non-SpLD people
- §12 benefits of recognising the problems
- §13 key elements of the stories in the book

3 Adaptations for children
- §3 age range
- §4 teachers and parents
- §5 is there a problem?
- §6 teaching an individual pupil
- §7 whole school approach
- §8 dyslexic/ SpLD friendly classroom teaching

4 A new paradigm
- §3 justification for philosophy of the series
- §4 methodology of the series
- §5 comments on current research
- §6 new paradigm
- §7 changes with time

Different, larger maps of each book: Book 3: p 37; Book 4: p 39

First published 2021
by Routledge
2 Park Square, Milton Park, Abingdon, Oxon OX14 4RN

and by Routledge
52 Vanderbilt Avenue, New York, NY 10017

Routledge is an imprint of the Taylor & Francis Group, an informa business

British Library Cataloguing-in-Publication Data
A catalogue record for this book is available from the British Library

Library of Congress Cataloging-in-Publication Data
Names: Stacey, Ginny, author. | Fowler, Sally (Dyslexia), author.
Title: Gaining knowledge and skills with dyslexia and other SpLDs /
Ginny Stacey with Sally Fowler.
Description: Abingdon, Oxon ; New York, NY : Routledge, 2021. | Series:
Living confidently with specific learning difficulties (SpLD) ; book 3 |
Includes bibliographical references and index. |
Identifiers: LCCN 2020049567 (print) | LCCN 2020049568 (ebook) |
ISBN 9781138202436 (hardback) | ISBN 9781138202443 (paperback) |
ISBN 9781315461137 (ebook)
Subjects: LCSH: Dyslexics--Life skills guides. | Learning disabled--Life skills guides.
Classification: LCC RC394.W6 S732 2021 (print) | LCC RC394.W6 (ebook) |
DDC 616.85/53--dc23
LC record available at https://lccn.loc.gov/2020049567
LC ebook record available at https://lccn.loc.gov/2020049568

ISBN: 978-1-138-20243-6 (hbk)
ISBN: 978-1-138-20244-3 (pbk)
ISBN: 978-1-315-46113-7 (ebk)

Typeset in Calibri
by Ginny Stacey

Publisher's Note
This book has been prepared from camera-ready copy provided by the author.

Visit the companion website www.routledge.com/cw/stacey

Gaining Knowledge and Skills with Dyslexia and other SpLDs

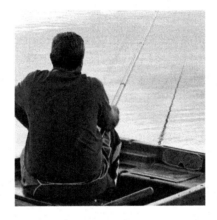

The fisherman recalls the saying:
'Give a man a fish and you feed him for a day;
teach a man to fish and you feed him for a lifetime.'

Ginny Stacey
with Sally Fowler

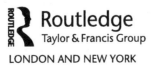
Routledge
Taylor & Francis Group

LONDON AND NEW YORK

'Having dyslexia/SpLD means thinking, learning and doing things differently. This is exemplified skilfully by the layout of the book. It both appeals to different reading styles and shows others that these styles exist. An expert, Ginny gives information, examples and explanations that are essential for anyone working to enable and support a dyslexic/SpLD individual. It is a comprehensive and practical guide, with skills and strategies that transfer to several contexts (studying, the workplace and everyday life).'
– *Henrietta Court MSc; OCR DipSpLD; TPC (PATOSS), Adult Dyslexia/SpLD specialist, UK*

'Ginny's zen-like understanding of the workings of the human mind has been laid bare in this book, which helped me to achieve far higher than I ever thought was possible in my studies.'
– *William Darby, MEng, MSC, former student of Ginny Stacey*

'I've often thought that publishing books to help dyslexic people is a bit of a paradox – that is until I read Ginny's book. Here at last is information that allows for the diversity of its readership's reading preferences; there's meaningful use of colour, chunked text, clearly isolated tips and insights, etc. Possibly best of all, there's an opportunity to guide one's personal reading interest at will so that interesting bits that appeal individually can be got at without a lot of bother. Awesome! Ginny advises that neurodiverse learners will benefit from "being careful, particularly at the beginning of something new" and this holds true for this book. Take time to orientate yourself in its Preface to learn how the book is set out and then dip in where your fancy takes you. The advice the book offers is based on years of experience and insightful expertise. Ginny is right to thank all her students; working through this book, her readers will thank her back tenfold.'
– *Tanya Zybutz, Dyslexia Co-ordinator, Royal Central School of Speech and Drama, UK*

Ginny Stacey did not realise she was dyslexic until her mid-20s. The challenge of learning to play classical guitar helped her to understand how her dyslexic mind works. Committed to helping other dyslexics achieve their potential, she developed a range of highly effective techniques for supporting dyslexic students in studying all subjects and coping with life in general. The techniques are widely used in universities and colleges. She has become a nationally-recognised expert in the field.

Sally Fowler stepped into the dyslexic world in her late 40s. It was a revelation to see the impacts of her dyslexia clearly. She became an approved teacher for the British Dyslexia Association with an M.A. in special education. She taught dyslexics, both children in schools and students at university. In Oxford, she met Ginny Stacey: the collaboration of two dyslexic minds has brought a wealth of experience to the *Living Confidently with Specific Learning Difficulties* series.

<u>Dedication</u>

Dear fellow dyslexics,

The laughter we've shared tells me I'm on the right lines with my understanding of dyslexia. So do:

- the tears some of you have shed as you tell me your story and you know I hear
- the courage you've shown as you reveal your vulnerable side
- the joy you've known as you find ways to take charge of your dyslexia and run with it, not against it.

I hope this book will help many others to find their way through the trials and tribulations of dyslexia/ SpLD so that they can come out the other side to enjoy some of the good parts of being dyslexic/ SpLD.

SpLD = Specific Learning Difficulty
       dyslexia
       dyspraxia
       AD(H)D
       dyscalculia
see Ⓖ p 573 for descriptions

Where to start:

- ### Linear readers, who like to read straight through:

In *USEFUL PREFACE*:

➤ Read *THIS BOOK: GAINING KNOWLEDGE AND SKILLS WITH DYSLEXIA AND OTHER SPLDS*.

➤ *THE SERIES: LIVING CONFIDENTLY WITH SPECIFIC LEARNING DIFFICULTIES (SPLDS)*, unless you have read another book of this series.

➤ Read sections marked with this book's icon.

Then read from Chapter 1.

- ### Non-linear readers, who prefer to move around a book:

A) Read the boxes in the *USEFUL PREFACE*
B) Choose one of these 5 suggestions:

1   Read the coloured boxes throughout the book and see what takes your interest.
2   Use the *INDEX* to find topics that interest you.
3   Use *DIPPING-IN TO TRY OUT IDEAS*, §1, in each chapter to find the most important topics.
4   Randomly move through the book to find what takes your interest.
5   Use the *EXERCISE: INITIAL PURPOSE FOR READING* to create your own list of what you want to read first.

THIS BOOK: GAINING KNOWLEDGE AND SKILLS WITH DYSLEXIA AND OTHER SPLDS:
p 26

THE SERIES: LIVING CONFIDENTLY WITH SPECIFIC LEARNING DIFFICULTIES (SPLDS):
p 31

USEFUL PREFACE:
p 0

EXERCISE: INITIAL PURPOSE FOR READING: p 17

Tip: Reading Styles

It is useful to think about how you read.
See *DIFFERENT WAYS TO READ*: p 12

---

§ = subsection

Ⓖ = *GLOSSARY*

= Companion website
www.routledge.com/cw/stacey

Tip: This is a book to dip into. Solid reading is not necessary.

About the coloured boxes

Meaning of Box Colours

There are coloured boxes throughout the book:

 orange for stories

orange for insights

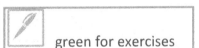 green for exercises

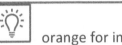 light blue for examples

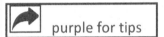 purple for tips

 chapter purple for key points and summaries

dark blue for text and diagrams

Contents of boxes:

     story: a narrative
     insight: story with added information; or an important point
     tip: contains a suggestion to help you make progress
     example: usually more general than a story; sometimes directly expanding
          on some part of the preceding text
     exercise: instructions to try out some idea(s)

Flow of boxes

The boxes are part of the text. They are often split across pages.

Tip: Finding Information

The *INDEX* is organised alphabetically, with some particularly useful groups of entries listed at the beginning.

The Glossary Ⓖ has all the acronyms and symbols, as well as explanations of words and phrases. Page numbers are given for the relevant sections.

Summary of the chapters

Chapter 1 Imparting Knowledge and Skills

The first part of the chapter deals with issues about individual dyslexic/ SpLD people that may need to be taken into account when imparting knowledge and skills to them. It then divides imparting knowledge and skills into: teaching, dialogue and indirect communication. It includes typical roles of people involved; what can go wrong when the impacts of dyslexia/ SpLD are ignored; and what changes can be made so that dyslexic/ SpLD people can gain knowledge and skills with minimum disruption from their individual dyslexia/ SpLD.

Chapter 2 Foundations for Knowledge and Skills

This chapter deals with basic elements of learning and dealing with information. It includes: where to start working with them; techniques for using the mind; comprehension; recognising goals; and planning.

Chapter 3 Guidance for Non-Linear Readers

Chapters 4 – 14 are practical discussions about helping dyslexic/ SpLD people. The guidance for non-linear readers, *DIPPING-IN TO TRY OUT IDEAS,* would be identical in all the chapters, so it has been put together in this chapter; it is a pattern for efficiently finding the information you want from any material. Individual chapters list important sections to read or scan.

Input Modes: Chapter 4 Reading   Chapter 5 Listening   Chapter 6 Doing

Chapter 4: Reading includes: reading mechanisms, with a section about reading electronic devices; reading effectiveness improved by pleasure in reading or a high level of interest; preparation; strategies; problems and proof-reading.
Chapter 5: Listening is covered in terms of experiences, preparation and strategies.
Chapter 6: Doing, as a mode of learning, is covered in terms of different attitudes (liking or disliking), preparation, strategies and problems.

Chapter 7 Taking and Making Notes

Taking notes is important for immediately capturing information; making them is for longer-term uses. The chapter discusses the processes involved; the uses of notes; and keeping them. It ends with examples of a wide range of styles for notes.

Output modes: Chapter 8 Writing   Chapter 9 Talking   Chapter 10 Taking-Action

The chapters include: **Chapter 8:** Writing: fluency; different forms of writing; proof-reading and language.
Chapter 9: Talking: fluency; preparation; consideration of listeners; the environment; structure and discussion.

Chapter 10: Taking-action to use knowledge and skills: review of processes involved; no stopping point; major projects; and applying and adapting skills.

Situations: Chapter 11 Exams   Chapter 12 Group Work: Meetings, Seminars and Debates Chapter 13 Driving   Chapter 14 Social Examples: travel, job application, eating out and finances

These chapters look at the various situations in terms of applying knowledge and skills to deal with them. Group Work, Chapter 12, is set out in a way that can be readily adapted to many other situations.

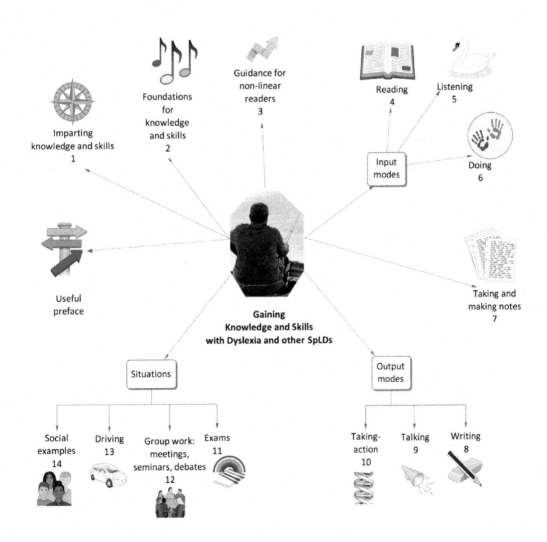

Acknowledgements

These books are the result of working with many, many dyslexia/ SpLD people since 1991. They have told me their stories; they have explored new ways of doing things; they have passed on the solutions they have found. I have worked with a few people with other disabilities or none. It has been a great adventure learning from them all.

I've also had conversations with many other people, sometimes deliberately, sometimes by chance – like a 20 minute conversation with a fellow passenger on a train. The books have benefitted from the ideas generated by the conversations.

My grateful thanks go to all these people.

I'd also like to thank colleagues in The Oxford SpLD Tutor Group, those at The University of Oxford and Oxford Brookes University for formal and informal exchange of ideas and experience. The network of support that we have between colleagues allows us to provide a high quality of support to the people we work with.

Several friends and colleagues have proof-read chapters for me in the final stages. Their comments have been very useful in clarifying the expression of my ideas. Sometimes their comments have re-enforced my view that the experience of dyslexia/ SpLD is foreign to the non-dyslexic/ SpLD world. If my expression occasionally seems strange to you, please wonder whether I'm saying something about dyslexia/ SpLD that is hard for a non-dyslexic/ SpLD person to understand since their minds simply don't give them the same experience.

I'm especially indebted to David Bullock who made 3 structures to lift my laptop, extended monitor, mouse and keyboard so that I worked standing and kept my brain's arousal system alert. Without these structures I would have struggled against the way words and my dyslexia send me to sleep. The final stages of preparing these books would have been months of awful struggle instead of the excitement I experienced.

I'd like to thank my family for their patience during the writing of these books. My husband deserves special mention for his encouragement, patience and his shed, which was my writing shed for many years.

Routledge and Taylor & Francis have been very patient with the time taken to convert the original single book into four standalone books. My commissioning editor, Lucy Kennedy, the assistant editor, Lottie Mapp, the production team leaders, Siân Cahill and Alison Macfarlane, and the proof-reader, Jackie Dias, have all done their best to understand and accommodate the unorthodox needs of dyslexic/ SpLD readers and my needs as a dyslexic author. My thanks to everyone who has been involved with this project.

I'd like to thank Carl Wenczek, of Born Digital Ltd, for tuition and much advice on dealing with my illustrations. I couldn't have managed all the visual components and figures without his guidance.

I have been extremely fortunate to benefit from Mike Standing's experience as a retired production manager of a printing company. He came and guided me through many details of the printing process as I undertook author typesetting of these books. Without his input, the typesetting process would have been a horrible struggle.

And finally, my thanks go to Sally Fowler who has accompanied me throughout the writing of the series. When I've been daunted or hit a blank patch, Sally's encouragement and enthusiasm have carried me through. Without Sally's belief in this work, the project would not have been finished.

Illustrations

Illustration acknowledgements and key to symbols

❖	Complete figures created using Inspiration® 9, a product of Inspiration Software®, Inc.
✍	Photos or drawings created by Ginny Stacey.
O	Material by Routledge/ Taylor & Francis.
☞	Other figures whose sources are acknowledged in the text.

Throughout the book

❖	Mind maps for *USEFUL PREFACE* and all the chapters
O	The icons for the series, books and chapters were created by Routledge/ Taylor & Francis and inserted into the mind maps or other diagrams as appropriate

Contents

 Useful Preface   This is worth reading

 Marks sections where some or all of the text is specific to this book.

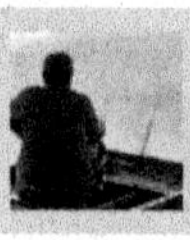

Chapter 1 Imparting Knowledge and Skills

➢ = Book 1; ♈ = Book 2; ♓ = Book 4

➢, ♈ and ♓ mark sections that are discussed more fully in other books of this series. Key ideas are included here to support suggestions made in this book.

Chapter 1 Imparting Knowledge and Skills *continued*

➤ = Book 1; ♈ = Book 2; ⚹ = Book 4

➤, ♈ and ⚹ mark sections that are discussed more fully in other books of this series. Key ideas are included here to support suggestions made in this book.

Chapter 2   Foundations for Knowledge and Skills

➤ marks sections that are discussed more fully in Book 1 of this series.
Key ideas are included here to support suggestions made in this book.

Chapter 2   Foundations for Knowledge and Skills   *cont'd*

➢ marks sections that are discussed more fully in Book 1 of this series.
Key ideas are included here to support suggestions made in this book.

Chapter 3   Guidance for Non-Linear Readers

Chapter 4   Reading

Chapter 4   Reading   *continued*

3   Mechanics of reading (visual strategies) 234

    3.1   Eye movement   234

    3.2   Meaning-related groups of words   237

    3.3   De-coding   237

    3.4   Colour   237

    3.5   Font   239

4   Reading from a computer, e-reading 240

5   Reading for pleasure 242

6   Preparation for reading 243

    6.1   Mind set before reading   244

    6.2   Thinking clearly   245

    6.3   Distractions   245

    6.4   Unfamiliar words   246

7   Strategies for reading 246

    7.1   Pay attention to small print   248

7.2   List of strategies involving *Thinking Preferences*   248

7.3   Verbal strategies   249

7.4   Searching for meaning   249

7.5   Kinaesthetic strategies   251

8   Reading problems 252

    8.1   Author's style   253

    8.2   Comments about grammar   254

    8.3   Punctuation   255

    8.4   Negatives can be complex   256

    8.5   Background to the material   258

    8.6   Mind engaged on another topic   258

    8.7   Other reading problems   259

9   Proof-reading   259

10   PhotoReading 260

References and website information 261

Chapter 5   Listening

Mind map and contents 262

List of key points and summaries 263

Templates on the website 263

Information for non-linear readers 263

1   Dipping-in to try out ideas: reading and scanning lists 263

    1.1   Key points: for policy-makers and general readers   264

2   Context 264

3   Different experiences 267

4   Mentally storing dialogue 269

5   Consequences from misinterpretation 269

6   Preparation for listening 271

7   Strategies for listening 275

8   Listening problems 276

9   Listening to body language 278

10   Summary: check-list for discussion about listening 279

References and website information 279

Chapter 6   Doing

 ## Chapter 7   Taking and Making Notes

Chapter 8   Writing

 # Chapter 9   Talking

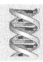

Chapter 10   Taking-Action

Chapter 11   Exams

Chapter 12   Group Work: Meetings, Seminars and Debates

 Chapter 13   Driving

 Chapter 14   Social Examples

Chapter 14   Social Examples   *continued*

 Appendix 1 Resources

 Appendix 2 Individual, Personal Profile of Dyslexia/ SpLD and Regime for Managing Dyslexia/ SpLD

Appendix 3 Key Concepts

Glossary

List of Templates on the Website

Index

Useful Preface
This is worth reading

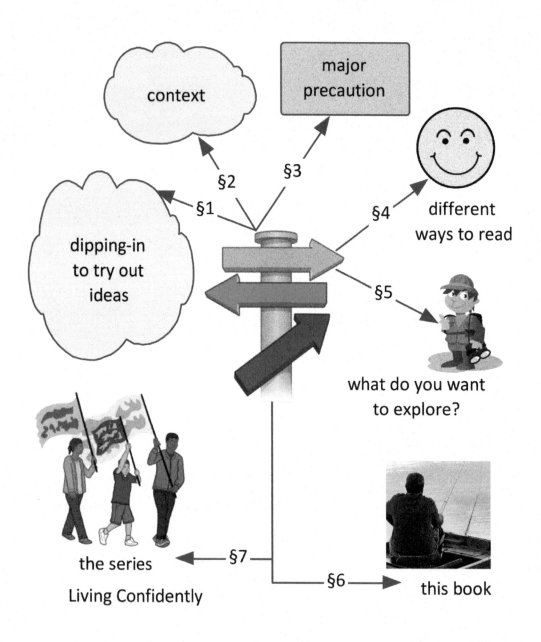

context

major precaution

§2

§3

§1

§4

different ways to read

dipping-in to try out ideas

§5

what do you want to explore?

the series

Living Confidently

§7

§6

this book

Contents

Ⓖ p 573: SpLD: specific learning difficulty of which dyslexia is the best known and most widely researched

Insight: What to expect from this book

A comprehensive discussion, with stories and suggestions, of how to enable dyslexic/ SpLD people:

- to gain knowledge and skills
- to maximise their individual potential
- to minimise the effects of their dyslexia/ SpLD.

The book covers teaching, dialogue and production of indirect materials as channels through which dyslexic/ SpLD people gain knowledge and skills.

The book includes education, employment and everyday life since dyslexia/ SpLD affects all areas of life. The dyslexic/ SpLD people you enable or encounter may be:

- your students
- your clients and customers
- your friends or family members
- your work colleagues or fellow hobbyists
- people for whom you make policies or programmes
- people for whom you produce materials
- people on behalf of whom you campaign
- people with whom you have one-off conversations.

Use of pronouns in this book

The books in this series are conversations. I don't know whether you, the reader, are dyslexic/ SpLD or not. For the sake of consistency, I am writing as if you are helping someone else. The usual question arises of what pronoun to use for the person you are helping; he, she, they and all the relevant variations (3rd person pronouns).

Dyslexic/ SpLD people are all very different. To refer to the whole group often doesn't fit reality. Sometimes, I need to refer to a single person, who may not be the person you are helping. Once it was thought there were 4 male dyslexics for every 1 female, but that ratio has not stood the test of time and a significant number of female dyslexic/ SpLDs have been identified.

My decisions for the 3rd person pronouns are:

- to avoid combinations such as he/ she, with one exception*
- to be consistent about the gender within one chapter
- to alternate genders (he and she) between chapters
- to use the plural (they) when appropriate.

*I have used he/ she in CHAPTER 3, GUIDANCE FOR NON-LINEAR READERS, because the chapter could be used with any of chapters 4 – 14.

GUIDANCE FOR NON-LINEAR READERS: p 222

Some of the boxes are addressed specifically to dyslexic/ SpLD people; it's the only way they make sense. They are marked with the green bar on the left hand margin. This information is also in the GLOSSARY, Ⓖ .

Ⓖ p 572

The phrase 'your student'

The dyslexic/ SpLD person you are helping, or thinking about, may not be a student. He/ she could be a friend, an employee, a colleague, family member or have any other relationship with you.

The language involved in keeping this wide range of possibilities in mind would be very clumsy and not easy to read. Therefore, the phrase 'your student' has been used in this book to signify a dyslexic/ SpLD person that you are thinking about or helping with the aid of the book.

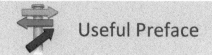

Useful Preface Summary

This preface is similar in the four books.

The book icon shows the sections that are particular to this book. The left margin blue line shows the length of these sections.

§1, *DIPPING-IN TO TRY OUT IDEAS,* suggests a quick way through.

§2, *CONTEXT,* shows my positive approach to dyslexia/ SpLD.

§3, *MAJOR PRECAUTION,* is about avoiding an increase in the effects of anyone's dyslexia/ SpLD.

§4, *DIFFERENT WAYS TO READ,* is a first look at some of the issues with reading and will help you to read in different ways.

§5, *WHAT DO YOU WANT TO EXPLORE?,* will help you decide how you want the book to help you.

§6, *THIS BOOK: GAINING KNOWLEDGE AND SKILLS WITH DYSLEXIA AND OTHER SPLDS,* sets the scene for this book.

§7, *THE SERIES: LIVING CONFIDENTLY WITH SPECIFIC LEARNING DIFFICULTIES,* gives a broad brush synopsis of the four books with details of the aims, outcomes and benefits.

Templates on the website

A1   *JOTTING DOWN AS YOU SCAN*
A2   *BOOKMARK – PURPOSE*
A4   *JOTTING DOWN AS YOU READ*
A5   *COLLECTING IDEAS THAT INTEREST YOU*
B1   *COLLECTING IDEAS THAT RELATE TO YOU* (specially for readers who are themselves dyslexic/ SpLD)

Use the recording templates to develop your use of the ideas in this book:
B5-8   *RECORDING TEMPLATES - 1-4*

TEMPLATES

COMPANION
@
WEBSITE

CHECK-LISTS FOR READERS describes the purposes of the following check-lists:

CHECK-LISTS FOR READERS: p 21

H2   *CHECK-LIST ABOUT GENERAL BACKGROUND*

H3   *AUDITS OF UNDERSTANDING AND SKILLS – FOR AN INDIVIDUAL DYSLEXIC/ SPLD PERSON*

H4   *CHECK-LIST FOR DIRECT SUPPORT*

H5   *CHECK-LIST FOR GENERAL TEACHING*

H6   *CHECK-LIST FOR PROFESSIONAL PEOPLE EXERCISING RESPONSIBILITY OR AUTHORITY*

H7   *CHECK-LIST FOR POLICY-MAKERS, CAMPAIGNERS AND MEDIA PERSONNEL*

H8   *CHECK-LIST FOR INDIRECT COMMUNICATORS*

Appendix 1   Resources

COLLECTING INFORMATION TOGETHER has ideas to help you be systematic about the way you gather information together.

COLLECTING INFORMATION TOGETHER: p 526

1   Dipping-in to try out ideas

Read *INSIGHT BOX: WHAT TO EXPECT FROM THIS BOOK,* above.

Read *§3, MAJOR PRECAUTION.*

§3: p 10

Ask your students to do the *EXERCISE: AVOID MORE PROBLEMS WHEN LEARNING NEW SKILLS.* Discuss their responses with them.

EXERCISE: AVOID MORE PROBLEMS ...: p 11

Read the 3 boxes in *§2, CONTEXT.*

Scan *§4, DIFFERENT WAYS TO READ,* then do the *EXERCISE: READING STYLE, §4.1.*

§2: p 6
§4: p 12
§4.1: p 14

Read *§4.2, SOMETHING GOES WRONG WITH READING.*

§4.2: p 14

Read *TIP: KNOW YOUR REASON FOR READING, §5.*

Do the *EXERCISE: INITIAL PURPOSE FOR READING* in *§5.1.*

§5: p 15
§5.1: p 17

2 Context

Story: Two dyslexic sailors

Scene: sailing on a yacht belonging to John. I had to learn the sequence for turning on the engine safely.

"I just can't do it that way! I know how my mind works. I've been teaching in the field for ages. You've got to listen to me! Let me ask my questions. Let me understand. Then I will be able to do it."

The frustration of being faced with another dyslexic person who WILL NOT LISTEN!

Both of us are fairly stubborn because we've individually worked out what we need to do to succeed and we're both teachers in different fields. We just don't happen to have the same thinking preferences.

In this situation, I'm slightly at a disadvantage because I'm the novice in John's field and there's no way either of us want me to go into my professional role to analyse his strategies.

We simply both want me to learn to switch the engine on.

If I hadn't found my voice, there was no way I could find my way through my friend's view of how to learn (but see *MARGIN NOTE*).

MARGIN NOTE:
I appreciated John's approach when he used it to help me up and down a 604m climb beside a Norwegian fjord.

As we learn we change the workings of our minds. There are changes at the neuron level of the brain. Efficient learning results in good neural networks. The following analogy helps you to think about neural networks.

Ⓖ p 575: neural networks

Insight: Park paths and pruning neurons

If a park has no fences round it, people will walk across in many different directions.

If a park has 2 gates on opposite sides of the park, people will walk across in a straight line between the gates. A definite path will show where the grass is worn away.

If the park has several gates either side, there will be a series of paths linking the various gates.

When a baby is born, the brain is like the unfenced park: few routes have been established through the brain to respond to the world around.

As a result of good learning, definite neuronal networks become established with use; this is the result of neuronal pruning. The single path is the analogy for non-dyslexia/ SpLD.

The park with several gates either side and many paths linking them is the analogy for dyslexia/ SpLD.

Ⓖ p 575:
pruning, neuron

Neuronal pruning:
Kolb (1995)

The philosophy of this series

The philosophy of this series of books is that we, dyslexic/ SpLD people, can work out how our minds work, we can direct our thinking so that it is as effective as possible and we can enjoy contributing to the situations that we find ourselves in (see *MARGIN NOTE*).

We then have ownership of our thinking and actions. We can achieve to the level of our individual potential. We can confidently take our place alongside everyone else in the situations in which we find ourselves.

MARGIN NOTE: As so often, this is good practice for everyone, but VITAL for dyslexic/ SpLDs.

We know how to *MANAGE OUR DYSLEXIA/ SpLD*. We can co-operate with others to minimise the effects of our dyslexia/ SpLD on our own lives and on the lives of those who live, work or engage in action with us.

REGIME FOR MANAGING DYSLEXIA/ SpLD:
p 540

Dyslexia/ SpLD is not seen as a static phenomenon, like short sightedness that only slowly changes with time. Dyslexia/ SpLD is seen as a collection of chaotic[1] neural networks that can exist alongside more useful networks.

Once the chaotic neural networks have established, dyslexia/ SpLD has developed. The chaotic neural networks are not destroyed when the more useful networks are established; they can lie dormant for a significant amount of time; they can be triggered into use in different ways. However well you manage it, you are always at risk of being as thoroughly dyslexic/ SpLD as ever.

The collection of chaotic neural networks will vary from person to person, even with the same dyslexia/ SpLD label.

ⓖ p 575:
neural networks

Underlying the networks is a constitutional level of difference, which, when ignored, leads to the establishment of the chaotic neural networks. The constitutional level of difference is the permanent part of dyslexia/ SpLD. The chaotic neural networks are the source of the observed, problematic behaviours.

A child born with the differences at the constitutional level is 'at risk' of dyslexia/ SpLD. When recognised early in the development of learned networks, the constitutional differences do not have to lead to chaotic neural networks, though it may be impossible to prevent all of them. The unorthodox thinking processes that many successful dyslexic/ SpLDs enjoy will still develop, since they

[1]Chaos theory: when asked to spell a word, many dyslexic people have a collection of possibilities, for example sense, sens, cens, sns, scens. Each of these possibilities is the product of neural networks that connect the prompt to spell the word to the action of spelling it. By practice of the 'correct spelling' these alternative spellings are expected to be reduced (pruned) to only one, resulting in a stable neural network to achieve the correct spelling. That dyslexics continue throughout life with the variable spelling, shows this pruning isn't working for them and the implied collection of neural networks behind the variations is what I mean by 'chaotic neural networks'. The idea comes from my understanding of chaos theory (Gleick, 1997).

ⓖ p 575: chaos theory

are needed very early in learning to prevent establishment of the chaotic neural networks.

John is typical of many successful dyslexic/ SpLDs who have got through life without any special attention. They may have used:

John is in *Two Dyslexic Sailors:* p 5

- hard work
- sheer determination (John: bloody-mindedness)
- winging it
- the gift of the gab
- secretaries, parents, spouse or partner, children, friends
- one or two teachers with just the right approach
- pot luck
- apprenticeships, or other routes to the top from the shop floor, etc.
- 'other' (always a necessary option; it's listed in the *Index*).

Index: p 589

Whatever the route, they succeeded and they don't see what all the fuss is about now. They are the lucky ones; they made it to success. Many of their contemporaries didn't achieve very much; they can be dissatisfied with life and what they contribute.

Dyslexia/ SpLD, education and beyond

The educational system used to have elements that suited dyslexic/ SpLDs better than current systems do, and it was possible to get promotion without having to produce certificates that showed what qualifications you had.

There are changes afoot, but not ones that look likely to take us back to a regime that will suit most dyslexic/ SpLDs.

Society, workplace practices and education may change to be more sympathetic to dyslexic/ SpLD people (and to those with other disabilities); assistive technology allows access to modern communication systems; but without finding her own voice a dyslexic/ SpLD person isn't fully the person she could be; in using that voice to communicate with others she needs listeners who can hear what she is saying: these last two objectives are the main aims of this series.

Proverb: 'Give a man a fish and you feed him for a day; teach a man to fish and you feed him for a lifetime.'

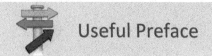

3 Major precaution

Protection from further dyslexic/ SpLD problems is an important aspect of managing dyslexia/ SpLD.

Insight: Anything 'new' needs care

Your student needs to be very careful in the initial stages of a subject, or situation, even before she starts to make sense of it. She can too easily create an unhelpful memory that interrupts her thinking for a very long time.

Example: A problem created at an initial stage

After some 20 years of playing the guitar, my sight reading is still impaired by an early mistake.

One note (B on the treble clef) is an open string for a beginner, i.e. no left hand finger is needed to play it. In musical notation, this note is a blob with a line through it (it is the middle line of the treble clef).

'Blob on a line' equated to 'finger on a string' when I first met it, and it still does. I still have to work really hard to remember the note is an open string; I have to work hard to stop myself putting a finger on a string.

I didn't know then how to manage my dyslexia. Now I know that I have to be careful, particularly at the beginning of something new.

Exercise for student: Avoid more problems
when learning new skills[2]

- What were the skills you learnt most recently?
- How did you learn them?
- What task was involved?
- How important are the skills to you?
- What made them easy to learn?
- What was hard about learning them?
- How easily have you been able to adapt the skills to other uses?

Reflection question: Is it a good idea to try out something new on tasks that are really important to you?

- It is OK if you can easily make changes to the way you do something later.

- It is not OK if you find the first way you tackle something leaves a strong impression.

- If this is your experience, try out new systems or skills on tasks that you don't mind about too much but that you are quite interested in.

- It is not OK if you are likely to think: "Can I trust this new approach? Will it muck up this task or topic?" Doubt like this will not allow you to explore the new approach freely.

- If in any doubt, use a task or topic that doesn't matter too much first; struggling with dyslexic/ SpLD tangles is such a pain, it's worth avoiding new problems.

- You won't give a new skill or system a fair trial, if you are worried about it or the task.

This green colour is recommended for colour blind people on the website of Okabe and Ito (Accessed 29 Jan 2017)

---

[2] The way many dyslexic/ SpLD people have to pay attention to learning may mean first learning makes more of an impression than it does for other learners.

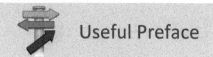
4 Different ways to read

You may be dyslexic/ SpLD and not like reading, many don't.
Do take notice of the message in *SOMETHING GOES WRONG WITH READING:*
the author's style can cause problems.

SOMETHING GOES WRONG WITH READING:
p 14

Tip: Margin

You can use the right-hand margin to jot down your ideas as you scan or read the book.

I have used it for cross-referencing and for references to help you find these when you want them.

The books in this series are written with several different styles of reading in mind.

You need to decide what your style of reading should be; do *EXERCISE: READING STYLE.* You may find a new style that suits you. Different styles might suit you at different times or for different purposes.

MARGIN NOTE: the different ways of reading relate to *THINKING PREFERENCES:* p 72 and in *INDEX*

EXERCISE: READING STYLE: p 14

The reading style is in green;
the writing styles in this book are in blue.

Linear readers People who read easily, starting at the beginning of a book.

The books are written with a flow of information that can be read from beginning to end.

Spatial readers People who would read best by moving about a book, finding the most relevant parts first.

Each chapter starts with a *DIPPING-IN* section that helps the reader choose the best way to dip-in.

Framework readers People who need an overview to be able to understand. Some people's brains don't retain information unless they have thought about the framework, or schema, that holds it all together.

Ⓖ p 575: framework schema

Framework readers *continued*	The *PHILOSOPHY OF THIS SERIES* is one framework of the series.	*PHILOSOPHY OF THIS SERIES:* p 7
	Each chapter has a contents list and a mind map at the beginning to help people understand the author's overview.	
	RATIONALE, OR FRAMEWORK outlines the importance of establishing a schema.	*RATIONALE OR FRAMEWORK:* p 563
Sense-oriented readers	Some people's understanding is dependent on the sense(s) they use. They may not use the senses equally. Vision, hearing and the kinaesthetic sense are the most commonly used ones in education. People vary: of these three senses, sometimes one or another is very much more used, or one may be decidedly less used than the other two. Smell and taste are also senses and may need to be considered.	Senses: visual, hearing, kinaesthetic
		Ⓖ p 575: kinaesthetic *MARGIN NOTE:* The kinaesthetic sense uses body perception and physical movement to good effect
	1) Visually: different layouts are used to indicate different types of information. For example: exercises for the reader are in green boxes. Cartoons and figures are used.	
		visual: p 74 and in *INDEX*
	2) Hearing related: the language is direct, not complicated, but elegant (at least that is the intention).	hearing (verbal): p 74 and in *INDEX*
	3) Kinaesthetic: there are exercises for the reader which should engage the kinaesthetic sense; as should the anecdotes about the actions of others.	kinaesthetic: p 74 and in *INDEX*
Interest-oriented readers	Some people use their strongest interests in order to understand; they cannot retain information if these interests are not actively engaged.	
	1) Some ideas about innate interests are listed in *MOTIVATION* in terms of Myers-Briggs Personality Type and Multiple Intelligences. Any reader for whom motivation is a key issue should use the ideas to work out what their particular motivation might be and deliberately use it while reading these books.	*MOTIVATION:* p 563

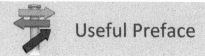
Interest-oriented readers *continued*	2) Material can be written bearing in mind different motivations by presenting different perspectives. The suggested *ROUTES* on the *WEBSITE* for various reader groups are examples of catering for different perspectives.

ROUTES

Further comment	If two or more people are using the book together, the different styles of reading should be accommodated.

4.1   Exercise: reading style

Exercise: Reading style

Consider which styles of reading might suit you:

    Why might they suit you?

    Which have you tried already?

    Which work most of the time/ sometimes/ never?

    Which sound worth experimenting with?

    What do you know already about your way of reading?

See examples in *DIFFERENT WAYS TO READ:* p 12

4.2   Something goes wrong with reading

If a dyslexic/ SpLD person is struggling with reading, it is important to check whether there is anything that can be done about it.

For example, going to sleep over reading can indicate that the brain is taking in too much material that has not been understood properly.

There are many approaches to make reading effective that do not involve the mechanics of reading. The full discussion is in *READING*. The discussion includes ways in which an author's style of writing is unhelpful to dyslexic/ SpLDs.

READING: p 230

Insight: External factors hamper reading

Reading difficulties can be made a lot worse by the way the text is written or presented. They aren't just from your dyslexia/ SpLD.

Insight: Word changes cause doubt

Some authors don't like to repeat the same word too many times, so they change the word even though the idea hasn't changed.

Do you ever find that you then start to doubt your reading ability? It's as if your mind is worrying because you may have missed some significant detail that the change of words indicates. Then gradually, your reading skill deserts you; you struggle; you end up sleeping over the text, even when you are very interested in it.

Sometimes in this series, I have deliberately not changed words, even though the repetition is rather tedious.

5 What do you want to explore?

One key tactic for making reading easier is to prime your mind, rather like warming up muscles. No serious sportsman would start their sport without warming up their muscles. The mind can be looked after in the same way.

>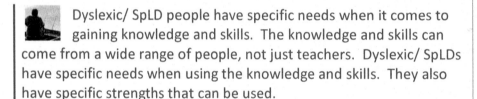
>
> **Tip: Know your reason for reading**
>
> When you identify your main purpose for reading anything, you give your mind some guidelines for understanding what you are reading.
>
> You then allow yourself to explore the text, looking to satisfy your purpose; reading is much easier.

Dyslexic/ SpLD people have specific needs when it comes to gaining knowledge and skills. The knowledge and skills can come from a wide range of people, not just teachers. Dyslexic/ SpLDs have specific needs when using the knowledge and skills. They also have specific strengths that can be used.

Ginny Stacey and Sally Fowler are both dyslexic, in different ways!

This book is worth reading because:

- it suggests how to explore the specific needs and strengths of individual dyslexic/ SpLD people in relation to gaining knowledge and skills
- it considers different means of assisting dyslexic/ SpLD people
- it sets out a wide range of people who assist
- it sets out a range of people who are interested in good practice and value for money
- it discusses fundamental aspects of learning knowledge and skills that assist dyslexic/ SpLD people
- it discusses strategies for, and problems with the major forms of communication:
    - reading and writing
    - listening and speaking
    - doing and taking-action (kinaesthetic communication)
- it discusses the problems and strategies for some everyday tasks, such as driving or dealing with finances

MARGIN NOTE: the kinaesthetic route is often neglected, therefore attention is drawn to it here.

- it discusses policies to enable the practices that are VITAL for dyslexic/ SpLD people and GOOD PRACTICE for all.

Any of these topics in the book could be part of your purpose for reading.

5.1 Initial purpose for reading

The following exercise is designed to help establish any reader's initial purpose: you are effectively creating your own dipping-in list.

Exercise: Initial purpose for reading

TEMPLATES

1 Use the *TEMPLATE: A1 - JOTTING DOWN AS YOU SCAN* to keep track of ideas.
  1.1 Remember you are scanning for this exercise, not reading. You are finding the sections most interesting to you now.

2 Scan the following places to find ideas that catch your interest:
  2.1 point 1.1 above, to remember to scan
  2.2 the orange insight boxes in this chapter
  2.3 the *TABLE OF READER GROUPS, §5.2*
  2.4 the themes in *§5.3, READING TO FIND OUT ABOUT A THEME*
  2.5 *§6, THIS BOOK: GAINING KNOWLEDGE AND SKILLS WITH DYSLEXIA AND OTHER SPLDS*
  2.6 *§7, THE SERIES: LIVING CONFIDENTLY WITH SPECIFIC LEARNING DIFFICULTIES (SPLD)*
  2.7 the *CONTENTS* of the book
  2.8 the *INDEX*.

§5.2: p 18

§5.3: p 23

§6: p 26

§7: p 31

CONTENTS: p xv

INDEX: p 589

3 For each idea that catches your attention:
  3.1 note where in the book the idea is
  3.2 why the idea interests you
  3.3 how important the idea is to you immediately and in the longer-term.

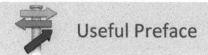

4   Think about your life:
   4.1   What issues to do with dyslexia/ SpLD do you want to
         understand or solve?
   4.2   What situations in everyday life, employment or study are
         affected by your dyslexia/ SpLD, or might be affected?

NB: you are creating your personal dipping-in list.

5   Look at the list of ideas you have made.
   5.1   Are there any common threads that could be grouped
         together? Use *TEMPLATES: A5 - COLLECTING IDEAS THAT INTEREST
         YOU* or *B1 - COLLECTING IDEAS THAT RELATE TO YOU* to gather the
         common threads.
   5.2   Number the ideas in the order that you would like to explore
         them now.
   5.3   Write the ideas on the *TEMPLATE: A2 - BOOKMARK – PURPOSE* in
         the order that you want to explore them. The *BOOKMARK –
         PURPOSE* will remind you what you have decided to explore.

TEMPLATES

6   Start reading. Use *TEMPLATE: A4 - JOTTING DOWN AS YOU READ*, or any
    other template, to capture insights as you read.

5.2 Reader groups

One way of giving your mind the guidelines that assist reading is to
recognise why you want to acquire any new information.

I have thought about different reader groups with different means of
imparting knowledge and skills to dyslexic/ SpLD people.

These are shown below in the *BOX: READER GROUPS,* together with the
sections in *IMPARTING KNOWLEDGE AND SKILLS* which discuss their
interactions with dyslexic/ SpLD people.

I have also included people who are using knowledge of dyslexia/ SpLD to affect society's attitude to dyslexia/ SpLD.

- Politicians and policy-makers need to know about the best ways to impart knowledge and skills to dyslexic/ SpLD people because they enable it to happen.
    - They need to listen accurately to what dyslexic/ SpLD people and their supporters are saying.
    - They need to make policies and regimes based on what actually achieves good outcomes; Peter Hyman's book, *1 Out of 10: From Downing Street Vision to Classroom Reality* (2005) makes this case very well in the education setting.

- People in the media and people concerned with disability issues also need to listen to dyslexic/ SpLD people and their supporters.
    - They need to bring to the attention of the general public the best ways of helping dyslexic/ SpLD people gain knowledge and skills.
    - They need to support those politicians and policy-makers who are working to enable best practice.

Hyman (2005)

Reader groups	Relevant section
specialist support tutors SENCOs ⓖ p 574 SENCO school subject teachers university and evening class teachers, etc. sports coaches, etc. teachers and parents of dyslexic/ SpLD children	*TEACHING:* p 85
professional people, people in authority or having responsibility people living with, working with, taking-action with dyslexic/ SpLD people	*DIALOGUE:* p 107

Reader groups	Relevant section
writers of public communications, e.g. exam writers people providing a service people dealing with indirect communication	*INDIRECT COMMUNICATION:* p 119
policy-makers, politicians, people in the media, people concerned with disability issues	*POLICY-MAKERS, CAMPAIGNERS AND MEDIA PERSONNEL:* p 112
readers in of all these groups could be dyslexic/ SpLD themselves	

Decide which reader group(s) you belong to.

Why do you choose the group(s)?

What information are you looking for? Use *READING TO FIND OUT ABOUT A THEME*, below, and *AIMS, OUTCOMES AND BENEFITS* to help you decide.

AIMS, OUTCOMES AND BENEFITS: p 27

Dyslexic/ SpLD readers

As well as belonging to one or more of the reader groups above, you may have a formal diagnostic assessment or you may suspect you belong to the dyslexic/ SpLD group. You will be both the reader who is helping and the dyslexic/ SpLD person being helped. Working with this book could provide you with the opportunity to recognise and understand what happens to you as a result of your dyslexia/ SpLD. Build any insights into your own *INDIVIDUAL, PERSONAL PROFILE OF DYSLEXIA/ SPLD* and your own *REGIME FOR MANAGING DYSLEXIA/ SPLD* and take the opportunity to become more autonomous.

INDIVIDUAL, PERSONAL PROFILE OF DYSLEXIA/ SPLD: p 540
REGIME FOR MANAGING DYSLEXIA/ SPLD: p 540

Ⓖ p 575
autonomous

5.2.1 Check-lists for readers

TEMPLATES

COMPANION @ WEBSITE

It is often useful to have a check-list of ideas to make sure you cover everything. The following reflect different situations in which you might be with dyslexic/ SpLD people or might want to know more about dyslexia/ SpLD.

Check-list and description	Sections of interest
H1: *CHECK-LIST FOR RESEARCHERS AND ASSESSORS* This check-list enables you to reflect on the wider impacts of dyslexia/ SpLD.	*INDIVIDUALS WITH DYSLEXIA/ SPLD:* p 57 *DIALOGUE:* p 107 *WHAT COULD HAPPEN AND USEFUL, RELEVANT SECTIONS:* P 464
H2: *CHECK-LIST ABOUT THE GENERAL BACKGROUND* This check-list is about understanding dyslexia/ SpLD issues and about using dyslexia/ SpLD-friendly approaches, in particular about the way you give information to dyslexic/ SpLD people.	*INDIVIDUALS WITH DYSLEXIA/ SPLD:* p 57 *WHAT COULD HAPPEN:* p 464-470 *GENERAL ISSUES ABOUT TEACHING:* p 85 *DIALOGUE SECTIONS §§6.4-6.8:* p 111-118 *MODEL OF LEARNING:* p 145 *GENERAL APPROACHES:* p 81
H3: *AUDITS OF UNDERSTANDING AND SKILLS – FOR AN INDIVIDUAL DYSLEXIC/ SPLD PERSON* I often do an audit with students whom I support to find out what they know about their dyslexia/ SpLD and how it affects them and what skills they can develop to be able to maximise their potential and minimise the disruption from the dyslexia/ SpLD. This check-list includes the areas I might cover. As with all things, not everything will be relevant to all dyslexic/ SpLD people.	*INDIVIDUALS WITH DYSLEXIA/ SPLD:* p 57 *GENERAL APPROACHES:* p 81 *GENERAL ISSUES ABOUT TEACHING:* p 87 *ACCOMMODATIONS:* p 128 *MODEL OF LEARNING:* p 145 *FOUNDATIONS FOR KNOWLEDGE AND SKILLS:* p 134 To select appropriate sections from the rest of the book, use: *INDEX:* p 589 *CONTENTS:* p xv
H4: *CHECK-LIST FOR DIRECT SUPPORT* This check-list is about approaches for delivering support in one-to-one situations. It should be used in conjunction with *H3: AUDITS OF UNDERSTANDING AND SKILLS.*	*BEHIND THE OBVIOUS:* p 64 *TEACHING:* p 85 *THINKING PREFERENCES:* p 72 *DIALOGUE:* p 107

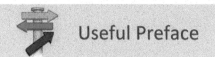

Check-list and description	Sections of interest
H5: CHECK-LIST FOR GENERAL TEACHING This check-list will help teachers to reflect on the way their teaching enables dyslexic/ SpLD students and how their materials can be dyslexic/ SpLD-friendly. It is based on an open approach to teaching dyslexic/ SpLD students in general settings.	*MODEL OF LEARNING:* p 145 *DIALOGUE:* p 107 *FOUNDATIONS FOR KNOWLEDGE AND SKILLS:* p 134 *THINKING PREFERENCES:* p 72 Summaries in chapters 4 - 12, from the list in *INDEX:* p 589
H6: CHECK-LIST FOR PROFESSIONAL PEOPLE EXERCISING RESPONSIBILITY OR AUTHORITY This check-list is about avoiding misunderstandings that could materially impact the lives of dyslexic/ SpLD people.	*DIALOGUE:* p 107 *BEHIND THE OBVIOUS:* p 64 *SUPPLEMENTARY ISSUES:* p 68 *THINKING PREFERENCES:* p 72 *BUILDING CONFIDENCE AND SELF-ESTEEM:* p 78
H7: CHECK-LIST FOR POLICY-MAKERS, CAMPAIGNERS AND MEDIA PERSONNEL This check-list covers the important issues for changes in society, rules and regulations to enable dyslexic/ SpLD people to contribute at the level of their potential, unhampered by the dyslexia/ SpLD.	*MODEL OF LEARNING:* p 145 *KEY POINTS: FOR POLICY-MAKERS AND GENERAL READERS,* see list in *INDEX:* p 589 *INDIVIDUALS WITH DYSLEXIA/ SPLD:* p 57 *GENERAL ISSUES ABOUT TEACHING:* p 87 *DIALOGUE:* p 107
H8: CHECK-LIST FOR INDIRECT COMMUNICATORS This check-list covers the issues that can make a significant improvement in the ease with which dyslexic/ SpLD people can access information.	*INDIRECT COMMUNICATION:* p 119 *MODEL OF LEARNING:* p 145 *INDIVIDUALS WITH DYSLEXIA/ SPLD:* p 57

B4:   *ACTION, RESULTS, NEXT STEP*

B5-8:   *RECORDING TEMPLATES - 1-4*

B11:   *MONITORING PROGRESS*

These templates can be used to develop the use of any ideas in the above check-lists. Suggestions for using these templates are given in the instructions for the check-lists.

5.3   Reading to find out about a theme

You may be a dyslexic/ SpLD reader and as such find it easier to read focusing on a particular theme of dyslexia/ SpLD that you want to explore first.

In thinking how a dyslexic/ SpLD person might approach the material, I put together several different themes. The themes relevant to this book are listed below. The full list of *THEMES* in the series is on the *WEBSITE*, along with where to find the discussions.

THEMES

The themes that are relevant to this book include:

- the individuality of dyslexic/ SpLD people

- exploring with each one:
    - learning needs
    - thinking strengths
    - core issues of problems and solutions

- different means of assisting dyslexic/ SpLD people
    - teaching
    - conversation and dialogue
    - indirect communication, e.g. written materials or online or signs

- a wide range of people who assist through contact
    - their roles
    - what can go wrong when the impacts of dyslexia/ SpLD are ignored
    - the approaches they can adopt to help dyslexic/ SpLD people learn knowledge and skills as effectively as possible with minimum impact from their dyslexia/ SpLD

- people who put in place the policies and systems that facilitate the practices which are VITAL for dyslexic/ SpLDs and GOOD for all

- people who publicise best practice for dyslexic/ SpLD people

- fundamental aspects of learning knowledge and skills that assist dyslexic/ SpLD people to:
    - learn and recall them
    - use and develop them

- strategies for the major forms of communication and the problems that can occur:
    - Input modes:
        - reading
        - listening
        - doing (kinaesthetic)

MARGIN NOTE: the kinaesthetic route is often neglected, therefore attention is drawn to it here.

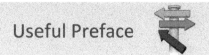

- output modes:
  - writing
  - speaking
  - taking-action (kinaesthetic)

MARGIN NOTE: see *MARGIN NOTE* on previous page.

- the problems and strategies for
  - making notes
  - exams
  - group work: meetings; seminars; debates
  - driving
  - social situations: travel; job application; eating out; finances

The themes for the rest of the series come under the general headings of:

Living with confidence:
- individual, personal profile of dyslexia/ SpLD
- regime for managing dyslexia/ SpLD

The impact of dyslexia/ SpLD on everyday life and resolving any problems

Problems arising from dyslexia/ SpLD:
- their persistence
- the manifest behaviours

Avoiding the development of problems
- teaching younger children
- a new paradigm for teaching programmes

6 This book: *Gaining Knowledge and Skills with Dyslexia and other SpLDs*

This book is about helping dyslexic/ SpLD people gain knowledge and skills to become autonomous, in study, employment and everyday life. It is also about helping them use the knowledge and skills.

Ⓖ p 575
autonomous

It is important to include everyday life because dyslexia/ SpLDs only have one brain and mind, so the effects noticed in study and employment also impact on all the activities of everyday life: shopping, hobbies, sport, gardening, socialising, to name but a few.

There is a wide range of professionals who might be helping dyslexic/ SpLD people; the level of understanding needed will vary. People who work or live alongside dyslexic/ SpLD people are also likely to contribute to the knowledge and skills gained. People who design or write indirect communications can help by using techniques that assist dyslexic/ SpLD people.

For simplicity of style, many sections are written as if you, the reader, are helping someone, 'a student', to become more proficient. It contains ideas that will help you to understand how to help your dyslexic/ SpLD student and why she might need the specific help; it also contains what you can teach her so that she can gain knowledge and skills more easily.

The green line in the left-hand margin indicates paragraphs that are predominantly ideas to teach or discuss with your student. This information is also in the GLOSSARY, Ⓖ. You will need to select those ideas that are relevant to her and will help her.

Ⓖ p 572

The people helping are often themselves dyslexic/ SpLD, so the methods of writing in this book still cater for non-linear readers.

Dyslexia and the other SpLDs can be problems, but then so can many other things in life. 'A problem shared is a problem halved' is an idiom you can look up in a dictionary or online. To do the sharing, both the speaker and the listener need to understand the issues.

Insight: From problems to solutions

One client came to talk over how she deals with her dyslexia.

She was clear about her problems and the ways she deals with them in practical terms, but she didn't have an overview of how her strategies fitted together and how to adapt to new situations.

At the end she told me, "It's great to be understood. Not to keep explaining yourself. To move on and find solutions."

Knowing How To Find Solutions
Leads To
Confident Dyslexic/ SpLD People.

6.1 Aims, outcomes and benefits

Aims

People teaching dyslexic/ SpLDs, or working with them, or living alongside them, will know how to help them:

- gain knowledge and skills
- become autonomous individuals in charge of their dyslexia/ SpLD
- maintain confidence and self-esteem.

Ⓖ p 575
autonomous

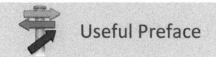

Policy-makers and politicians will recognise the value of the approaches that help dyslexic/ SpLD people to maximise their potential and minimise the effects of their dyslexia/ SpLD.

People in the media and concerned with disability issues will understand the approaches that help dyslexic/ SpLD people; they will be willing to promote them and support people using them and putting them in place.

Insight: Ultimate aim for an individual

A dyslexic/ SpLD person knows how and when to look for ways to deal with any situation that occurs in her life in the confidence that she can maximise the use of her innate potential and minimise the effects of her dyslexia/ SpLD.

Her general attitude at the end of the process is almost:

- OK, I'm dyslexic/ SpLD; I really enjoy the way I process information, the way I am;

- everyone has some problems, mine just happen to have a label;

- there's no big deal; I'll do well 'with a little help from my friends'.

Insight: Ultimate aim for society

Conversations about dyslexia/ SpLD that result in changes of attitudes and policies will involve:

- informed policy-makers and informed people in society
- confident dyslexic/ SpLD people with good self-esteem however reliably they manage their dyslexia/ SpLD.

'Nothing about us without us' or 'Talk to us and with us' will be easier to achieve with knowledgeable people on both sides of the majority-/ minority-group divide.

Outcomes

Those helping, supporting and interacting with dyslexic/ SpLD people will:

- know the potential undesirable outcomes from the impacts of dyslexia/ SpLD

- know what to do to establish and maintain good communications whether
    - by teaching
    - in dialogue with
    - by producing materials for indirect communication

- be better equipped to talk openly with dyslexic/ SpLD people about problems and solutions

- know how to help dyslexic/ SpLD people use their best potential and minimise the effects of their individual dyslexia/ SpLD.

Policy-makers, politicians, people in the media and people concerned about disability issues will:

- recognise that much of the VITAL practice for dyslexic/ SpLDs is GOOD practice for all
- understand that it is cost effective for these practices to be in place throughout education and that, as a result, there are savings in other sections of society.

Policy-makers and politicians will:

- be willing to put the policies and systems in place that will embed the VITAL practices so that they become the norm.

People in the media and people concerned about disability issues will:

- be willing to promote the policies and systems
- support those who put them in place and who use them.

Benefits

Dyslexic/ SpLD people who have been helped in a way that's individually right for them will confidently:

- use their best potential to study and to contribute to work and everyday life
- manage the effects of their dyslexia/ SpLD by
    - taking prompt action to contain the effect at the level of glitch
    - using strategies to deal with hazards
    - negotiating accommodation to deal with insuperable obstacles.

Ⓖ p 575 glitch, hazard, obstacle

Misunderstandings arising from the effects of dyslexia/ SpLD will be easier to resolve.

The financial and emotional costs to society will be reduced.

The full benefits will come from using the other books in this series, too.

7 The Series: *Living Confidently with Specific Learning Difficulties (SpLDs)*

7.1 Readership/ audience

Living Confidently with Specific Learning Difficulties (SpLDs) is a series of books that look at the whole of the experience of living with these Specific Learning Difficulties.

Descriptions in Ⓖ
p 573 of 4 SpLDs:
dyslexia
dyspraxia
AD(H)D
dyscalculia

The ideas described in this series draw on work over 25 years helping individuals to find out how their minds work and how to use them effectively in study or everyday life.

Finding Your Voice with Dyslexia and other SpLDs and *Organisation and Everyday Life with Dyslexia and other SpLDs* are both written addressing dyslexic/ SpLD people.

Gaining Knowledge and Skills with Dyslexia and other SpLDs and *Development of Dyslexia and other SpLDs* both address people in roles alongside a dyslexic/ SpLD person.

Each book can be used on its own, but there are some concepts that spread over the four. The KEY CONCEPTS are summarised in APPENDIX 3.

APPENDIX 3: p 554

7.2 Summary of the series

Life is a journey. We need to find our way through it.

We need our own voice to help us navigate.

Living Confidently with Specific Learning Difficulties (SpLDs) is about living life to the full and enjoying the journey, each person using her maximum potential and minimising the effects of her dyslexia/ SpLD.

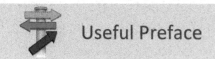

Book 1: *Finding Your Voice with Dyslexia and other SpLDs* (Stacey, 2019)

The book is written for dyslexic/ SpLD people and contains:

- building a personal, individual profile
    - thinking preferences
    - pitfalls
    - ways to pause well
    - accommodations

- four steps for managing dyslexia/ SpLD
    - recognising your pitfalls
    - pausing
    - using your thinking preferences
    - knowing your goal

- ideas from physiology and psychology that
    - relate to dyslexia/ SpLD
    - help make sense of some effects of dyslexia/ SpLD

- techniques for using the mind well
    - mind set
    - chunking
    - recall
    - memory consolidation
    - concentration
    - metacognition
    - objective observation
    - reflection
    - making connections
    - prioritising

- thinking preferences
    - sense-based: visual, verbal, kinaesthetic
    - framework or rationale
    - holistic vs. linear thinking
    - Myers-Briggs Personality Type, especially motivation
    - Multiple Intelligences

- thinking clearly: techniques for using maximum mental capacity
    - emotional hi-jacking
    - emotional states of mind
    - confidence
    - self-esteem
    - breathing
    - relaxation
    - Brain Gym
    - Neuro-Linguistic Programming (NLP)
    - the art of pausing and maintaining clear thinking

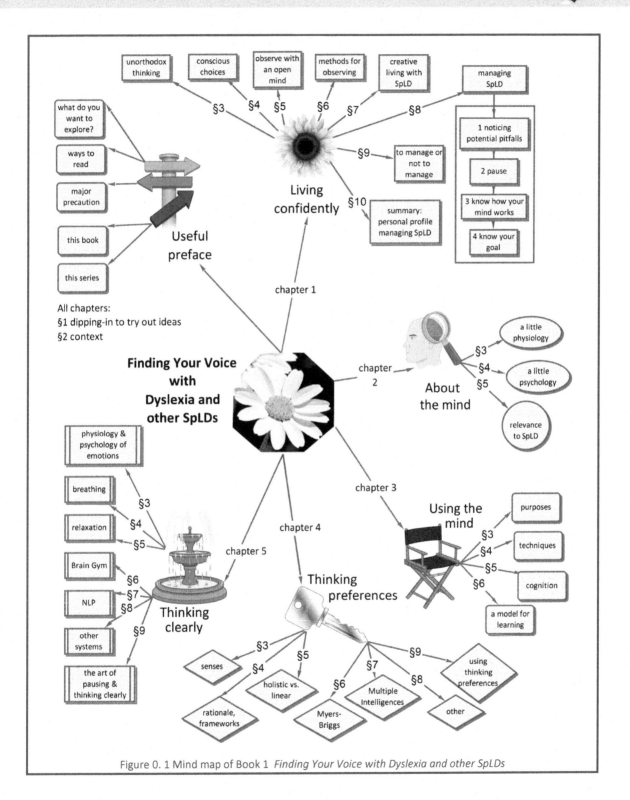

Figure 0. 1 Mind map of Book 1 *Finding Your Voice with Dyslexia and other SpLDs*

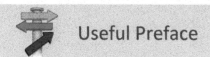

Book 2: *Organisation and Everyday Life with Dyslexia and other SpLDs* (Stacey, 2020a)

The book is written for dyslexic/ SpLD people and contains:

- a model for working out issues to do with organisation
    - materials and methods for working on any ideas
- general problem solving
- solutions applied to
    - time and time management
    - space, place and direction
    - everyday life
    - study peripherals
    - employment.

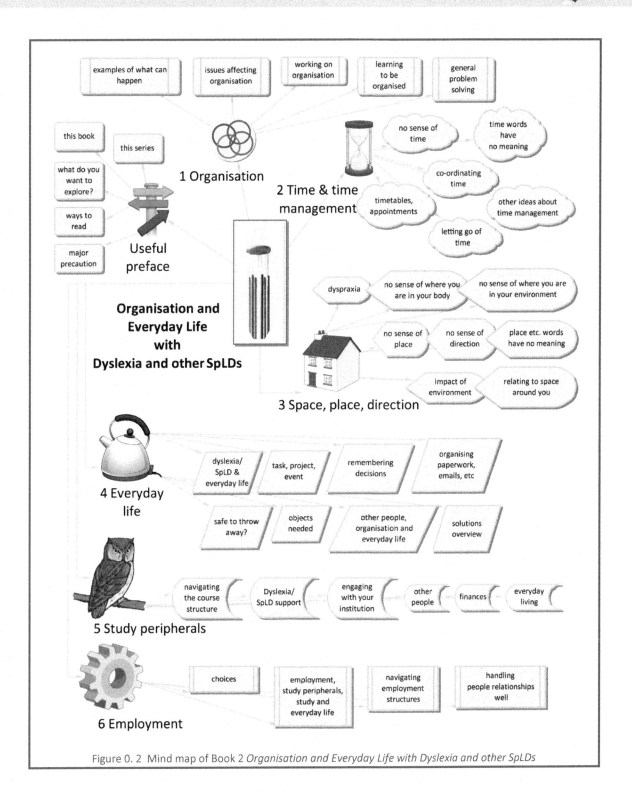

Figure 0. 2 Mind map of Book 2 *Organisation and Everyday Life with Dyslexia and other SpLDs*

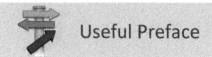

Book 3: *Gaining Knowledge and Skills with Dyslexia and other SpLDs* (Stacey, 2021)

The book is written for people who assist dyslexic/ SpLD people to gain knowledge and skills, which includes everyone:

- when you tell someone the time of day or how to cook an egg, you are passing on knowledge and skills
- you can't immediately tell whether the person you are talking to is dyslexic/ SpLD.

The book contains:

- different roles people have:
    - 1-1 support teachers, subject teachers and lecturers
    - employers, managers and supervisors
    - professionals in positions of influence and authority: healthcare, legal, financial
    - family, friends, acquaintances, work colleagues,
    - designers and producers of indirect communications
    - policy makers
    - people in the media
- imparting knowledge and skills:
    - general approaches
    - teaching
    - dialogue
    - indirect communication
    - accommodation
    - policies and systems
- foundations for knowledge and skills:
    - model for learning
    - comprehension
    - knowing the goal
    - planning
- input modes: reading, listening, doing
- taking and making notes
- output modes: writing, speaking, taking-action
- situations: exams, group work (meetings, seminars, debates), driving
    - social examples: travel, job applications, eating out, finances.

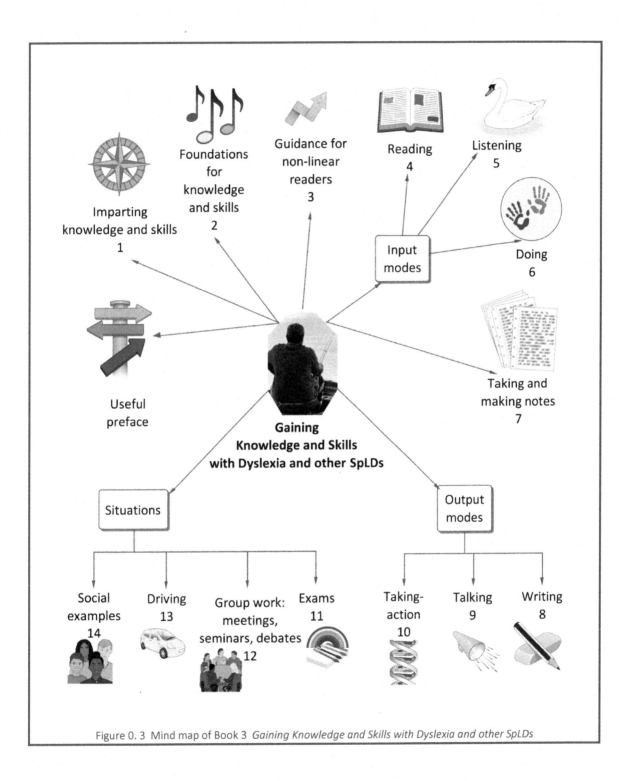

Figure 0. 3 Mind map of Book 3 *Gaining Knowledge and Skills with Dyslexia and other SpLDs*

Book 4: *Development of Dyslexia and other SpLDs* (Stacey, 2020b)

The book is written for those alongside dyslexic/ SpLD people and contains:

- ideas about the persistence of dyslexia/ SpLD and reasons to take dyslexia/ SpLD into account earlier rather than later, including:
    - learned confusion
    - neurons firing together, wire together
    - the persistence of dyslexia/ SpLD
    - problems masked by average language skills
    - levels of compensation
    - degrees of severity
- what goes wrong
    - discussion about the different SpLDs
    - discussion about similar problems experienced by non-dyslexic/ SpLD people
- adaptations of the ideas for younger children
- how to approach matching an individual's learning to what they are good at.

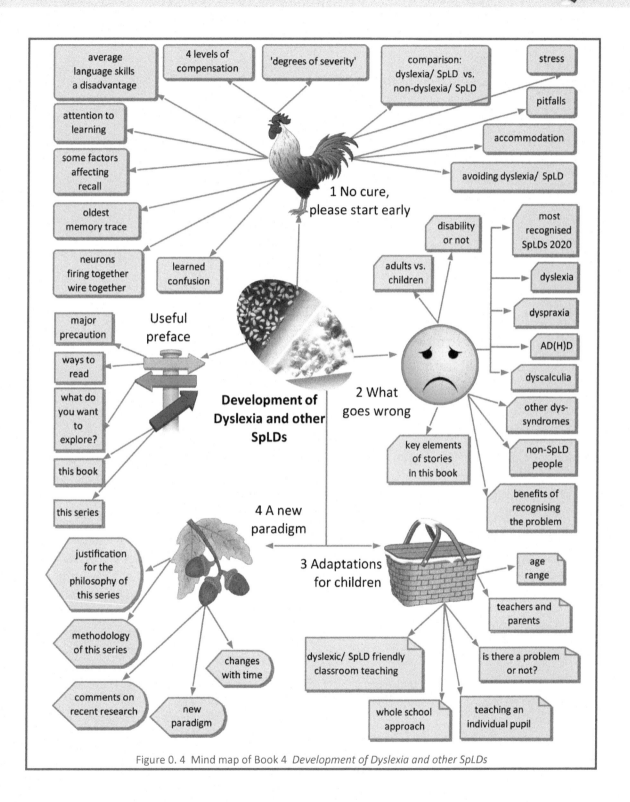

average
language skills
a disadvantage

4 levels of
compensation

'degrees of severity'

comparison:
dyslexia/ SpLD vs.
non-dyslexia/ SpLD

stress

pitfalls

accommodation

attention to
learning

some factors
affecting
recall

avoiding dyslexia/ SpLD

oldest
memory trace

neurons
firing together
wire together

learned
confusion

1 No cure,
please start early

disability
or not

most
recognised
SpLDs 2020

adults vs.
children

dyslexia

major
precaution

Useful
preface

dyspraxia

ways to
read

AD(H)D

what do
you want
to
explore?

Development of
Dyslexia and other
SpLDs

2 What
goes wrong

dyscalculia

other dys-
syndromes

this book

key elements
of stories
in this book

non-SpLD
people

this series

benefits of
recognising
the problem

4 A new
paradigm

justification
for the
philosophy of
this series

3 Adaptations
for children

age
range

teachers and
parents

methodology
of this series

changes
with time

dyslexic/ SpLD friendly
classroom teaching

is there a problem
or not?

comments on
recent research

new
paradigm

whole school
approach

teaching an
individual pupil

Figure 0. 4 Mind map of Book 4 *Development of Dyslexia and other SpLDs*

Applicable to all books in the series

Series Website

- has material to assist with using the books:
    - templates and check-lists
    - different ways to select the material most useful to you.

Useful Preface

- is mostly the same for each book
- the sections particular to each book are marked by the book icon and a blue line on the left hand margin.

It contains:

- the philosophy of the series
- a warning to avoid further dyslexic/ SpLD traits developing as new things are learnt
- some suggestions to make reading easier
- information about the book in question
- information about the series.

Appendix 1 Resources (The same in all 4 books except for referencing.)

will help you collect information together, decide on priorities and monitor progress.

Appendix 2 Individual, Personal Profile and Regime for Managing Dyslexia/ SpLD

(The same in all 4 books except for section 1 and referencing.)
will help you build the information about your dyslexia/ SpLD and how you manage it.
Section 1, *LIVING CONFIDENTLY*, starts by stating the aim for dyslexic/ SpLD people to be as autonomous as possible. In books 2 - 4, a summary of the material in book 1 is included so that these books can be used independently of each other.

Appendix 3 Key Concepts (The same in all 4 books except for referencing.)

In order to allow the separate books of the series to be used on their own, summaries of the key concepts of the individual books are given in *APPENDIX 3*. These are the concepts I think are most important for living confidently with dyslexia/ SpLD.

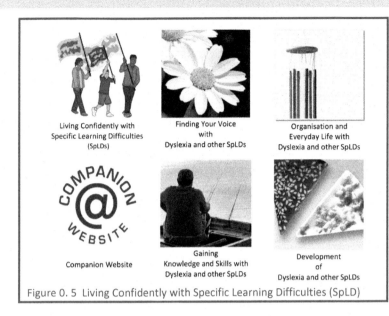

| Living Confidently with Specific Learning Difficulties (SpLDs) | Finding Your Voice with Dyslexia and other SpLDs | Organisation and Everyday Life with Dyslexia and other SpLDs |
| Companion Website | Gaining Knowledge and Skills with Dyslexia and other SpLDs | Development of Dyslexia and other SpLDs |

Figure 0. 5 Living Confidently with Specific Learning Difficulties (SpLD)

The book cover images:

The daisy represents growth.

Wind chime music represents life flowing well when organisation suits the individual concerned.

The fisherman recalls the saying: 'Give a man a fish and you feed him for a day; teach a man to fish and you feed him for a lifetime'.

The slices of cake represent changing 'That's the way the cookie crumbles' to 'It's a piece of cake'.

7.3 Aims and outcomes

The first group of aims of this series is that dyslexic/ SpLD people can:

- find out what their best ways of thinking are, how to use them and maintain their use
- understand how their specific learning difficulty affects them
- be able to pause when they recognise a pitfall has occurred
- know how to deal with the pitfall
    - o by using best ways of thinking
    - o knowing what needs to happen
- negotiate with those around them so that they are able to fulfil their potential in any situation and so that the dyslexic/ SpLD effects are minimised.

The general attitude at the end of the process is almost:

- OK, I'm dyslexic/ SpLD; I really enjoy the way I process information and the way I am;
- everyone has some problems, mine just happen to have a label;
- it's no big deal; I'll do well 'with a little help from my friends'.

In order to achieve this group of aims, a group of specialist support providers will need in-depth knowledge of dyslexia/ SpLD. Their knowledge and experience are usually a major contribution to the progress made by any dyslexic/ SpLD person.

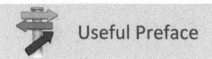

The second group of aims is that:

- non-dyslexic/ SpLD people can understand better what the issues are for the people with dyslexia/ SpLD

- communication between the two groups can be improved to the benefit of all parties.

These two sets of aims produce different outcomes depending on whether you are dyslexic/ SpLD or alongside a dyslexic/ SpLD person. The *WEBSITE* has *OUTCOMES* for various reader groups more finely classified.

OUTCOMES

They have been divided into:

- the Skills and Knowledge,

- the Benefits, including changes of behaviour

- and some thoughts about the Potential Possibilities

There can be a lot of laughter and joyful living once good communication is established across the differences of dyslexia/ SpLD.

7.4   Distinguishing between different SpLDs

Most of the series is not marked as more or less relevant to a particular SpLD. People are so varied even when their problems are given the same labels. The clearest separation I know is that organisation is the major problem for dyspraxic adults when it comes to thinking (the motor side of dyspraxia is not covered). But even in this group, I'm aware of one student with no dyslexic problems who needs to be aware of his thinking preferences in order to do justice to his knowledge.

Out of respect for the overlap of experiences (problems and solutions), this book makes no distinction between the different SpLDs, with one exception. The exception is *RESPECTING THE LEARNING NEEDS OF THE FOUR SPLDS* which outlines learning needs for people with the different SpLDs.

RESPECTING THE LEARNING NEEDS OF THE FOUR SPLDS: p 60

TEACHING LANGUAGE: p 94

Teaching language and maths to dyslexic/ SpLDs is covered, but not in a way that is specific to dyslexia and dyscalculia respectively.

SUPPORTING MATHS LEARNING: p 102

7.5   The way forward

The whole series is about the autonomy that allows dyslexic/ SpLD people to get out from under the difficulties. These difficulties have a label, may have various labels, but they aren't the only difficulties that people face. Negotiating accommodations should be done with understanding of the issues for all parties involved. The way forward could benefit many groups of people.

Ⓖ p 575: autonomy

What I hope people will get from the series:

Dyslexic/ SpLD people:

> a systematic way of observing strengths and weaknesses and using the strengths to help them manage the problems they face because of their dyslexia/ SpLD; the confidence to contribute to work, life, in their study, in a way that fulfils their innate potential and which is not masked or hampered by their dyslexia/ SpLD.

Those in supporting roles, whether in a 1-1 relationship or in a more general type of relationship:

> resources to understand the impact of dyslexia/ SpLD on the whole lives of dyslexic/ SpLD people and ways of making necessary adjustments to facilitate better communication.

Those who have to think about public communication and use of public spaces:

> an understanding of the difficulties encountered by dyslexic/ SpLD people and a recognition that making communication and access easier for them will also help many other people.

Politicians, other policy-makers and people in the media:

> an understanding that dealing with dyslexia/ SpLD effectively as early as possible is the right thing for society to do; that done well it has cost benefits in many different ways and is therefore worth carrying through properly; that mutual respect and consideration between all members and levels of society are enhanced through the best approaches to dyslexia/ SpLD.

What I hope will happen for dyslexic/ SpLD children:
> that adults will listen to them and observe them so that they can grow up with maximum autonomy and management of their dyslexia/ SpLD; that many of the recognised problems might not develop for them.

What I hope will happen in general education is that the new paradigm I have put forward (Stacey, 2020b) will be seen as teacher-friendly, effective, sensible, satisfying and cost saving.

Ⓖ p 575: paradigm Stacey (2020b)

The new paradigm is:

- that systems are developed, and used, to explore how individuals, children and adults, learn
- that learners have the opportunities to tailor their learning tasks so that they can achieve the knowledge and skills being taught
- that teaching programmes are flexible enough to accommodate all learner approaches.

Final comment

When people are confident of their skills and not afraid to own and manage their weaknesses, they have many of the tools necessary to face the various situations in their life, see the *TOOL BOX FOR LIVING CONFIDENTLY*.

TOOL BOX FOR LIVING CONFIDENTLY: p 545

The voice is found; the potential is unlocked; living with dyslexia/ SpLD is done with confidence.

References

Gleick, James, 1997, *Chaos, The Amazing Science of the Unpredictable*, Minerva, London

Hyman, Peter, 2005, *1 Out of 10: From Downing Street Vision to Classroom Reality,* Vintage, London

Kolb, Bryan, 1995, *Brain Plasticity and Behaviour,* Lawrence Erlbaum Associates, Mahwah, NJ

Stacey, Ginny, 2019, *Finding Your Voice with Dyslexia and other SpLDs,* Routledge, London

Stacey, Ginny, 2020a, *Organisation and Everyday Life with Dyslexia and other SpLDs*, Routledge, London

Stacey, Ginny, 2020b, *Development of Dyslexia and other SpLDs,* Routledge, London

Stacey, Ginny, 2021, *Gaining Knowledge and Skills with Dyslexia and other SpLDs*, Routledge, London

Website information

Okabe, Masataka, Ito, Kei, 2008, *Color Universal Design (CUD) – How To Make Figures and Presentations That Are Friendly to Colorblind People*,
http://jfly.iam.u-tokyo.ac.jp/color/ Accessed 3 January 2017
Series website: www.routledge.com/cw/stacey

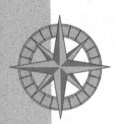

1 Imparting Knowledge and Skills

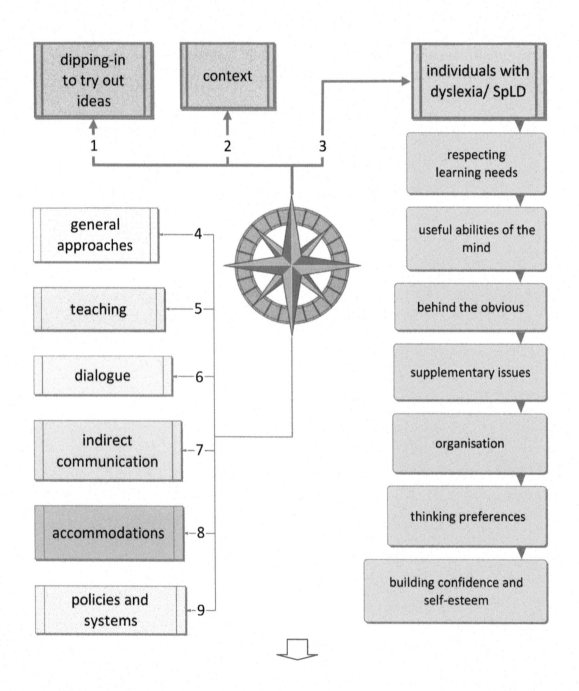

dipping-in to try out ideas

context

individuals with dyslexia/ SpLD

1

2

3

respecting learning needs

general approaches — 4

teaching — 5

dialogue — 6

indirect communication — 7

accommodations — 8

policies and systems — 9

useful abilities of the mind

behind the obvious

supplementary issues

organisation

thinking preferences

building confidence and self-esteem

Contents

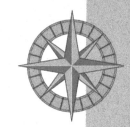

➢ = Book 1;   ϒ = Book 2;   ✂ = Book 4

➢, ϒ and ✂ mark sections that are discussed more fully in other books of this series. Key ideas are included here to support suggestions made in this book.

THINKING PREFERENCES are highlighted in orange in the book. They can be found using the *INDEX*: p 589

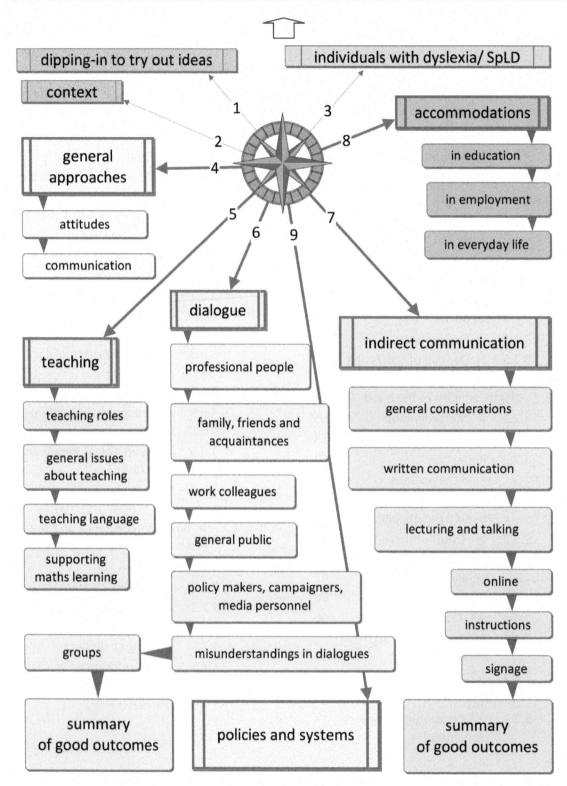

Contents *continued*

List of key points and summaries

K = key points
S = summaries

Working with the chapter

The table *WHAT CAN GO WRONG – WHAT CAN GO RIGHT* describes outcomes in different situations depending on whether communication is working for dyslexic/ SpLD people or not. From this chapter, you should:

WHAT CAN GO WRONG – WHAT CAN GO RIGHT: p 54

- become aware of the ways an individual's dyslexia/ SpLD hampers communication in a variety of situations

- become aware of what can be done to promote good communication

- realise that there are some situations when lack of clear communication leads to seriously wrong outcomes for the dyslexic/ SpLD person

- recognise that approaches that are VITAL for dyslexic/ SpLD people are good practice for all.

The green line in the LH margin indicates those paragraphs that predominantly contain ideas to be discussed with or taught to your student. The meaning of the green line is also in the *Glossary*.

Ⓖ p 575

Other ideas in the chapter are to help you understand more about the whys and hows of helping dyslexic/ SpLDs.

Some of the boxes are addressed to dyslexic/ SpLD people; it's the only way they make sense. They are marked with the green strip in the left hand margin. The meaning of the green strip is in the *Glossary* too.

Templates on the website

Templates
COMPANION @ WEBSITE

A1 *Jotting Down as You Scan*
A2 *Bookmark – Purpose*
A4 *Jotting Down as You Read*
A5 *Collecting Ideas That Interest You*
B1 *Collecting Ideas That Relate to You* (specially for readers who are themselves dyslexic/ SpLD)

The following templates can be used for working with your student:
B2 *Know Your Own Mind*
B3 *Compare Expectations and Reality*
B4 *Actions, Results, Next Step*
B5-8 *Recording Templates - 1-4*
B11 *Monitoring Progress*
E1 *List of Options for Thinking Preferences*
E7 *The Box 'Other'*

The following templates can be used for working on language:
G1 *The Functions of 'Round' and Other Words*
G2 *The Functions of Words*
G3 *Constant Content to Demonstrate Language Function*
G4 *Basic Sentence Pattern*
G5 *Basic Sentences from a Complex One*

Check-lists for Readers describes a set of check-lists available on the website to help different reader groups engage with the ideas in the book. It also lists the most relevant sections of the book.

Check-lists for Readers: p 21

All the *Templates* suggested in this chapter are shown in the *List of Templates*.

List of Templates: p 582

Appendix 1 Resources

APPENDIX 1: p 524

This appendix will help you and your student collect information about the way he does anything and how his dyslexia/ SpLD affects him. It collects together some of the general skills he will need in order to make progress.

If you are dyslexic/ SpLD, this appendix will help you gather the information you want from this book.

Appendix 2 Individual, Personal Profile of Dyslexia/ SpLD and Regime for Managing Dyslexia/ SpLD

APPENDIX 2: p 538

If you are supporting a dyslexic/ SpLD student, as you understand how to help dyslexic/ SpLD people better, you can help your student build his PROFILE and REGIME.

Appendix 3 Key Concepts

APPENDIX 3: p 554

This appendix has a summary of the key ideas I cover when doing an audit of skills and knowledge with a dyslexic/ SpLD student. They fall into the categories of:

> THINKING CLEARLY
> USING THE MIND WELL
> THINKING PREFERENCES
> USEFUL APPROACHES
> ASPECTS OF DYSLEXIA/ SPLD.

THINKING PREFERENCES, p 72, are highlighted in orange in this chapter. Examples of their use are listed in the INDEX: p 589

The appendix shows which of the 4 books in the series covers each idea in full.

1 Dipping-in to try out ideas

IMPARTING KNOWLEDGE AND SKILLS can be as simple as telling someone what time the next bus will come and how to chop an onion, so no one is excluded from this chapter.

Read the CONTEXT.
Scan INDIVIDUALS WITH DYSLEXIA/ SPLD and note the suggestions for uncovering 1) an individual's strengths and 2) anything that needs solving.

CONTEXT: p 53

INDIVIDUALS WITH DYSLEXIA/ SPLD: p 57

Scan the rest of the chapter to identify all the ways you impart knowledge and skills to anyone else.

Read the *KEY POINTS* and *SUMMARY BOXES,* see the *LIST* for page numbers.
Reflect:

LIST OF
KEY POINTS AND
SUMMARY BOXES: p 50

> How well do people generally understand what you tell them?
> How well can you pass a skill on to someone else?

> Do you know anyone who is dyslexic/ SpLD? Or is there
> anyone you think might be?

Scan the chapter to find sections that relate to the ways you impart
knowledge and skills to others.

Work with these sections to explore your interactions with dyslexic/
SpLD people. Use the appropriate *TEMPLATES ON THE WEBSITE*.

TEMPLATES ON THE
WEBSITE: p 51

2 Context

We gain knowledge and skill from a variety of people. Some are
officially teachers, many are not. Most of the time, we expect people
to process information in the same way as ourselves and we expect
that the way we express ideas or information will fit into their minds
quite easily. As a society, we don't usually compare how we think our
way through a task or an idea. When I run workshops, I include an
exercise which allows people to compare how they think about
something and the participants are surprised at the different ways
people have of doing even the simplest task (Stacey, 2005, 2019).

Stacey (2005, 2019)

Dyslexic/ SpLD people often process information in significantly
different ways and the ways their dyslexia/ SpLD impacts on their
thinking often makes processing information hazardous.

Dyslexia/ SpLD is not an indication of low overall intelligence: there
are people at all levels of intelligence who have dyslexia/ SpLD, but
they need to gain knowledge and skills using the processes that work
for them. One of the key factors in enabling them to use their full
potential is teachers and communicators who:

- understand the approaches that will enable dyslexic/ SpLD people
  to learn knowledge and skills
- are willing to adapt to the needs of dyslexic/ SpLD people,
  recognising that what's VITAL for them is often GOOD PRACTICE
  for everyone
- are able to accommodate particular needs when general
  adaptations don't quite meet the need of an individual.

The following table contrasts some problems from lack of shared understanding with some benefits from good shared understanding between a dyslexic/ SpLD person and those around him.

What can go wrong	What can go right
The widespread impact of dyslexia/ SpLD can be missed. Dyslexic/ SpLD people's potential qualities are not fully used.	A person's full potential is used and the disruption from dyslexia/ SpLD is minimised with tolerance.
The dyslexic/ SpLD person doesn't learn.	Learning is not much harder than for any other group and sometimes is easier.
The dyslexic/ SpLD person gives up.	The dyslexic/ SpLD person contributes at his best potential.
The professional assessment doesn't describe the experience known by the dyslexic/ SpLD person.	The dyslexic/ SpLD person recognises the descriptions in the assessment and trusts it as a document.
The effects of dyslexia/ SpLD are misinterpreted: judgements and decisions are based on wrong assumptions.	Judgements, decisions and plans are well grounded and beneficial.
Counsellors looking for psychological signs are following the wrong insights and their work is off target.	Counselling is seeing a fuller picture and helps the dyslexic/ SpLD person through problems.
General communication is confusing and leads to hassle for everyone concerned.	Communication systems work well for the vast majority of people.

There is tension, frustration and significant miscommunication within homes, workplaces and social settings.	There are still miscommunications, but the response is more sympathetic; there is more laughter and fun.
The ways dyslexic/ SpLD people do tasks is regarded as annoying.	The ways dyslexic/ SpLD people do tasks are at least tolerated by others, at best seen as being very suitable and worth adopting.

Key point: Success – internal sources

One dimension in finding out what makes the difference between success and lack of it, is to explore:

- what each individual does well
- how to transfer these strengths to tasks that are not going well
- what the root cause is for tasks that are proving difficult.

This is an internal dimension because you are exploring with each individual what is happening for him. The process includes reviewing suggestions and modifying them in the light of experience.

Key point: Success – external sources

A second dimension is the right external conditions that allow dyslexic/ SpLD people to gain knowledge and skills. There are 3 main channels for the processes involved:

- teaching
- dialogue
- materials, or indirect communication.

There are some approaches that apply to all 3 channels above. Many of the ideas are suitable for all people and could be brought into mainstream teaching and general communication so that the needs of dyslexic/ SpLDs are catered for naturally.

Accommodations may still be appropriate in some very individual circumstances. Policies and systems will be necessary to ensure the changes are brought into being.

The internal sources are reviewed in:

- *Individuals with Dyslexia/ SpLD, §3*

The external sources are discussed in:

- *General Approaches, §4*
- *Teaching, §5*
- *Dialogue, §6*
- *Indirect Communication, §7*
- *Accommodations, §8*
- *Policies and Systems, §9.*

Key point: The gift of your understanding

When you understand more about the problems dyslexic/ SpLD people have with gaining knowledge and skills, you lift a layer of burden from them. They no longer have to explain their ways of doing anything or justify them. They can get on with finding the solutions that allow them to gain knowledge and skills to the best of their abilities and then to contribute to society to their full potential.

3 Individuals with dyslexia/ SpLD

This section is a brief résumé of ideas from the other three books of the series (Stacey 2019, 2020a, 2020b). The ideas are included here because they are fundamental to managing dyslexia/ SpLD and to *Gaining Knowledge and Skills with Dyslexia and other SpLDs.*

➢ indicates book 1; ⋎, book 2; and ✻, book 4.

The *METHODS FOR EXPLORING BEHIND THE OBVIOUS* are given with sufficient detail for them to be used from this book. Many of the other subsections indicate areas to explore for strengths or problems

Stacey (2019, 2020a, 2020b)

METHODS FOR EXPLORING BEHIND THE OBVIOUS: p 65

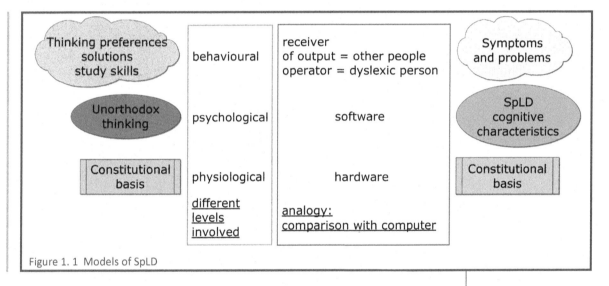

Figure 1. 1 Models of SpLD

FIGURE 1.1 shows two *MODELS OF SPLD* based on Morton and Frith's work (1995).

The left-hand version is used in *Finding Your Voice with Dyslexia and other SpLDs* (Stacey, 2019) with the focus of attention being to find out how a dyslexic/ SpLD person maximises his potential.

The right-hand version is used in *Development of Dyslexia and other SpLDs* (Stacey, 2020b) which is about the persistence of dyslexia/ SpLD into adulthood and reasons to deal with the syndromes early in a child's life.

Morton and Frith (1995)

Stacey (2019)

Stacey (2020b)

The following three stories illustrate elements of these two models.

In the first story, the woman knew her unorthodox strengths; in the second, the man didn't know either his strengths or his problems but had energy to get where he wanted. In the third the woman was disabled by her SpLD cognitive characteristics.

Story: I know how I learn

During a lengthy consultation process, I was watching the consultant put data into a computer. She was using so many tactics that I teach dyslexic/ SpLD students that I eventually asked if she were dyslexic.

- She had grown up in a Hampshire town.
- At the age of 6, her school had tested the learning styles of the class.
- She found out she learnt best visually and kinaesthetically and she'd used these processes all her life.
- Spellings were not secure, but she could write down all the possible options, look at them and decide which to use.

Knowing how they learn and think is a major element in dyslexic/ SpLD people taking control of their lives. This woman sounded like an 'at risk' child whose school had helped her avoid any serious problems.

Story: Just bash on

One dyslexic is worried that the label becomes a problem you get stuck with. He says, "You just bash on. Don't give in." He's a feisty dyslexic. He can upset people.

Bashing on is easier when you have ideas as to what will work.

58

Story: Don't worry, we know you can't do this

One student needed help with writing a major report. We went through the standard collection of received wisdom for dealing with major projects. We used different types of technology, programs and recording devices. We drew up plans for the report, timetables and various lists for dealing with all aspects of getting the report written.

She was making a little bit of progress. There were many issues to do with the work that had gone wrong and which undermined her writing fluency.

She was dyslexic and known to have mental health problems.

There was one session at which she had decided to face up to the enormous task she was trying to complete. Gradually we could see that she was crippled by the legacy of kindly meant reactions from her childhood: "Don't worry, we know you can't do this."

She has a deep-seated belief that she can't do anything and any time there was a difficulty with her writing, this belief got activated. It is so deep it is going to take this student many years to be free of its influence.

The people in her childhood were doing the best they could, but the outcome was far from good and a huge burden for the student.

In the first story, a child has probably been diverted from developmental dyslexia through good policies in her school. In the second, the man is successful but there is a cost to other people and little deliberate understanding on his part. In the third, well-meaning but uninformed kindness has demoralised the woman.

This section is looking at the software and operator components of the two models in *Figure 1.1*. The rest of the chapter looks at how the receiver of output can contribute to good outcomes. The whole book is about finding, testing and refining solutions for many different tasks and situations.

Figure 1.1: p 57

This section has

- a summary of dyslexia/ SpLD issues, §3.1
- a brief outline of three *Useful Abilities of the Mind*, §3.2
- suggestions for exploring *Behind the Obvious*, §3.3
- a summary of *Supplementary Issues*, §3.4
- some important themes relating to *Organisation*, §3.5
- key ideas relating *Thinking Preferences* to dealing with dyslexia/ SpLD, §3.6
- suggestions for *Building Confidence and Self-esteem*, §3.7.

§3.1: p 60

§3.2: p 63

§3.3: p 64

§3.4: p 68

§3.5: p 70

§3.6: p 72

§3.7: p 78

A final thought: often the strategies for dealing with a situation or task that dyslexic/ SpLD people devise to help themselves is adopted by the non-dyslexic/ SpLD people around them. These people weren't struggling sufficiently to develop any system, they could muddle by, but then found the dyslexic/ SpLD's system was better than muddling by.

✄ 3.1 Respecting the learning needs of the four SpLDs

Finding solutions to the problems of dyslexia/ SpLD often has to start by respecting the core learning needs.

Dyslexic people usually need to be allowed to think in different ways, so exploring their *Thinking Preferences* is one of the first tasks of support.

Thinking Preferences: p 72

Dyspraxic people need help with organisation, whether of ideas or more everyday tasks. Some of them have no concept of organisation, so that, however often you have worked together on organisation they never remember that this stage is very helpful.

AD(H)D people don't pay attention to one thing for very long; their attention switches impulsively between different topics or areas of their life. When their minds switch away from a topic they don't hold the information relating to that topic, so when the mind switches back, they have to start again. Solutions start with ways their minds can hold information better and how they can capture it so that it is still available when they come back to the topic.

For dyscalculic people you need to find the root of the problem. I find the best way is to watch them working and to ask questions to find out how they are mentally processing the material and how they are organising the practical working out of any maths problem. Finding the solutions may involve:

- exploring how their minds work well
- organising the mechanics of maths working
- showing how the maths is useful in everyday situations that they know about and are interested in
- uncovering gaps in their knowledge.

Key point: Lack of flexibility

For most dyslexic/ SpLD people, there is little flexibility in the way they learn:

- they have to do it the way that works for them
- they need to be disciplined to keep to that way
- trying someone else's way often leads to no learning
- the determination to learn in their own way can be misinterpreted as bloody-mindedness.

�֍ 3.1.1 Core issues

- The core problems are
    - dyslexia: language is not automatic in the same way it is for non-dyslexics
    - dyspraxia: problems with fine and gross motor control
    - AD(H)D: attention is not kept on one topic since the mind switches impulsively between topics
    - dyscalculia: there are problems with maths, either with basic numbers or with maths concepts
- the core difficulty has impaired development of the basic skills in childhood
- it will continue to cause difficulties for the adult learning higher-level thinking skills:
    - organisation of ideas
    - comprehension
    - organisation of self
    - management of time
    - management of place
    - all forms of spoken and written language.

✖ 3.1.2 Overlap of SpLDs and variability of effects

The following are worth bearing in mind:

- the core problems of the different SpLDs are different, but the behaviour can be affected in very similar ways
- frequently people have difficulties from two core problems, or more, i.e. there is overlap of syndromes
- you can't look at a person and know they have dyslexia/ SpLD
- the manifest behaviours will be different from one person to another, even with the same label
- for a single person, the effects of the syndromes will vary from one time to another
    - predictably from known difficulties
    - facing new challenges of whatever kind
    - under stress
    - randomly

- however well a person usually manages the impacts of his dyslexia/ SpLD, it is always possible for a situation to develop that makes his management as bad as it can be.

3.2 Useful abilities of the mind

The following three abilities of the mind are fundamental in the process of noticing what is happening under the influence of dyslexia/ SpLD and making any changes to the way your student manages his dyslexia/ SpLD.

➢ 3.2.1 Metacognition

- Metacognition is the skill whereby a person becomes aware of what they are doing as they do it.
- It can be developed through various exercises in this book by your student switching to being aware of what he is doing while doing the exercise:
    - *BREATHING*
    - *RELAXATION*
    - the mind exercise in *METHODS FOR EXPLORING BEHIND THE OBVIOUS*
    - *EXERCISE FOR STUDENT: MEMORISING EXERCISES*
- As part of managing dyslexia/ SpLD, metacognition allows your student:
    - to notice when his dyslexia/ SpLD is affecting him
    - to make choices as to how to deal with the situation.
- As part of study, employment and life in general, metacognition allows your student to keep his mind on the task in hand, i.e. it allows him to focus his mind.

BREATHING: p 557

RELAXATION: p 558

METHODS FOR EXPLORING BEHIND THE OBVIOUS: p 65
EXERCISE FOR STUDENT: MEMORISING EXERCISES: p 160

➢ 3.2.2 Objective observation

Ⓖ p 575
objective

- Both you and your student should try to be as objective as possible.
- You may need to let go of your own ideas and expectations.
- He may need to let go of any emotions attached to his dyslexia/ SpLD.
- It helps to be curious about the ways he does things and the way he thinks.

3.2.3 Reflection

- As your student gathers objective observations about the way he does anything, he can reflect on the data to see what it is telling him.

- Reflection is very useful in order to make progress.

- It needs to be constructive and focus on positive outcomes.

➢ 3.3 Behind the obvious

Insights: Some unobvious problems

- I couldn't spell 'develop' or 'development' without an 'e' after 'p' until I recognised the confusion with the similar pattern in 'envelope'.

- A student wanted writing strategies; it turned out that worry about a family problem was undermining his considerable stock of strategies; recognising the worry sorted out the essay writing.

- A student being treated for panic attacks in exams, over many years, just needed a pattern for dealing with exams.

- A dyspraxic student, who asked about keeping on task and using time well, didn't need time management strategies; she needed to recognise that her self-criticism over dyspraxic incidents was putting her into a depressed state so that she couldn't access any strategies.

These are just a few examples when working with the presented behaviour did not produce a solution and that probing behind the obvious was necessary in order to find out the root cause of the problem.

An intractable problem sometimes emerges, but at least then the student is not investing energy and other resources and still not finding a way forward.

♈ 3.3.1 Methods of exploring behind the obvious

As you work to explore behind the obvious, be mindful of the boundaries between support work and counselling.

Use any insights into things that don't help your student; they are also telling you both about the way his mind works.

The following are the basic ways I work with students when we need to find out more about how they think, what strategies they use and what problems they face.

Mind exercise: *TEMPLATE B2 - KNOW YOUR OWN MIND*

- o ask your student to collect ideas about a simple topic for 1½ minutes
- o ask how the ideas came to him, i.e. what links there are for him between the different idea
- o interpret the links in terms of the *THINKING PREFERENCES*.

TEMPLATES

THINKING PREFERENCES:
p 72

- • *EXERCISE FOR STUDENT: MEMORISING EXERCISES* allows you:
  - o to monitor the way your student's mind is linking information together
  - o to suggest what he might do to link missing information more securely.

EXERCISE FOR STUDENT:
MEMORISING EXERCISES:
p 160

- • Record what your student says about any situation or problem:
  - o I use A3 paper and as my student speaks I group what he says into related issues
  - o I ask questions to understand what's happening
  - o the student can alter my choices as to where to write anything
  - o we are both able to reflect on all he's said
  - o we discuss suggestions that I make as to whether the student thinks they will work
  - o we draw up a plan of action, and both keep a copy
  - o we discuss next time what has happened as a result and modify anything as need be; *TEMPLATE: B4 - ACTIONS, RESULTS, NEXT STEP* is useful for this step.

TEMPLATES

- Get your student to teach you:
    - let him choose something he knows well
    - observe how he sets about it
    - listen to the language he uses, especially in terms of *THINKING PREFERENCES*
    - discuss the insights you gain with him and how he might use them for other tasks.

THINKING PREFERENCES: p 72

FIGURE 1.2: p 66

- Use a mind map, such as *FIGURE 1.2*, or use a list of similar questions
    - accept what your student says without judgement
    - pitfalls of dyslexia/ SpLD can be divided into:
        - glitches, that need a moment to deal with
        - hazards, that need strategies to be used
        - obstacles, that have no solution and need to be avoided
    - let your student range as widely as necessary to look for anything influencing what he is trying to do
    - progress is the key that lets you know you have identified the root and have found the right way forward.

Ⓖ p 575
pitfall, glitch, hazard, obstacle

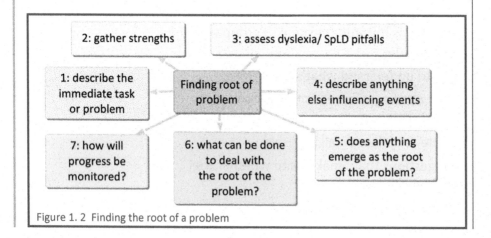

Figure 1. 2 Finding the root of a problem

- *MONITORING PROGRESS* is also part of the exploration:
  - o progress gives assurance that the insights gained fit your student
  - o your student's confidence and self-esteem will increase as his success increases
  - o anything that doesn't yield results should be used positively: it tells you more about the way your student's mind works.

MONITORING PROGRESS: p 535

➢ 3.3.2 'Other'

- Other: there is a need for openness to other possibilities.
- Sometimes I have the impression that a student has definite ways of thinking but these don't seem to fit any pattern I already know.
- I don't want to lose the information, but trying to make it fit a known way of thinking is not going to be productive.
- I use the *TEMPLATE: B7 - Box 'OTHER'* to capture this information.

TEMPLATES

3.3.3 Check-lists for exploring behind the obvious

The following check-lists summarise exploring behind the obvious.

Insights will emerge as you work with your student.

As insights are confirmed by experience, help your student add them to his

  - *INDIVIDUAL, PERSONAL PROFILE OF DYSLEXIA/ SPLD*
  - *REGIME FOR MANAGING DYSLEXIA/ SPLD*, both in *APPENDIX 2.*

APPENDIX 2: p 538

Check-list 1: Approaches to exploring

- Different methods for exploring.
- Willingness to search behind the obvious.
- Remember the whole of life is vulnerable.
- Remember the variation between people and for one person at different times.

OBJECTIVE OBSERVATION: p 63

- Skills for exploring: *OBJECTIVE OBSERVATION, METACOGNITION AND REFLECTION.*

METACOGNITION: p 63
REFLECTION: p 64

Check-list 2: Possible sources of difficulties

WHAT CAN HAPPEN AND USEFUL, RELEVANT SECTIONS describes the impact of various difficulties.

- Check for
    - difficulties arising from *CORE ISSUES* of each SpLD
        - at basic skills level
        - at advanced skills level
    - difficulties arising from
        - *TIME* and time management
        - *SPACE, PLACE AND DIRECTION*
        - the *ENVIRONMENT*
        - *ORGANISATION*
    - anything new.
- Are *THINKING PREFERENCES* being used and encouraged?
- Do confidence and self-esteem need to be built up?
- Use the category 'Other' to record any insight that doesn't fit into existing categories.

WHAT CAN HAPPEN AND USEFUL, RELEVANT SECTIONS: p 464

CORE ISSUES: p 62

TIME: p 69

SPACE, PLACE AND DIRECTION: p 69

ENVIRONMENT: p 70

ORGANISATION: p 70

Check-list 3: Finding the root of any problem

- Use the *MODELS OF SPLD* in *FIGURE 1.1* and *FINDING THE ROOT OF A PROBLEM* in *FIGURE 1.2*:
    - look for anything your student does well and how he shows intelligence
    - use anything he is good at or interested in
    - find out the root of any problem and use what he does well, or is interested in, to find solutions
    - keep reviewing insights and developing them
    - focus on what can be done and what can be got round
    - as a last resort, have a positive acceptance of anything that really is intractable.

FIGURE 1.1: p 57
FIGURE 1.2: p 66

3.4 Supplementary issues

Time, time management, space, place, direction and the environment can all contribute to dyslexic/ SpLD people's hassles with life, study and employment. The following subsections list the main issues.

Some of the issues are shared with the non-dyslexic/ SpLD population, but the effects of dyslexia/ SpLD add to the difficulties and can often result in quite a different order of magnitude to the experience.

'Inconsistency is easy to achieve; consistency in getting the answer wrong is not.' (Miles, 1993) This quote is in reference to confusion about left and right. It also applies to many of the ways in which dyslexic/ SpLDs attempt to deal with time, space, place and direction.

Miles (1993)

♈ 3.4.1 Time

- No sense of time.
- Words for time do not have secure meanings.
- Emphasis on one element of time can disrupt dealing with time.
- Working out timetables, in the short term and the longer term, i.e. for a day, a week, a year or more.
- No mental time triggers to alert a dyslexic/ SpLD person to something he should remember at a specific time.
- Saving time by being organised.
- Being prepared saves time and energy.
- A dyslexic/ SpLD person can work very hard and still arrive precisely at the wrong time or in the wrong place.

♈ 3.4.2 Space, place and direction

- Your student may have no sense:
    - of his own body
    - where he is in relation to the place around him
    - of direction.
- The words for space, place and direction may have no secure meaning despite your student having a good sense of each.
- Moving the head during any task can interrupt processing, whether side to side or up and down.
- Pen grip can influence writing skills.

♈ 3.4.3 Environment

- The environment may have an impact on how well he can think or do anything ; it can help or hinder through:
    - light levels
    - surrounding colours
    - noise levels
    - how much he can spread out, e.g. his work.
- The environment can influence:
    - recall of memories
    - fluency with
        - reading or writing
        - listening or speaking
    - confidence in doing or taking-action.
- The layout of the equipment during a talk can disrupt processing, whether your student is a listener or speaker.
- The style of clothing for different environmental settings may have an impact on your student's confidence and hence his ability to manage his dyslexia/ SpLD.

♈ 3.5 Organisation

- Organisation is a frequent difficulty, especially for those with dyspraxia.
- Use the MATERIALS AND METHODS that suit your student.
- Cover:
    - name of the task to be organised
    - assess strengths for the task
    - assess dyslexia/ SpLD pitfalls
    - describe what has to be organised
    - recognise any insuperable obstacles, whether from dyslexia/ SpLD or otherwise
    - develop constructive ways forward.

MATERIALS AND METHODS: p 565

Ⓖ p 575
pitfall, obstacle

♈ 3.5.1 Decision-making and remembering

- Decisions can be influenced by
    - priorities of time, money and other resources
    - interest
    - expectations of other people
    - your student's own wishes and well being.
- It is very easy to make one set of decisions one day and another set a day or two later; both could work, but a combination could be unworkable.
- Decisions need to be recorded where they will be useful and where they can be remembered when required.

♈ 3.5.2 Objects needed

- If objects needed for a task have to be found part way through a task, it can be frustrating or it can prevent completion.
- One tactic frequently used is to take absolutely everything that might be useful.
- Developing a system to deal with objects for a task and making sure it doesn't get disrupted.
- Using imagination to think through all objects that might be used is one good way of remembering everything.
- Choosing when to collect items together is important.
- Making sure everything gets taken.

♈ 3.5.3 Paperwork, including filing

- Dealing with paperwork promptly and efficiently is the most productive approach to adopt.
- Develop reading skills and questioning skills to deal with paperwork.
- Have a system that minimises the amount of reading necessary.
- Record any decisions where they will be found again easily.

- A good filing system can be set up to satisfy the answers to the following questions:
  - How will your student be looking for something when he wants to find it?
  - How will he decide what is important?
  - How long does he need to keep important paperwork?
  - How can he throw away papers without having to re-read them?

♈ 3.5.4 Stages in big projects

- Big projects broken into smaller stages
  - don't look as daunting
  - can be seen more clearly for what is involved
  - are much easier to handle.

♈ 3.5.5 Course structures and employment processes

- These can be regarded as big projects.
- They are worth setting out and analysing.
- Anything new can be identified.
- The skills and knowledge needed can be identified.
- Any gaps can be seen in advance and provision made to fill them.
- The impacts of dyslexia/ SpLD are likely to be better managed with advanced assessment and accommodations.

➢ 3.6 Thinking preferences

- *THINKING PREFERENCES* provides a framework for describing how any individual thinks well.
- Thinking preferences can make a significant difference to the successful thinking approaches for many dyslexic/ SpLD people.
- For others they are no more important than they are for the rest of the population.

THINKING PREFERENCES are highlighted in orange in most chapters.

Examples of their use are listed in the *INDEX*: p 589

- Baddeley (2007, p263) discusses Eysenck's theory of processing efficiency in which people's minds automatically switch between ways of thinking
  - some dyslexic/ SpLD people need to make the switch deliberately.

Baddeley (2007, p263)

Dyslexic/ SpLD people who have unorthodox thinking preferences:

- need to deliberately find out how they think well
- can add the insights to their *INDIVIDUAL, PERSONAL PROFILE OF DYSLEXIA/ SPLD* and their *REGIME FOR MANAGING DYSLEXIA/ SPLD*.
- have to give themselves permission to think in their best ways and so allow their minds to make good connections
- need to recognise problems caused by not using their best ways of thinking and then be able to switch into these better ways.

INDIVIDUAL, PERSONAL PROFILE OF DYSLEXIA/ SPLD: p 540

REGIME FOR MANAGING DYSLEXIA/ SPLD: p 540

Key point: Suggestions for *THINKING PREFERENCES*

TEMPLATE: E1 - LIST OF OPTIONS FOR THINKING PREFERENCES gives ways the different preferences can be used.

Examples of their use are listed in the *INDEX*.

TEMPLATES

thinking preferences, examples
in *INDEX:* p 589

➤ 3.6.1 Input, output and motivation

- When *THINKING PREFERENCES* are important, they need to be considered at all stages of the *MODEL OF LEARNING*, but especially when new information is presented to the mind and when material is being recalled from memory.
- At the input stage of the *MODEL OF LEARNING*, the visual, verbal, kinaesthetic thinking preferences and the need for a rationale or framework all need to be covered by the way the information is presented.
- The motivation, or driving force, of a person can be influenced by his *THINKING PREFERENCES*.

MODEL OF LEARNING: p 145

- If the right motivation is not being used for a task, a dyslexic/ SpLD person can find his dyslexia/ SpLD problems are enhanced, sometimes to the point of not being able to function with words at all. *MYERS-BRIGGS PERSONALITY TYPE* and *MULTIPLE INTELLIGENCES* are two useful systems for exploring motivation. *EXAMPLE: GOAL FOR ENGAGING WITH PRACTICAL WORK* shows motivation for a task being altered.

MYERS-BRIGGS PERSONALITY TYPE: p 76

MULTIPLE INTELLIGENCES: p 78

EXAMPLE: GOAL FOR ENGAGING WITH PRACTICAL WORK: p 186

➢ 3.6.2 Senses

- The senses receive signals from the environment. The 5 physical ones are: sight, hearing, touch, smell and taste.

ⓖ p 575
senses

- In these books, touch has been expanded into kinaesthesia which includes:
    - touch
    - knowing where your body is
    - movement
    - experience
    - concrete objects.

- Being able to choose between the three senses, sight, hearing and kinaesthesia, is important for learning and communication.

- There is a range of balances between them:
    - sometimes one is much stronger than the other two, which are equally balanced
    - sometimes one is weaker than the other two, which are equally balanced
    - sometimes all three have different strengths
    - I have never seen all three equal, but it is a possibility.

- Sometimes sight and hearing don't work together: one works and the other doesn't register very much at all.

- Sometimes people lip-read in order to hear the spoken word well.

- People can have preferences in the way they use sight, hearing and kinaesthesia.

➢ 3.6.3 Sense-based thinking preferences

- The visual thinking preference includes the way the mind uses a spatial awareness to process signals from the sight sense. There are many different visual devices used in learning and communication. Also, a person uses sight to read what another has written.

- Language originally developed using sound, involving the hearing sense and the ability to produce sounds. The verbal thinking preference is based on using language. The hearing sense is involved when a listener hears what a talker says.

- Kinaesthetic thinking skills are based on the kinaesthetic sense. Some people have a preference for these thinking skills.

- The kinaesthetic learning can be ignored in education, which denies some people their best way of learning.

➢ 3.6.4 Rationale or framework

- Knowing the rationale behind a topic or task provides the links that keep the information together and allows the mind to learn, see *CAPACITY OF WORKING MEMORY*.

- A schema or framework might be necessary.

- Recognising the logical procedures of a task or topic might provide the necessary links.

- For some dyslexic/ SpLDs, the lack of such structure leaves information unconnected and the mind cannot work with it.

ⓖ p 575 rationale schema, framework

CAPACITY OF WORKING MEMORY: p 157

➢ 3.6.5 Holistic vs. linear thinking

- The difference between linear and holistic thinking can be important, especially for those who process information in a holistic way.

- Linear thinking processes the first idea, then the second, then the third. Each idea is completed before the next occupies the mind.

- In holistic thinking, many ideas are present in the mind at the same time and linked in a holistic way.

- Holistic thinking is very rich.

- Holistic thinkers can go off at a tangent very easily.

- Holistic thinkers can move on to a new idea before finishing a sentence.

- Language may cause problems for holistic thinkers.
- Language is a linear process and holistic thinkers need to learn to convert linear language into their holistic processing and then convert back again to communicate with other people.
- Using language can feel like using a second language to holistic thinkers.

➤ 3.6.6 Myers-Briggs Personality Type (MBPT)

Myers-Briggs Personality Type is a framework for discussing differences between the approaches that people adopt.

- Four attitudes in the theory are, with signifying letters:
  - Perceiving – P
  - Judging (decision making) – J
  - Introversion – I
  - Extroversion – E.

- Four mental functions in the theory are:
  - Sensing – S
  - Intuiting – N
  - Thinking – T
  - Feeling – F.

Table: **MBPT mental functions and motivation**

Mental function	A few characteristics showing motivation
S	respond to practical, functional tasks "Can this teacher and subject show me something useful?" "Will I learn skills I can master and put to good use?" think best with their hands get lost when steps are missed out
N	crave inspiration find routines dull want their imagination to be fired with intriguing ideas and plans when bored they will seek out something to relieve the boredom

T	energised by logically organised material thrive on things that can be analysed resent material to be learnt that fits no logical structure resent and resist a teacher with non-logical organisation when logical orderliness is absent, no way is open for them to use their best energies
F	"Does this teacher care about me?" "Can I give my heart to this subject?" caring about the teacher carries them over boring tasks caring about the teacher and subject brings out their best when unable to care, lose their primary motivation and nothing is gained by changing instructional procedures or physical conditions

- If the prime motivation for the mental functions is not engaged in a task, a dyslexic/ SpLD person may find his language fluency has deteriorated, even to the point of language skills not functioning at all.

Other issues relating to MBPT characteristics:

- Acquiring information concerns decision-making by different P and J types; persuading them to alter their approach can be quite difficult:
  - o Judging (deciding) types don't want to stop to gather information; they want to get into action immediately.
  - o Perceiving types want to keep gathering; they are reluctant to move on to the next stage.
  - o For Judging (deciding) types, the breadth of their acquired knowledge could be too narrow.
  - o For Perceiving types, the amount of acquired knowledge could be too great for them to sift out details, so moving towards making an evaluation or going into action can take a long time.

Many practical people have S in their personality type. They find doing easy, but often relating what they do to the theories or guidelines of their discipline is daunting or impossible.

➤ 3.6.7 Multiple Intelligences (MI)

There is considerable overlap between MBPT and Multiple Intelligence theory. The *Naturalist Intelligence* was a late addition to the original set of MI and I was pleased when it was added as it covered several characteristics that were sitting in my collection of '*OTHER*' stories.

'*OTHER*': p 67

- Naturalist Intelligence includes:
    o   recognising and categorising species
    o   classifying and charting out relationships.

- This group of people are very good at seeing links between disparate systems and they can use this strength in many different ways in study, everyday life and employment.

➤ 3.7 Building confidence and self-esteem

The *STORY: DON'T WORRY, WE KNOW YOU CAN'T DO THIS* shows the importance of helping your student succeed. Usually success increases confidence and self-esteem. Sometimes, it is necessary to teach your student how to switch on these mental attitudes and how to maintain them. The level of stress is also an important factor in dealing with confidence and self-esteem. This section starts with some ideas about stress and continues with summaries of processes that I use with my students.

STORY: DON'T WORRY, WE KNOW YOU CAN'T DO THIS: p 59

3.7.1 Stress

- Stress can make the problems of dyslexia/ SpLD very much more difficult to manage.
- Any new situation or task can be a source of stress until what needs to be done has been practically run through.
- When language is not secure, your student will find it hard to talk his way out of difficult situations.
- Stress can be caused by internal expectations or worries or many other kinds of thoughts.
- There are chemical reactions in the body related to stress and these take time to reset to normal levels.
- Emotional hi-jack is a fast response in the brain and can produce states like panic very quickly.

- Stress is not always undesirable, some people need a certain level to keep energised.
- Your student needs to know his best level of stress and how to keep it at that level.

➢ 3.7.2 **Thinking clearly**

- Good breathing and panic are not states that coexist in a person.
- Good breathing:
    - ○ switches off panic
    - ○ is a way to keep thinking clearly
    - ○ enhances mental capacity.
- Learning to pause and take control of breathing, and hence mental functioning, is seen as a fundamental part of the *INDIVIDUAL, PERSONAL PROFILE OF DYSLEXIA/ SPLD* and *REGIME FOR MANAGING DYSLEXIA/ SPLD*.
- Teach your student *BREATHING* and *RELAXATION* exercises; one of each can be found in *APPENDIX 3*.

INDIVIDUAL, PERSONAL PROFILE OF DYSLEXIA/ SPLD: p 540

REGIME FOR MANAGING DYSLEXIA/ SPLD: p 540

BREATHING: p 557
RELAXATION: p 558

➢ 3.7.3 **Neuro-Linguistic Programming (NLP)**

I have found several processes from NLP very useful when helping dyslexic/ SpLD students. *RECORDINGS* of the processes can be found on the *COMPANION WEBSITE*.

RECORDINGS

- I have shown them:
    - ○ how quickly one can change from negative thinking to positive thinking
    - ○ how this change from negative to positive has an immediate effect on the physical state of their bodies.
- I have taken them through exercises that:
    - ○ allow them to see the characteristics of their internal thinking
    - ○ help them to see and alter their belief systems about themselves and any particular situation they face.
- The students then have an understanding that helps them look for positive ways to deal with the challenges of being dyslexic/ SpLD.

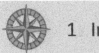

➢ 3.7.4 Using challenges

Using challenges is based on the NLP exercises.

- I talk a student through an experience which:
    - o was a challenge at the time
    - o came to a successful conclusion.
- The student then reflects on the qualities that enabled him to succeed.
- We discuss how those qualities could be adapted to apply to a present situation that is causing problems.
- Transferring skills from the successful situation to a present challenge often has very good results.

➢ 3.7.5 Self-referenced vs. other-referenced

- In NLP, there is discussion about the origin[1] of a person's thinking:
    - o self-referenced have the origin at themselves
    - o other-referenced people have the origin with other people.
- Self-referenced is not the same as being self-centred and only thinking of oneself.
- If you are working with a self-referenced person, you may have to find ways to express any new experience or information in ways that are relevant to your student.

3.7.6 Exercise

- Some dyslexic/ SpLD people are good at some form of sport and the confidence and self-esteem they gain can be an important part of being able to face the challenges of dyslexia/ SpLD.
- Going running or going to the gym is often a way to give space for thinking.
- Short breaks can be used for a few exercises; this way they don't turn into long breaks because your student has forgotten what he was doing and has become distracted.

---

[1] Origin: 'A fixed point from which measurement or motion commences' ('origin, n. 2c' OED Online, 2018 Accessed 8 Feb 2018)

4 General approaches

Other people impart knowledge and skills to dyslexic/ SpLDs and do so in particular settings. Imparting knowledge and skills has been divided into *TEACHING*, *DIALOGUE* and *INDIRECT COMMUNICATION*. This section discusses approaches that apply to all three. They are listed in the table below with the discussion indicated in the margin. A few of the ideas are résumés of fuller discussions in the other three books of the series: ➢ indicates book 1; ♈, book 2; and ✂, book 4.

The table *WHAT CAN GO WRONG – WHAT CAN GO RIGHT* gives some indication of the benefits of the right approaches.

TEACHING: p 85

DIALOGUE: p 107

INDIRECT COMMUNICATION: p 119

WHAT CAN GO WRONG – WHAT CAN GO RIGHT: p 59

Summary: General approaches

Attitudes

- To be open-minded
- To listen well
- To be tolerant of differences
- To be willing to negotiate through the differences
- To be willing to negotiate accommodations

discussed in this section

Communication

- To know there could be problems with communications
- To know how fundamental the problems are
- To explore different interpretations

discussed in this section and also
TEACHING: p 85
DIALOGUE: p 107
INDIRECT COMMUNICATION: p 119

Knowledge of dyslexia/ SpLD

- Understanding that people have different capabilities for managing their dyslexia/ SpLD
- Accept that dyslexia/ SpLD are not static syndromes; they vary from time-to-time for one person and from one person to another
- Know that anything new is likely to make a person more vulnerable to his dyslexia/ SpLD
- Recognise the different profiles of dyslexic/ SpLDs

gained from using suggestions in
INDIVIDUALS WITH DYSLEXIA/ SPLD: p 57

4.1 Attitudes

These attitudes represent flexibility in communication and a courtesy to pay attention to other people. They are VITAL for communication about dyslexia/ SpLD because the differences are so deep-seated, and they are GOOD PRACTICE for all.

Being <u>open-minded</u> implies letting go of preconceived ideas as to how another person thinks and takes-action[2]; it is a component of listening well and helps to diminish the friction and difficulties caused by differences between people.

Ⓖ p 575
take-action

Key point: Check with your student

If you are working with a student, remember that initially you don't know how the student thinks. 'Working with him to find a solution' is a process of you both exploring; you are not steering your student towards a solution that you already think will work for him.

Even when you know a lot about how he thinks, you always have to check with him that your insights still fit with his current experience.

<u>Listening well</u> to another person requires attention being paid to what he is saying, what he is feeling and experiencing, what his perspective is and letting him know that you have heard what he says. You don't have to agree with him or try to talk him out of his experience; you have to hear what a particular situation is like for him. The same applies to listening well to yourself. In the initial stages of working with dyslexia, I knew I wouldn't believe what I was saying if I couldn't see what was happening in my mind; I had to let my mind show me the effects of my dyslexia: I had to listen well to myself.

---

[2] Grammatically, the hyphen in 'takes-action' may seem unacceptable but in the context of these books it expresses a concept that is key to kinaesthetic learning.

Tolerance of differences can result from good listening with an open mind.

There seems to be a strong human impulse to want to be with people who are the same as you and to comment about anyone who has different characteristics.

Story: Being different

I am a person who feels the cold. I need to wear many layers of clothes in order to be warm. Wherever I go and however long people have known me, there are always comments about the number of layers of clothes I wear.

If the temperature goes up and I take a layer off, there are often immediate comments.

One group I've known for 13 years, still has to comment.

Differences are not easy.

Genuine interest in someone else's different experience and way of being is an important part of being able to tolerate the differences between dyslexic/ SpLD people and non-dyslexic/ SpLD people.

Negotiating through differences is helped by tolerance.

There are many ways in which people can be different and sometimes the differences have quite an impact on the relationships between people. Co-operative, harmonious relationships can be fostered between people who are different when they want to communicate and are able to negotiate.

<u>Accommodation may be needed</u>

Sometimes there are obstacles due to dyslexia/ SpLD that an individual person cannot manage without assistance from those around them; in this case ACCOMMODATIONS need to be negotiated. It is important to have open discussion about the negotiations. It is all too easy to slide into a way of doing things that 1) becomes a burden for those around the dyslexic/ SpLD person and 2) leaves the dyslexic/ SpLD person taking others too much for granted.

Ⓖ p 575
obstacle

ACCOMMODATIONS:
p 128

♈ 4.1.1 Declaring dyslexia/ SpLD or not

The attitudes of those around will influence people's choices about declaring their dyslexia/ SpLD. The choice can be very important for employment.

- Your student has to be comfortable with his choices.
- It is not a legal requirement for dyslexia/ SpLD to be disclosed.
- No employer can make reasonable adjustments for a condition she doesn't know about, even during an interview.
- Typical worries are:
  - there will be no interviews or job offers if dyslexia/ SpLD is disclosed
  - being 'found out' once on the job.
- Some people feel comfortable discussing issues once a job has been offered.

♈ 4.1.2 Dyslexia/ SpLD and interesting jobs

Your student needs to choose his career path carefully. Avoiding the effects of his dyslexia/ SpLD may hinder the evolution of encouraging attitudes in those around him.

- An interesting job is likely to be beneficial:
  - the interest will provide structure that assists with dyslexia/ SpLD pitfalls

Ⓖ p 575
pitfalls

  - the interest will probably result in greater productivity and engagement with the job
  - management will be more likely to value the contributions made out of the interest.

- Accepting a boring job:
  - often done by opting for a job with fewer challenges to dyslexia/ SpLD
  - the lack of stimulus can make the problems of dyslexia/ SpLD worse
  - the lack of enthusiasm will not lead to job satisfaction
  - management are less likely to value an uninterested employee.

4.2 Communication

People who deal with communication systems need to:

- know there could be problems with communications
- know how fundamental the problems might be
- explore different interpretations of words and conversations.

It can be very liberating to realise that there are likely to be problems with communication as a result of dyslexia/ SpLD. It isn't anybody's fault. Nobody is deliberately causing a break in communications. Once you can work in an objective way to solve a problem in communication you are likely to enhance the communication to the benefit of all.

Ⓖ p 575
objective

It should come as no surprise to think that different minds will have different interpretations of exactly the same words, see DIFFERENCES IN THOUGHT PROCESSING. Jokes and comedy are based on these kinds of differences and in such situations can be very enjoyable. With dyslexia/ SpLD, the interpretations can be different when nobody is expecting it and nobody is double-checking for consistency. So it is very necessary to explore the possible different interpretations that can interfere with good communication. Good communication is the aim of TEACHING, DIALOGUE and INDIRECT COMMUNICATION.

DIFFERENCES IN THOUGHT PROCESSING: p 114

TEACHING: p 85

DIALOGUE: p 107

INDIRECT COMMUNICATION: p 119

5 Teaching

TEACHING ROLES shows a wide range of people who might be imparting knowledge and skills. GENERAL ISSUES ABOUT TEACHING briefly discusses factors that hinder or support learning.

TEACHING LANGUAGE and SUPPORTING MATHS LEARNING have some ideas about teaching language and maths.

TEACHING ROLES: p 86
GENERAL ISSUES ABOUT TEACHING: p 87

TEACHING LANGUAGE: p 94
SUPPORTING MATHS LEARNING: p 102

DIALOGUE and *INDIRECT COMMUNICATION* are also part of teaching and the discussions in these sections are relevant to teaching.

DIALOGUE: p 107
INDIRECT COMMUNICATION: p 119

There are some aspects of thinking well that are usually not taught explicitly, but students are expected to pick them up as they learn different subjects. Very often dyslexic/ SpLD students don't pick these skills up; they need to be taught them explicitly. They need to recognise what they are learning and focus their attention on it. These aspects are covered in *FOUNDATIONS OF KNOWLEDGE AND SKILLS*.

FOUNDATIONS OF KNOWLEDGE AND SKILLS: p 134

Story: Not realising what you are doing

"You are so busy asking the question, you don't realise that's what you are doing" is the way one of my dyslexic colleagues describes her lack of grasp of what is happening when she is using words.

Key point: Mental on/off switch

It is important to recognise that students are not wilfully switched off from learning; and to recognise that their brains and minds need switching on in a different way in order for learning to happen.

5.1 Teaching roles

People actively engaged in teaching dyslexic/ SpLD people include:
 specialist support tutors, SENCOs
 subject teachers, university lecturers, evening class teachers
 head teachers
 trainers, sport or hobbies or otherwise
 librarians
 employers, managers
 parents, spouses, other family members, friends
 assessors and researchers
 teachers and parents of younger children
 anyone helping dyslexic/ SpLD people to learn.

Ⓖ p 574
SENCO

Teachers and coaches of any kind need to :

- understand the problems of dyslexia/ SpLD

- help their students find the solutions that work well for them

- use teaching methods that cater naturally for dyslexic/ SpLD students

- give their students the tools to find and develop solutions in the future for themselves.

There are significant numbers of adults who have struggled at school but not enough to be assessed as dyslexic/ SpLD. Their struggles can become major issues in adulthood because what is expected of them is beyond their ability to manage their unrecognised dyslexia/ SpLD. Teachers and coaches who recognise the patterns of behaviour and problems are often able to talk to these students and encourage them to be assessed for dyslexia/ SpLD.

Key point: Widening competences in learning

"If this child doesn't learn the way we teach, can we teach him the way he learns, and then develop and widen his competences in learning?" This question was posed by Harry Chasty in 1989.

Chasty (1989)

The first part of the quote can be found in many places on the internet. The second part has often been overlooked, but it is even more important. By helping your student to develop and widen his competences you should be giving him the tools to become an autonomous learner and to contribute using his full potential to anything else he endeavours in adult life.

5.2 General issues about teaching

NEURONS FIRING TOGETHER, WIRE TOGETHER outlines an important aspect of changes in the brain that are part of learning. The subsections from *SUBLIMINAL LEARNING* to *BEING ALERT, §§5.2.2 - 5.2.6,* outline different ways that learning is hampered in dyslexic/ SpLD minds. These subsections are brief résumés of ideas from books 1 (➤) and 4 (✂) of

§5.2.2: p 88
§5.2.3: p 89
§5.2.4: p 89
§5.2.5: p 90
§5.2.6: p 91

the series (Stacey, 2019, 2020b). *Static Material and Constant Content* discusses the importance of not varying too much at once. *IT Solutions* briefly touches on deciding what's best. *Helpful Teaching Practices* contains a summary of influences on dyslexic/ SpLD people's learning.

Stacey (2019, 2020b)
Static Material and Constant Content: 91

IT Solutions: p 93

Helpful Teaching Practices: p 93

✖ 5.2.1 Neurons firing together, wire together

As part of learning, neural networks are established, see *Insight: Park Paths and Neural Pruning*. The important point for the present discussion is that, to make the networks that belong to learning, the neurons involved need to be operational at the same time, they need to 'fire together'. When they have fired together once, they are more likely to do so again, which means they have been connected: they have 'wired together' (Stein and Stoodley, 2006; Stacey, 2020b). In dyslexic/ SpLD students' learning, there are some situations that seem to prevent the 'firing together, wiring together' process; the *Techniques for Using the Mind* help it.

Insight: Park Paths and Neural Pruning: p 7

Stein and Stoodley (2006)
Stacey (2020b)

Techniques for Using the Mind: p 156

Key point: The starting point matters

You need to work with the most pressing task that your student is facing. If you decide you will work on a skill or topic unrelated to his task, he is unlikely to be able to learn. Even if he tries to pay attention, the task will be lurking in his mind and preventing the right neurons from firing together, see *Where to Start* for several suggestions.

Where to Start: p 144

✖ 5.2.2 Subliminal learning

Subliminal learning takes place without conscious thought. If you read a lot, you are expected to learn how words are spelled. If you listen to radio programmes, you learn how words are spoken. You don't deliberately pay any attention, your brain and mind put together the right components and you learn. At a higher level of skills, you can subliminally learn about other people by reading books or watching TV.

ⓖ p 575
subliminal learning

Subliminal learning is very unreliable for dyslexic/ SpLD people: the right networks are not connecting up. The dyslexic/ SpLDs need to learn many of the skills for thinking and understanding as lessons in their own right and not alongside other topics; these skills are discussed in *FOUNDATIONS OF KNOWLEDGE AND SKILLS*.

FOUNDATIONS OF KNOWLEDGE AND SKILLS: p 134

5.2.3 Rote learning

Rote learning is not as useful for dyslexic/ SpLD students as it can be for others. It seems as if anything that is learnt by this method is learnt as a whole package that cannot be used in parts. Even though someone has learnt the whole alphabet, he doesn't know where individual letters come: a letter and its place are not being directly connected. He will either have a rough idea where a letter comes and he will start a little bit before to find the exact place or he will have to start at 'a' and carry on until the letter arrives. Reciting times tables or days of the month can similarly not lead to learning the parts within the whole.

Ways round are not difficult to introduce. Work or games that involve more randomness will lead to attention being paid to the detail that needs to be connected in, e.g. connecting each letter directly with its place in the alphabet.

5.2.4 First learning becomes fixed

There are a couple of other considerations that are important about the way information is registered in dyslexic/ SpLD minds: it can become 'set in stone' and it is very difficult to add anything to it later.

Insight: Set in stone

A prime example of this is that 'verbs are doing words'. When teaching grammar to groups of dyslexics/ SpLDs, the comment was frequently made that "sleeping and thinking are not doing, they can't be verbs!" Once verbs are identified with doing words, it is really hard for some to add abstract concepts to the list of verbs and to work with the patterns of verbs.

I have also heard dyslexic/ SpLD students complain when the initial information about something has not given the complete picture. "I have worked so hard to grasp that idea. Now I'm told it wasn't complete and the new stuff changes everything I've put together."

For situations similar to the verbs case, you need to make sure you fill in the steps when going from the initial simplified set of information to a more complex set.   For other situations, it is probably worth saying that the initial information is partial. If you know your student works with *RATIONALE OR FRAMEWORK*, let him know the overview before he starts learning anything in that topic.

RATIONALE OR FRAMEWORK: p 75

5.2.5 Out of sight is out of mind

It can be astonishing how quickly something is no longer available to your student's mind when the source has gone out of sight.

Insight: Out of sight, out of mind

Looking from the vertical plane of the computer screen to a horizontal piece of paper that I want to write on, I can't keep very much in mind. I have to go backwards and forwards very carefully to make sure I am taking down text or numbers correctly. Often, my mind is not connecting anything together.

One colleague could only remember the information in the book on the top of a pile. All the other books might as well not have existed.

Find out whether your student is bothered by this problem and work out solutions with him. Just being able to acknowledge the problem often opens the way for him to find the solution. This is an example of sight being an important part of making connections.

sight being a visual process

➤ 5.2.6 Being alert

If your student's mind is not using his best way of thinking, he is unlikely to process any words easily, even for a subject he's really keen to study. His mind will get switched off; he might daydream; he will probably struggle to stay awake. There are neurological reactions that shut down the arousal system (Stein and Stoodley, 2006; Stacey, 2019).

One technique that helps to keep the arousal system alert is to stand while working, even working at a computer. It is very important that you work with your student to find those *Techniques for Using the Mind* and thinking processes that will enable him to stay alert and function well. Use suggestions from *Behind the Obvious* to look for solutions.

Stein and Stoodley (2006)

Stacey (2019)

Techniques for Using the Mind: p 156
Behind the Obvious: p 64

5.2.7 Static material and constant content

Sometimes, an assessment of dyslexia/ SpLD will state that the person needs 'static material': material that doesn't shift around. You can help by leaving main points in view, either while you are talking about them or while students use them in an exercise.

One way material shifts is when details are changed just because keeping them the same would be boring. For example, authors use a variety of words for one concept. Many a dyslexic/ SpLD reader becomes insecure as a result. They worry in case they have missed some subtle change of meaning. It can take a while to mull over possible nuances and finally come to the conclusion that it is only a stylistic change with no significance. Such puzzling just adds to the frustration of reading.

In teaching situations, changing the content while teaching a skill or concept can obscure that skill or concept. You need to keep the content constant so that the desired connections have the best possible opportunity to be made.

Exercise: Constant content

Knowing the difference between facts, arguments and evaluations is part of *SKILLED THINKING*. To get students to see the difference, I asked them to plan three different essays. The context of the essay was kept constant so that the point of the exercise was obvious to them. They also needed to do the exercise; I couldn't use it as a demonstration. It is a good exercise for group work.

Object of the exercise: for your students to understand the difference between those essay titles, and exam questions, that require:
   a) facts
   b) arguments
   c) evaluations.

How would the essays be different in response to the following:
Facts level:
     Analyse the skills involved in study at university and their relevance to the work place.
Argument level:
     What arguments can be made for and against the view that the skills involved in study at university are relevant to the work place?
Evaluation level:
     Evaluate the skills involved in study at university and their relevance to the work place.

The exercise works best as a discussion between several students about what to include and why, and how to plan the essay.
Moving on to writing an essay would lose the distinctions you want the students to learn.
The distinction between these levels could be re-enforced by using a different topic to generate three similar essay titles, always keeping the content constant.

KNOWLEDGE: FACTS, DISCUSSION, EVALUATION: p 152

SKILLED THINKING: p 167

5.2.8 IT solutions

This book doesn't cover IT solutions. They play an important part, but in selecting which ones to use, the way each person works best needs to be taken into account.

The best selection process is for your student to try out anything on a task that is representative of what he needs to do.

5.2.9 Helpful teaching practices

The box below includes some practical measures that you can take which will help dyslexic/ SpLD students, as well as any other students. The measures address several of the difficulties dyslexic/ SpLDs have and they encourage the students to use their minds well. If you have a distinct teaching style, make sure you also include the preferences of others who have a different style. An organised teacher is often easier to follow than a disorganised one.

Summary: Influences on dyslexic/ SpLD people's learning

'Neurons firing together, wire together' is a crucial part of learning.

Beware of:
- expecting subliminal learning to happen
- rote learning
- out of sight being out of mind
- the effects on learning of:
  o space, place and direction
  o the environment
  o time
- your student's mind getting switched off because his innate learning style is not being used.

Techniques that help:

- various *TECHNIQUES FOR USING THE MIND* need to be taught explicitly

- unorthodox thinking preferences need to be encouraged

- keeping content static while teaching skills

- use *TEMPLATE: E7 - THE BOX: 'OTHER'* when a student's way of processing information doesn't fit into anything you know already.

FOUNDATIONS OF KNOWLEDGE AND SKILLS to teach overtly:

- comprehension

- identifying any goal

- planning

- organisation

- prioritising.

Teaching practices that help:

- clear framework and rationale

- handouts for lectures given in good time to allow preparation

- reading lists annotated to show core texts and clear, straightforward texts

- handouts for coursework or homework

- clear deadlines

- annotated model answers for guidance

- unambiguous feedback

- positive, encouraging use of mistakes.

TECHNIQUES FOR USING THE MIND: p 156

TEMPLATES

FOUNDATIONS OF KNOWLEDGE AND SKILLS: p 134

5.3 Teaching language

It is often a mistake to think that because a dyslexic/ SpLD person cannot learn to spell simple words he cannot learn grammar, other more advanced language skills or another language. I've heard many dyslexic/ SpLD students tell me that their own language made sense once they learnt a foreign language, especially when the foreign language is taught systematically or they go abroad and are immersed in the language.

My purpose for teaching grammar to university dyslexic/ SpLD students was to give them a tool that helps reading: when reading is not working, knowing how to fit the building blocks of language together can help your student to understand the text.

Example: Using building blocks of language as
a tool for reading

An example of complex writing:

> 'Evidence to support the argument that dyslexic people who have become successful readers, sometimes referred to as compensated dyslexics, make heavy use of semantic codes comes from a study by Lefly and Pennington (1991), who investigated the performance of compensated dyslexic people and other adults on silent reading and reading aloud.' (from McLoughlin et al. (2001)

McLoughlin et al. (2001)

The main sentence is 'Evidence comes from Lefly and Pennington (1991)' with 'evidence' as subject and 'comes' as verb. There are 24 words between the subject and the verb. Many times it is really useful to be able to break a sentence up in order to understand what is being said.

The above text can be reconstructed as:

> Dyslexic people can become successful readers. When they do, they are sometimes referred to as *compensated dyslexics*.

> It has been argued that they make heavy use of semantic codes.

> Evidence supporting this argument comes from a study by Lefly and Pennington (1991). They investigated the performance of compensated dyslexic people and other adults on silent reading and reading aloud.

English language was part of a module that I ran over 8 years for dyslexic students at Oxford Brookes University. I found some grammar books with different styles that students could use to re-inforce the teaching, including *Grammar Made Easy* by Barbara Dykes (1992) and *Usborne Book of Better English* by Robyn Gee (2004).

Dykes (1992)
Gee (2004)

- I taught the function of words:
  - ○ I had a table which showed how a word changes its function in different sentences

MEANINGS OF WORDS: p 98

- ○ I taught the functions as the relationships between words in a sentence
- ○ I used the names of the parts of speech: nouns, pronouns, adjectives, verbs, adverbs, prepositions

TEMPLATES

See:
G1 - THE FUNCTIONS OF 'ROUND' AND OTHER WORDS
G2 - THE FUNCTIONS OF WORDS

- ○ using the idea of constant content, the names and the functions were always visible once they had been taught
- ○ we focused on the way a word was being used in a sentence rather than which group it belonged to.

TEMPLATES

SEE
G3 - CONSTANT CONTENT TO DEMONSTRATE LANGUAGE FUNCTION

- I taught the patterns of verbs:
  - ○ the spelling changes
    - with tense
    - with 1st, 2nd, 3rd person and singular or plural
  - ○ and all the possible auxiliary verbs.

Blissett and Hallgarten (1992)

- I taught sentence structure:
  - subject, verb, 'everything else'
  - complex sentences and how to break them into basic sentences.

TEMPLATES

 See:

G4 - BASIC SENTENCE PATTERN
G5 - BASIC SENTENCES FROM A COMPLEX ONE

- I used text with no copyright restrictions, including newspaper articles.
- I sought to make the language work as easy as possible for them by having something interesting after it and by including good *BREATHING*, *RELAXATION* and other mentally calming exercises during the sessions (Stacey, 2019).

BREATHING: p 557
RELAXATION: p 558

Stacey (2019)

Some students liked it; some never liked it. Some of my one-to-one students have asked to be taught language.

My difficulty as a teacher is that examples never flowed easily into my mind when I needed them and that is always a problem. However, I could demonstrate the problems of reading text and how I use my knowledge of language to unravel the meaning.

THINKING PREFERENCES can affect how fluently a student can write. For example, practical dyslexic/ SpLDs can find theories and models of good practice more difficult to write about than the practical work they do.

THINKING PREFERENCES: p 72

When I read a student's work, any language-based comments are opportunities to teach good use of language. I collect them together on a separate sheet. I don't use red pen or pencil.

I explain any language comment. If a student just makes corrections because you have said so, there is unlikely to be any subliminal learning and the same errors will come again and again.

5.3.1 Meanings of words

Dyslexic/ SpLD people are often good at computer languages because there are stricter rules and less ambiguity. The subtle changes in words often cause considerable problems.

Comments about words in this book can be found in:

- *STATIC MATERIAL AND CONSTANT CONTENT*: discussion about words being changed for stylistic purposes.

- The *STORY: A WORD LOSING ITS CONTEXT*: an incidence when a familiar word was disconnected from its meaning.

- *SCHIZOPHRENIA: COLOURED SPELLING*: keeping families of words together to see their patterns.

- *UNFAMILIAR WORDS*: how the lack of meaning of words interferes with reading.

- *THE ORDER OF WORDS*: discussion of word order changing the meaning of a sentence.

- The *MAIN IDEA OF A SENTENCE*: discussion of clarity and the position of the main idea in a sentence.

- *COMMENTS ABOUT GRAMMAR*: discussion of several ways lack of understanding can be caused by the way words are used.

It is worth teaching about words systematically.

The *TABLE: THE FUNCTION OF 'ROUND'* demonstrates how a word can have different meanings depending on the way it is used in a sentence.

STATIC MATERIAL AND CONSTANT CONTENT: p 91

STORY: A WORD LOSING ITS CONTEXT: p 268

SCHIZOPHRENIA: COLOURED SPELLING: p 325

UNFAMILIAR WORDS: p 246

THE ORDER OF WORDS: p 356

MAIN IDEA OF A SENTENCE: p 357

COMMENTS ABOUT GRAMMAR: p 254

Crystal (1997)

Table: The function of 'round' (adapted from Crystal, 1997)		
Noun	It's your round. I'll have whisky.	It's your turn. I'll have whisky.
Adjective	Mary bought a round table.	Mary bought a folding table.
Adverb	We walked round to the shop.	We walked back to the shop.
Verb	The yacht will round the buoy soon.	The yacht will reach the buoy soon.
Preposition	The car went round the corner.	The car went past the corner.

This table demonstrates the fluidity of words and the importance of context.

There is a framework to words and sentences and often understanding that framework in its own right is a necessary part of helping a dyslexic/ SpLD person to use language well.

The *TEMPLATE: G1 - THE FUNCTIONS OF 'ROUND' AND OTHER WORDS* is a useful practice sheet in this context.

TEMPLATES

5.3.2 Spelling

There are many reasons why spelling is difficult and variable for dyslexic/ SpLD people; mal-sequencing is just one of them.

Story: Mal-sequencing in spelling

Michael Newby (1995) persuaded Tim Miles[3] that some spelling errors were mal-sequencing, or mistiming, rather than not knowing how to spell a word.

Certainly many students have described their writing problems as the mind racing ahead with thoughts while the hand lags behind.

The result is often that words the mind is thinking about get written into the text the hand is writing and the words look jumbled up.

Newby (1995)

---

[3] Prof Tim Miles was a highly distinguished dyslexia expert. He was joint editor of the book that contains Michael Newby's chapter. There is a footnote by the editors explaining that Michael Newby had 'argued that the word 'mal-sequencing' aptly describes the distinctive difficulties of the dyslexic'.

99

Does your student check a word's spelling by

- the movement of an imaginary pen
- saying the word
- sounding out the letters
- thinking how he's seen it
- thinking of the logic of the word?

Sound and spelling

- Has he got the right pronunciation for the word?
- Will he recognise the word correctly when he hears it, and relate the sound to the correct word?
- Would a dictionary, online or paper, with a useable guide to pronunciation help?

Learning issues

- Is he using his best way of learning, including his *Thinking Preferences*, to learn spelling?
- Would it help to shut his eyes and get the movement into his motor memory without interference from sight? See *Insight: Sight Interfering with Learning Movement*
- Does he practise little and often?
- Is he trying to use rote learning when that isn't going to work for him?
- Would colour coding as in *Schizophrenia: Colour Coding* help or *Creating Blocks by Adding Borders*?
- Does it help to understand how words change from one to another, e.g. schizophrenia, schizophrenic and schizophrene have the same initial letters, belong to the same context and have different sounds at the end?

Thinking Preferences: p 72

Insight: Sight Interfering with Learning Movement: p 148

Schizophrenia: Coloured Spelling: p 325

Creating Blocks by Adding Borders: p 331

Using correct spelling

- Many dyslexic/ SpLD people cannot think about spelling at the same time as focusing on the ideas they want to put across.
- Even in proof-reading, incorrect spelling may not be noticed.
- No collection of strategies to recall the correct spelling can solve this problem.

Confidence and self-esteem

- Does he understand why he in particular is having problems with spelling?
- Does he feel OK about those times when his spelling feels random[4], or do you need to help him with his confidence and self-esteem?

Other issues

- Can he spell a word in isolation but not when concentrating on putting his ideas across?
- Can he learn words now as an adult but not get words he 'learnt' as a child right?
- Can he give himself permission to not spell correctly when the writing is only for himself?

5.3.3 Punctuation

- It is worth teaching punctuation as a tool that is helpful rather than as an arbitrary set of conventions.
- Punctuation provides pauses between words and contributes to meaning.
- Text that is well punctuated is easier to read because it is easier to recognise meaningful groups of words.

---

[4] Random spelling: sometimes a dyslexic/ SpLD person will roughly know which letters ought to be in a word, but how to arrange them can feel like a process of random selection.

5.4 Supporting maths learning

One significant consideration about learning maths is the way it builds on previous knowledge.

Many other subjects have a linear progression; for example, history's progression through the centuries. You can learn about history out of order but it is very difficult to learn maths out of order. So the way your student has learnt maths in the past may have a considerable effect on his ability to use maths now and to continue learning more of it.

The *General Issues About Teaching* and *Experience and Episodic Memory* have significant insights which may help you to understand why your student's mind is not constructing the memories that constitute learning maths.

General Issues About Teaching: p 87

Experience and Episodic Memory: p 156

The most important part of supporting maths learning is to find out the root of the problem.

- Your student may be struggling with maths concepts.
- There may be a gap in his maths knowledge.
- He may be using inadequate techniques.
- Your student could be adopting the wrong approach for himself, e.g. trying rote learning when he is someone who needs to understand every step.
- It could be that the style of teaching doesn't suit your student:
  o the pace could be wrong
  o the balance of verbal, visual and kinaesthetic work could be unsuitable
  o the role of logic and organisation (rationale, framework) might have different importance for teacher and student.

There are many other stages which can be causing the problem, including not seeing the sense of doing maths.

Story: Maths is stupid

The problem set was:
Bath water runs in from the tap at 10 litres per minute. It runs out through the plug hole at 7 litres per minute. How fast does the bath fill?

One child's reaction was: "Don't they know to put the plug in? This is stupid. I'm not doing it." At which point, he disengaged from maths.

If maths concepts are at the heart of his problems, your student needs to be helped by someone who understands the maths very well. The tutor also should be willing to listen to the dyslexic/ SpLD problems of the student and know how to adapt to them. *The Trouble with Maths: A Practical Guide to Helping Learners with Numeracy Difficulties* has many suggestions about finding the right approach (Chinn, 2017).

Chinn (2017)

If maths problems are not at the heart of his problems, you don't need to understand the maths in order to be helpful though you should be comfortable[5] with symbols.

I often watch my student working and ask questions. I'm trying to find out
- where there is a gap in his knowledge
- whether learning the maths is holding up his progress
- whether there is any organisation of concepts that would help him
- whether short-term memory is a problem
- how he deals with vocabulary and the words involved
- how good his problem-solving skills are
- how he sets out his maths working

---

[5] I have 2 degrees in physics. Although it is a long time since I used maths professionally, I am comfortable with discussing maths.

- whether his spatial awareness is causing problems
- whether there's confusion from reading numbers left-to-right but working out sums right-to-left
- how he copies from one line to another
- and anything else; this list is not exhaustive.

Solutions are quite individual when it comes to resolving problems that have built up. Good organised teaching and learning from the beginning is the best solution. The suggestions set out here are those that have evolved while supporting my varied students.

Dyspraxic students often need special help with organisation of the maths concepts and how they work.

There can be solutions that come from your student's *THINKING PREFERENCES*:

THINKING PREFERENCES: p 72

- he may need to find the right *MATERIALS AND METHODS* to work with

MATERIALS AND METHODS: p 565

- if he is a logical thinker who likes a *RATIONALE OR FRAMEWORK*, he may need to start with a syllabus and break it into component parts that he can see coming together into a whole, as he progresses through a topic

RATIONALE OR FRAMEWORK: p 75

- as a logical thinker (possibly a linear thinker or using MBPT-T), he may also need to have explanations about the maths before doing any problems will help him to understand it
- if he is a kinaesthetic thinker (see *SENSE-BASED THINKING PREFERENCES*), he is likely to be well suited by the way maths work is repeated

SENSES-BASED THINKING PREFERENCES: p 75

- as a visual thinker, he may be helped by colour coding diagrams or process words or the working of processes
- he could use the suggestions relating maths formulae to vocabulary techniques using a verbal strength
- he may find a particular colour of paper helps him to read.

Encourage him to explore various options to find the ones that help him.

TECHNIQUES FOR USING THE MIND will all help with learning maths. Working on expanding the *CAPACITY OF WORKING MEMORY* makes a considerable difference. *RECALL AND MEMORISING EXERCISES* help to establish the maths in long-term memory so that it can be accessed again when needed.

TECHNIQUES FOR USING THE MIND: p 156

CAPACITY OF WORKING MEMORY: p 157

RECALL AND MEMORISING EXERCISES: p 159

Preparation is useful. Concentration can be maintained when the meanings of unfamiliar words are found before reading or doing problem sheets. Such preparation can be done the day before a period of work.

Handling the maths can be helped by:

- getting an overview of the topic being studied by using key words in a layout that shows the way one concept depends on another; the overview can come from a syllabus, lecture notes, book contents, etc.

- treating formulae, the symbols and their meanings as vocabulary to learn little by little through repeated *RECALL AND MEMORISING EXERCISES*; including the shape of symbols and their names

RECALL AND MEMORISING EXERCISES: p 159

- knowing what each symbol stands for in formulae

- understanding any science that is behind a maths problem

- distinguishing between *PROCESS AND CONTEXT WORDS*

PROCESS AND CONTEXT WORDS: p 189

- making a list of common processes and seeing how they fit into the syllabus

- knowing exactly what the process words tell him to do

- colour coding different concepts: red for proofs, green for examples, blue for theorems, etc.

- colour coding different elements in diagrams.

Mechanics of maths working

The comments above, about preparation, apply to doing problem sheets and homework.

Working memory is assisted by reading the whole set of problems to be done before starting the first one.

Underline or highlight the process words in all the problems.

If maths is set out well, it can be much easier to understand and much easier to do problems. Organising the way he puts his working on to a page can benefit your student. This could be by:

- spreading equations that occupy more than a single line over three lines of the page:
    1)   the top line of the equation,
    2)   any division lines that are part of the equation,
    3)   the bottom line of the equation
- using one side of the page so that all working can be seen at the same time
- not squashing work at the bottom of a page to avoid turning over
- tracking over equations as they are transferred to the next line of working; the tracking covers the symbols that have been used in the second line; it can be done by finger, pencil or piece of card
- finding the size of lines that help him transfer the maths from one line to the next without missing out any symbol or number.

Accommodations for maths

There are times when the way a student learns maths needs specific accommodations to enable him to show his capabilities. *EXAMPLE REQUEST FOR ACCOMMODATION* uses the situation for one maths student who needed special accommodation for stepwise learning. A few different accommodations for exams are discussed in *MATHS AND SCIENCE EXAMS*.

EXAMPLE REQUEST FOR ACCOMMODATION:
p 574

MATHS AND SCIENCE EXAMS: p 432

Summary: Teaching language and supporting maths

Systematic language teaching can provide a framework that allows your student to understand language and use it well.

Maths teaching involves finding out the root of the problem and observing your student working through his maths.
To what extend is there a problem with maths concepts? Is a maths teacher needed?

To what extent are other factors causing the problems? Can they be resolved so that the maths can be learnt?

Observe him working to find out where his problems lie and to suggest solutions. Monitor his progress, using progress and mistakes positively to let him develop his best way of learning maths.

6 Dialogue

DIALOGUES and conversations are carried out in many different settings, from formal ones to informal. Sometimes important information is exchanged, but not always. The way the information is conveyed may use incomplete sentences.

Story: Not finding words

In a group of dyslexics, person A was giving directions to B. It was a conversation, but neither was using words very well. They were using hands and diagrams to 'speak' to each other. At one point the rest burst into laughter. "You aren't using words! But B knows where to go!"

In this conversation there was no misunderstanding between the two involved and among the whole group. But if either A or B hadn't had a mind that worked without words, there would have been difficulty in exchanging the information. Then the conversation would have needed to be a dialogue: 'a discussion between representatives of different countries or groups, esp. with a view to resolving conflict or solving a problem' (OED Online, 2020). The problem being addressed in this section is misunderstandings that arise because of the effects of dyslexia/ SpLD during conversations.

('dialogue, n.2c' OED Online, 2020)

Misunderstandings and difficulties in the communication may be obvious to both sides but they can also be hidden because nobody is paying any attention to differences in thinking styles and different interpretations during the communication.

This section is about:

- the people involved in situations when dialogue is needed
    - professional people
    - family, friends and acquaintances
    - work colleagues
    - general public
- misunderstandings that could have serious consequences
- misunderstandings that add unwelcome tensions in life or study or work
- underlying differences in thought processing that contribute to the misunderstandings
- suggestions for dialogue to unravel the misunderstandings.

N.B. Dyslexia/ SpLD are not the only reasons for misunderstandings and other people also bring problems with them.

6.1 Professional people

There are people whose communication and dealings with dyslexic/ SpLD people can have long-reaching affects on the lives of the dyslexic/ SpLD people[6]:

- employers, managers, HRM staff
- job centre advisors, all other advisors
- social workers, medical and dental professionals
- counsellors, therapists
- legal professionals, bank managers and staff
- people in TEACHING ROLES
- anyone in a position of authority and responsibility
- retail, leisure industry, travel industry, etc.
- researchers, librarians
- diagnostic assessors
- needs evaluators.

Margin notes:

MARGIN NOTE: see WHAT CAN HAPPEN AND USEFUL, RELEVANT SECTIONS, p 464-470, for problems that dyslexic/ SpLD people experience that could underpin misunderstandings

HRM: human resource management

TEACHING ROLES: p 86

---

[6] The dyslexic/ SpLD people will not necessarily be students; for simplicity of language the phrase 'your student' is used to refer to anyone you might be thinking of or helping. see BOX: THE PHRASE 'YOUR STUDENT' p 3.

Misunderstandings involving these groups of people can be very serious.

Insight: Assumptions in counselling

If a person doesn't arrive for a counselling session, the assumption is that he is reluctant to engage with the process.

For a dyslexic/ SpLD client, it may be simply that he has no mental trigger for time; he has been looking forward to the session but at the last minute all thoughts about getting to it have just evaporated.

Interpreting late arrival as reluctance could be the exact opposite of the person's real attitude.

Counselling that involves wrong interpretations will not help the client.

People in these roles need to be aware that:
- a dyslexic/ SpLD person may not interpret words in the way intended
- direct questions are sometimes very unlikely to trigger recall of important information, see the story below
- the wrong work can be done between 2 meetings; considerable effort and care can be put into the work, but it is still off target
- a dyslexic/ SpLD person may be much more capable than his words indicate
- a dyslexic/ SpLD person may have very low self-esteem and low confidence; he may down-play the skills and knowledge that he has
- open-minded encouragement and confidence boosting may be needed to allow the dyslexic/ SpLD person to show what he is capable of.

Story: Why have you been sent to me?

One dyslexic was sent to a clinic for investigation of an intermittent, extreme pain. At the time of the consultation, the pain was absent. None of the consultant's questions triggered the memory of the pain. It was only the puzzled look on her face as she asked, "Why have you been sent?" that made the patient realise he had answered most of the questions incorrectly.

There can be a considerable contrast between the initial absence of memory of a given situation and the details that emerge when the information does come back. It can look as if the person is lying and making up a huge story. Professional people need to be very careful not to make judgements based on the likely reactions of non-dyslexic/ SpLD people.

Some of the professional roles will only involve short-term contact, with only one or two opportunities for dialogue. Others will continue over months or years and there will be time to resolve misunderstandings and unpick any unwanted consequences, providing they are noticed.

6.2 Family, friends and acquaintances

People living with dyslexic/ SpLD people often have problems:

- anticipating what is important for the dyslexic/ SpLDs
- finding out why they do the things they do
- what they mean in conversation.

The same is true for others who don't live with, but who have long-term relationships with dyslexic/ SpLDs. People included in this group are:

- spouses, siblings, families in general
- others living with dyslexic/ SpLD people
- friends, peers, co-hobbyists, house mates
- co-members of any organisation.

There can be misunderstandings because:

- the way thoughts are processed is different
- behaviour patterns can be different
- the way tasks are carried out is different.

Examples of these differences can be found in MISUNDERSTANDINGS IN DIALOGUES.

MISUNDERSTANDINGS IN DIALOGUES: p 113

Any misunderstandings can be accepted with love or tolerance. They may create irritation or serious tension. If the relationship between people is long-term, it is probably worth finding a comfortable reaction to the misunderstandings.

6.3 Work colleagues

Work colleagues and team members are people who are in positions of equality with a dyslexic/ SpLD colleague. They usually need to get on well with each other for the whole enterprise to succeed. The misunderstandings are the same as for FAMILY, FRIENDS AND ACQUAINTANCES, above, with the addition of those around:

Organisation and Everyday Life with Dyslexia and other SpLDs (Stacey, 2020a) deals with issues at work in detail.

- the special accommodations put in place without work colleagues knowing why
    - including acceptance of a slower work rate
- particular strategies which dyslexic/ SpLDs use to manage their dyslexia/ SpLD and which cause problems for those who work with them.

It is important to deal with misunderstandings in the workplace so that they don't build into bigger problems.

6.4 General public

There are enough dyslexic/ SpLD people for everyone to have contact with several, whether you know it or not. Dyslexia/ SpLD are hidden: you cannot look at one of this group of people and say, "That person has dyslexia/ SpLD, I need to be aware of that."

The attitudes that help dialogue with dyslexic/ SpLD people are also good when dealing with other people. So, people offering a service of any kind could find difficult situations are easier to manage if they understand the attitudes that help dyslexic/ SpLDs.

People offering a service include:

- shopkeepers, supermarket staff
- leisure centre staff
- hospitality staff
- travel industry staff
- librarians, public officers, local government officers
- etc.

When someone tells you he is dyslexic/ SpLD:

- don't take that to mean he has a low intelligence
- accept his description of his problem or his need
- ask what you can do to help
- if you feel it would help to write something down, try not to take no for an answer. I'm lucky in that respect, I can grin and say, "I would forget by the time I was out of the door, if I didn't write things down."
- find out whether words or diagrams work best
- if you can't provide the help requested, say so – politely.

SOCIAL EXAMPLES and *GROUP WORK: MEETINGS, SEMINARS AND DEBATES* give further insights into the problems dyslexic/ SpLDs face during everyday discussions.

SOCIAL EXAMPLES: p 492

GROUP WORK: MEETINGS, SEMINARS AND DEBATES: p 446

6.5 Policy-makers, campaigners and media personnel

The dialogue about dyslexia/ SpLD involves various groups of people who are speaking about and making plans on behalf of dyslexic/ SpLD people. The groups include:

- policy-makers of all kinds
- politicians
- disability campaigners
- media people.

People in all these groups need to have a positive attitude that is promoting the practices that are VITAL for dyslexic/ SpLD people and GOOD for all.

Their positive attitude can make a significant difference to the self-esteem and confidence of dyslexic/ SpLD people, which in turn enables the dyslexic/ SpLDs to contribute to society.

This attitude should underpin dialogue:

- with dyslexic/ SpLD people in getting to understand the syndromes better
- with many other people in promoting the right policies and attitudes.

6.6 Misunderstandings in dialogues

Dialogue contains uncertainty when you can't predict what another person will do – it could be a source of delight, but often it isn't. If you are wrong-footed because you can't predict, difficult emotions can get in the way and produce serious tension. Misunderstandings can multiply when they are not noticed and when they are not unpicked.

Misunderstandings are going to be particular to the people involved. Certain factors that would lead to good exchange of information between one couple could cause considerable confusion for a different couple, but it is worth discussing a few of the more prevalent causes. I've divided them into ones arising from:

- different thought processes
- curious behaviour
- tasks done differently.

6.6.1 Differences in thought processing

The various THINKING PREFERENCES can lead to different internal interpretations and you can hear these differences in the language used to carry on a conversation.

THINKING PREFERENCES: p 72

"You can see more sea gulls inland these days."
Possible internal responses from different THINKING PREFERENCES:

Verbal	prose or poetry relating to sea gulls and landscapes
Visual	mind's eye pictures of sea gulls in landscapes
Kinaesthetic	physical memory of walking through a field full of sea gulls
MBPT intuitive	thoughts about global climate issues, fishing issues
MBPT feeling	concern for a person having a sandwich snatched by a sea gull
MI naturalist	the different species of sea gulls and which ones are coming inland.

Ⓖ p 574 MBPT

Ⓖ p 574 MI

The different responses to the initial sentence will bring a different flavour to the conversation. Misunderstandings can follow when no-one is aware of the different way minds are interpreting the information.

Some characteristics of holistic thinking can cause difficulties. Holistic thinkers often think without words. If they need to describe their thoughts or actions:

HOLISTIC VS. LINEAR THINKING: p 75

- o finding all the words can be difficult
- o to say anything is too slow, holistic thinking is much faster
- o they may miss out important words
- o they may miss out important steps

- o they may miss out links between ideas
- o they may not complete one idea before starting on the next
- o they have so much in their head, they go off at a tangent very easily
- o too many thoughts come into their heads from a single idea, they produce too much for anyone else to keep up with.

Holistic thinking has many riches to contribute, but holistic thinkers need to be aware that others can be confused by the way they speak.

The Senses may not work together during a conversation. If a conversation involves words and pictures together, one or other sense may not register the information.

SENSES: p 74

If the Rationale or Framework is missing from the conversation, someone who has a preference for these may have no way to remember what is being said to him.

RATIONALE OR FRAMEWORK: p 75

Some dyslexic/ SpLD people's minds do not store enough spoken words in working memory, see *CAPACITY OF WORKING MEMORY.* During a conversation, their comprehension is restricted and they often don't have access to all the information that has just been given to them. It is difficult to keep asking others to repeat what they have said; it may be difficult to make notes during the conversation. Again misunderstandings will happen.

CAPACITY OF WORKING MEMORY: p 157

There are times when unspoken messages are completely ignored by dyslexic/ SpLDs. The *STORY: AN UNDERLYING MESSAGE MISSED* is an example of feedback to a student being understood as sympathetic encouragement when it meant, "Your work is no good."

STORY: AN UNDERLYING MESSAGE MISSED: p 266

If you have a mind that doesn't work reliably, consistently or
fluently with words, it is very easy to misinterpret a
conversation. The interpretation in your head can be
internally consistent; it just isn't what others expect.

Understanding jokes can also be a problem: you have so much
work to do to sort out the words that the essence of the
joke evaporates.

6.6.2 Curious behaviour

Story: Noticing curious behaviour

Often groups of students live together in a house. They select
their group because they all get on well together. One student in
such a group came to ask to be assessed for dyslexia. The others
in her house were dyslexic and already putting together ways to
manage their dyslexic traits. They had watched her using the
same kinds of strategies so then they all discussed the problems
they faced. The others were convinced she was also dyslexic and
that their shared experiences were why they all got on. On
assessment, she also turned out to be dyslexic.

Some of the curious behaviour includes:

- keys in the fridge with lunch box so that keys won't be left behind
- bike locked in the garage so that keys can't be left behind
- note-pads everywhere, since a thought will evaporate if it is not
  captured immediately
- objects left where they have to be tripped over so that they work
  as reminders (kinaesthetic)
- Post-it notes all over the place, e.g. on inside of front door with list
  of things regularly needed (visual)
- clothes pegs with notes on bags and clothes with reminder notes
- need for everything to be in its own place
- everything taken to a meeting just in case it will be useful.

Dealing with any of the issues that stem from the ideas in *Individuals with Dyslexia/ SpLD* can lead to different strategies that those around regard as curious.

Individuals with Dyslexia/ SpLD: p 57

There are effects on conversations and dialogue caused by the curious behaviour because there is a lack of shared experience.

- People will be making incorrect assumptions about other people's perspectives.
- Conversations can become more complicated with more explanations that seem unnecessary to one or other party.
- Unhelpful emotions can get into the conversation.

6.6.3 Tasks done differently

The way anyone does a task will depend on what exact problems they face and what their strengths are. To try to make a list of characteristics in this book would probably be unhelpful.

> As you understand more about your dyslexia/ SpLD and how it impacts on your life you can become more open about the ways you do tasks. You can make your own list of your characteristics. You can help other people to accept your ways as being right for you, even though they may not fully understand.

You may find dyslexic/ SpLD people being very determined to do tasks in their own particular way. I have watched students doing something in a completely bizarre, to me, way; I have made suggestions as to how it could be done more easily, but I have had to recognise that the way they are tackling the task is the only one that is going to work for them.

By accepting my students' perspectives of how they want to do a particular task, while gently questioning why it is like that for them, I can keep their trust and be able to support their endeavours. Nothing would have been gained by pushing beyond their willingness to try something different. I know from my own experience that chaos can quickly result from trying another person's way of doing something when it really doesn't fit my mind's requirements.

6.7 Groups

Dialogue in groups will have all the possibilities for misunderstandings mentioned above. The self-esteem and confidence of a dyslexic/ SpLD person will be an important factor in both his ability to ask questions when he knows he doesn't understand something and his willingness to contribute to the conversations. *Listening* and *Group Work: Meetings, Seminars and Debates* discuss the issues further.

Listening: p 262

Group Work: Meetings, Seminars and Debates: p 446

6.8 Summary: good outcomes for dialogue

Summary: Good outcomes for dialogue

- Professional people will recognise how important it is that any impact of the dyslexia/ SpLD is clearly and fairly dealt with.

- People in authority or having any kind of responsibility towards others will be aware of misunderstanding and the potential for wrong decisions based on them, see *Insight Box: Assumptions in Counselling*.

- People living with, working alongside, taking-action with dyslexic/ SpLD people will have a better understanding of the issues and problems faced by dyslexic/ SpLD people and hence a greater tolerance of many odd things that happen.

- Colleagues at work will accept any special accommodations put in place.

- People in the general public will have an understanding that allows them to be more open to helping.

- Policy-makers will be able to design useful, constructive policies.

- Media people will understand the wide impact of dyslexia/ SpLD and support the work designed to lessen the impact and to enable dyslexic/ SpLDs to use their full potential.

Insight Box: Assumptions in Counselling: p 109

(G) p 575
taking-action

7 Indirect communication

Indirect communication includes sign writing, manuals, exam papers, online information, notices (public, workplace, education, health), letters (official, legal, banking, tax, health, etc.), anything that is giving information without direct contact between the giver and receiver.

The lack of contact means the receiver cannot seek immediate clarification from the giver and the giver doesn't get the direct feedback as to where there are difficulties. Most of the time information is important and needs to be understood correctly.

People dealing with indirect communication include:

- writers of public communications
- writers of manuals
- public sign designers
- lecturers, exam writers
- shopkeepers, web designers
- and many similar roles involving writing or talking or designing material for general communication.

Good indirect communication will alleviate the problems of dyslexia/ SpLD and incorporate the most widespread solutions. Many problems and solutions are described in the rest of this book, together with underlying causes or resources, respectively. It would double the size of the book to repeat them all here to explain the bullet points in this section. Some useful sections are listed in the margin. As you consider the problems and solutions, anticipate the situations your readers or listeners will find themselves in and what experiences they are likely to bring while accessing your material.

From my own work, I know it is not possible to satisfy the particular needs of every dyslexic/ SpLD person with a single way of presenting the indirect communication, but there are a lot of elements that will make comprehension very much easier. Showing that effort is being made will also help.

INDIVIDUALS WITH DYSLEXIA/ SPLD: p 57 especially *INPUT, OUTPUT AND MOTIVATION:* p 73

READING PROBLEMS: p 252

LISTENING PROBLEMS: p 276

PROBLEMS RELATING TO DOING: p 297

WHAT COULD HAPPEN AND USEFUL, RELEVANT SECTIONS: p 464

Story: Someone knows about dyslexia

At my first role as university support tutor, the students had to fill in a form to request exam provisions every time they had exams. The exams office were frustrated that the forms from dyslexic students were so badly filled in. I told them to put example answers on the back of the letter that went with the exams form. I stressed that the students needed to see the blank form and the answers at the same time, otherwise there would be no improvement. The forms were then filled-in correctly.

One student told me the example being on the back of the letter told her that someone in the university knew the problems of dyslexia. The knowledge reassured her to the point that she relaxed about her difficulties and found her own ways round them.

Most organisations will have dyslexic/ SpLD people in them. It would be worth forming a group with different dyslexia/ SpLD profiles to tryout any new indirect communications that are going to be widely used. Smaller organisations could be helped by the local university or dyslexia/ SpLD adult groups.

This section is presented as bullet points which you can use either to guide your research into problems and solutions or as a check-list of what to bear in mind.

Key point: Be aware of difficulties

People who design public documents, notices and signs should:

- remember the user, usually, cannot contact you for clarification
- be well aware of the difficulties encountered by those who are dyslexic/ SpLD

- realise how fundamental the problems can be
- remember, one size does not fit all: cover widespread needs and allow for flexibility where possible
- try out their products with people who have different dyslexic/ SpLD profiles.

Key point: Universality of clarity

- When it is a question of suiting many different people, the aim should be for a clarity of style that can easily convey the complexity of ideas that are being put across.
- 'Style' includes the way language is used, the layout and the physical presentation of the material.
- The system for British road signs is a good example of simplicity being used to convey very complex information: as simple as possible and as complex as necessary.

- The clarity that helps dyslexic/ SpLD people will also help others, including people in a state of stress, e.g.:
  o   people short of time
  o   people living through a difficult time of life.

The first section below has some general ideas. The following sections cover a variety of indirect-communication methods.

For each, there is:

- list of things for designers to bear in mind
- list of good practice
- list of things to avoid.

7.1 General considerations

Bear in mind:

- ideas in *Summary: Influences on Dyslexic/ SpLD People's Learning*
- the problems and solutions in chapters 4 - 14
- clear communications reduce stress levels and will be easier to understand and follow
- visual images help words to be understood; words will often be needed too, but they should not obscure the visual images
- that many people need to understand a topic, or situation, in order to remember any information; bald facts on their own may not be registered in a reader's mind
- unfamiliar words will need explanations
- underlying messages are likely to be missed
- materials are needed early so that they can be used effectively for preparation.

Good practice:

- straightforward overview of material
- clear fonts without serifs
- left justification, words neither squashed up nor spread out
- fonts that have space between the words and between the lines
- good definition of words with sufficient ascenders and descenders to the letter shapes
- meaning-related words and phrases kept together
- direct sentences, because they are easier to understand
- materials made available well in advance.

Avoid:

- ambiguity
- complex and double negatives
- negative language: 'don't forget' can easily be registered as 'forget'; 'remember' is a better alternative
- talking down: recognise you may be addressing intelligent people who simply lack knowledge

- superfluous information that is not part of holding the facts together
- changing details too often, especially just before action is required
- making written materials available just before they are to be used.

7.2 Written communication

Bear in mind:

- people use filters to help their reading: changes of background colour may be unhelpful, unless they are part of deliberate colour coding, which can be very helpful
- give prominence to main ideas
- *GOOD PARAGRAPH STRUCTURE* is important
- good, specified overall structure is extremely useful.

see also: *GENERAL CONSIDERATIONS*: p 122

GOOD PARAGRAPHS STRUCTURE: p 250

Good practice:

- paper: pale/ pastel colours are best to cater for the majority
- feedback on work that has been submitted to you: clear writing; clear comments in complete sentences
- for work that is to be submitted: annotated examples showing good practice
- large tables: colour coding in both directions, i.e. the vertical columns alternating in 2 tones of, say, green and the rows alternating in 2 tones of, say, blue.

Avoid:

- black on white
- long paragraphs
- convoluted sentences
- for exams and forms: any layout that increases a dyslexic/ SpLD person's reading problems.

7.3 Lecturing and talking

Bear in mind:

- understanding speech can be difficult for some dyslexic/ SpLDs, see *A Range of Listening Experiences*
- *Mind Set* assists good listening
- handouts, work sheets, papers for meetings made available early allows for good preparation to be undertaken
- visual aids can make words easier to understand
- obvious, spelled-out overall structure helps comprehension
- that people have different internal representations of words, and may not have the same understanding, see *Meet You at the Top of the Road*
- if you say a string of numbers or letters, they may be remembered in the wrong order
- different accents are difficult to understand: speak more slowly if your accent is unusual for your audience.

see also: *General Considerations:* p 122

A Range of Listening Experiences: p 267

Mind Set: p 158

Meet You at the Top of the Road: p 367

Good practice:

- defined sections in medium-to-long talks or lectures
- good slides or other visual aids help people to listen
- leave any visual material in view for some time
- handouts and paperwork available well before a lecture or meeting
- handouts and paperwork in formats that can be annotated during the lecture or meeting.
- allow recording devices to be used
- clarity of speech, including a slower speed, helps people to listen and register what is being said.

Avoid:

- slides with a lot of text or numbers
- reading your slides verbatim
- reading script, if at all possible
- speaking too fast
- cramming in material at the end because time is running out.

7.4 Online

Bear in mind:

- *OUT OF SIGHT IS OUT OF MIND*
- problems arising from *CAPACITY OF WORKING MEMORY* being reduced by dyslexia/ SpLD
- clear navigation tools are needed.

Good practice:

- allow the use of assistive technology
- direct routes back to the main page
- succinct overview of pages
- for forms:
    - enable scrolling backwards and forwards
    - enable seeing different parts simultaneously
    - provide a pdf of any form to be filled in
    - allow entries to be changed
    - allow forms to be saved for later completion.

Avoid:

- clutter on the page
- dense text in early parts of a search process
- unnecessary distractions.

7.5 Instructions

Handouts, minutes of meetings and agendas for meetings are similar to instructions; the ideas set out here are relevant to all these types of written documents.

Bear in mind:

- diagrams and pictures can help people make sense of words
- good use of symbols assists understanding
- overview or list of sections helps efficient processing
- the sequence of the instructions or sections needs to be logical
- clarity is really important

see also: *GENERAL CONSIDERATIONS*: p 122

OUT OF SIGHT IS OUT OF MIND: p 90

CAPACITY OF WORKING MEMORY: p 157

see also: *GENERAL CONSIDERATIONS*: p 122

Good practice:

- for meetings: repeat the details of full date and day, time, place, reason or title of meeting on all communications, especially when one detail is changed

- for meetings: a layout that can be used for notes during meetings

- clear list of any parameters: deadlines, tools required for a construction project

- for projects with time elements: instructions given early enough for there to be time to work with them, but not so early they can be put aside till later

- for forms: instructions visible at the same time as the sections to be filled in.

Avoid:

- parameters (e.g. length of time for a talk) only being given in the middle of a paragraph of text

- giving details of time, place, date and title of meeting in a piecemeal fashion.

7.6 Signage

Bear in mind:

- clear signage can significantly help the people who use it

- other people being able to understand information is more important than a design that artistically satisfies the designer

- what people will be looking for when using signs; for example, train notices that only give directions to the final destinations can confuse people who only know the mid-way station they are going to

- words should keep their standard shapes

- difficulty in noticing differences, such as distinguishing between letters with similar appearance (e.g. b and d, u and n, m and w): so the different directions of the arrows in FIGURE 1.3 may well be missed.

see also: GENERAL CONSIDERATIONS: p 122

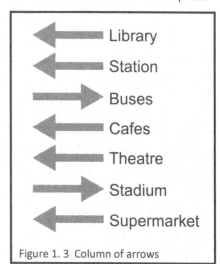

Figure 1. 3 Column of arrows

In talking to a designer about such signs, I suggested various ways the grouping could be changed:

- left-pointing arrows to the left; right to the right

Good practice:

- simplicity of design

- visual images

- clear separation of different categories: e.g. when the same information is given in 2 different languages, separate them on different backgrounds and keep the backgrounds consistent.

- different colours for the two directions

- the left and right ones separated into 2 groups.

I was told the design came first!

Avoid:

- unhelpful complication; the London Underground map is an example of avoiding complications from the streets above

- inconsistency; details changing purely for design reasons adds an unhelpful complication.

7.7 Summary: good practice for indirect communication

Summary: Good practice for indirect communication

People who write material for general use:

- need to recognise that appropriate communication and signage styles can make a significant improvement to the ease with which dyslexic/ SpLD people can gain information

- need to design effective materials that will assist dyslexic/ SpLD people and minimise any problems

- should know the techniques, often simple, that improve the clarity of communication for dyslexic/ SpLD people

- should try out a variety of styles with dyslexic/ SpLD people to find out what works well and what causes slow processing or miscommunication.

People who give public talks or lectures:

- need to choose a speed which most people can follow

- have a clear introduction and a clear final summary

- use visual aids when possible

- avoid too much information on any visual aids.

8 Accommodations

Elizabeth Henderson was a primary schoolteacher. There was one pupil whom she could not teach to read so she trained to teach dyslexic children. She went on to be head of 2 primary state schools where she established regimes that catered naturally for dyslexic pupils (Henderson, 2003). Henderson found there were very few children who needed a statement of Special Educational Need. The 'at risk' children left primary school with the knowledge and skills they needed. Like the woman in STORY: I KNOW HOW I LEARN, the 'at risk' children from Henderson's schools had the same opportunities as non-dyslexic/ SpLDs to progress through the rest of education to employment and adult life. They didn't need accommodation.

Henderson (2003)

STORY: I KNOW HOW I LEARN: p 58

While we wait for this desirable state of affairs to be widely established, there are children and adults who are not using their full potential because of the needs caused by their dyslexia/ SpLD. These people need accommodation to learn and contribute to society.

People in authority considering requests for accommodation should listen carefully to the presented case and remember that their own experience is not the same as that of the person making the request.

If you are helping a student to negotiate accommodation, you can use the ideas in BEHIND THE OBVIOUS to:

- find out the root of the problem that needs accommodation

- describe how the dyslexia/ SpLD is contributing to the difficulties

- describe solutions that have been tried, and possibly give evidence as to why they failed

- give evidence about your student's capabilities

BEHIND THE OBVIOUS: p 64

- describe what accommodation is required and how its success will be monitored.

An example can be found in *Negotiating Accommodation*.

Negotiating Accommodation: p 550

Accommodations can be general ones that cater for a wide range of needs or tailored to a particular dyslexic/ SpLD person when his needs can't be met in any other way. The lists below include just a few accommodations. What is put in place may be very individual.

8.1 Accommodation in education

- acceptance of different learning styles and needs catered for
- appropriate exam provisions
- handouts well constructed, see *Indirect Communications*
- note taker for lectures
- use of recording device for lectures and meetings
- unambiguous, clear feedback on work
- annotated examples of good practice
- opportunities to check that instructions have been properly understood
- difficulties explored openly so that mistakes are used positively.

Indirect Communications: p 119

8.2 Accommodation in employment

- recognition of the employee's best way of working, and any necessary adaptations put in place
- particular problems of employee's dyslexia/ SpLD accepted and managed
- management support to be sure that procedures and new instructions, etc., are fully understood
- own space allowed; hot desking is very difficult for dyslexic/ SpLD people
- noise levels to suit
- interruptions managed to the most suitable times and frequency
- rest of workforce given sufficient knowledge about accommodations to promote smooth working relationships.

8.3 Accommodation in everyday life

- curiosity and acceptance about the way dyslexic/ SpLDs do anything
- recognition that misunderstandings
  - can occur
  - need to be sorted with friendliness
  - are no-one's fault
- encouragement for a dyslexic/ SpLD person to engage with any task using his best ways of going about it
- help given to find ways to manage any problems with time, directions, space, organisation.

9 Policies and systems

Key point: Policy and systems to embed good practice

Much is known about the GOOD PRACTICE that helps dyslexic/ SpLD people.

Policies and systems are needed to embed them in mainstream education and society.

The groups of people who can bring about the change include:
policy-makers and politicians
media personnel
people concerned with disability issues and equality.

I hope policy-makers and politicians will realise the cost effectiveness of the approaches that are VITAL for dyslexic/ SpLDs and GOOD PRACTICE for all.
I hope media personnel will value and promote the general GOOD PRACTICE that is VITAL for dyslexic/ SpLDs.
I hope people concerned with disability issues and equality will understand the value of the GOOD PRACTICE that is VITAL for dyslexic/ SpLDs and will promote its adoption in mainstream educations and society.

Policy-makers and politicians, especially, need to be well informed at a general level of interest because policies built on incomplete knowledge can be harmful and expensive.

Peter Hyman was a speech writer for Tony Blair; he covered education. He wanted to know more about the reality of teaching, so he left politics and went to help at a school. He wrote about his experience in *1 Out of 10: From Downing Street Vision to Classroom Reality* (2005). The overriding message of his book is that progress won't come until politicians engage with those carrying out the work: they need to listen and to ask for solutions – which the workforce can often produce.

Hyman (2005)

In the case of dyslexia/ SpLD and appropriate teaching for young children, I hope politicians and policy-makers will:

- understand the issues facing dyslexic/ SpLD children and adults
- realise that the problems of dyslexia/ SpLD need not develop when the teaching and learning approaches suit the child
- enable the GOOD PRACTICE for all that is VITAL for dyslexic/ SpLD children
- recognise that the earlier the needs of dyslexic/ SpLD children are met, the less the cost in wasted human potential and the lower the financial cost
- recognise that minimising dyslexic/ SpLD problems early reduces the support needed by adult dyslexic/ SpLD people.

In the case of policies relating to secondary school pupils and adults, I hope politicians and policy-makers will:

- accept that there are cohorts of adults for whom early help has been missing
- accept that dyslexic/ SpLD learners and workers are different to non-dyslexic/ SpLD learners and workers
- recognise that systems and models that work for non-dyslexic/ SpLD people can't simply be adapted for dyslexic/ SpLD people
- accept that the different, unorthodox thinking processes of dyslexic/ SpLD learners and workers warrant new models and systems

- recognise that many of the practices and systems that help dyslexic/ SpLD people also help others
- recognise that resources of human potential and money are not being diverted from the majority to cater for a minority.

Much of the general approach to dyslexia/ SpLD is about courtesy between people. Responding with understanding to the needs of dyslexic/ SpLDs could become the default approach between many other groups of people. Policies probably won't help; people need to feel a change has some benefit for themselves. Maybe, people will find that the courtesy that helps dyslexic/ SpLD people also helps themselves to be happier and more fulfilled, in which case the attitudes that help dyslexic/ SpLDs will be beneficial to society at large.

Key point: Why waste human beings or money?

The GOOD PRACTICE proposed should increase satisfaction and human potential and reduce costs, both financial and resource.

References

Baddeley, Alan, 2007, *Working Memory, Thought and Action*, Oxford University Press, Oxford

Blissett, Celia, Hallgarten, Katherine, 1992, *First English Grammar*, Language Teaching Publications, Hove

Chasty, Harry , 1989, *The Challenge of Specific Learning Difficulties*, in Hales, Gerald, (ed.), 1989, *Meeting Points in Dyslexia*, Proceedings of the 1st International Conference of the BDA, Reading

Chinn, Steve, 2017, *The Trouble with Maths: a Practical Guide to Helping Learners with Numeracy Difficulties* , Routledge, Abingdon, 3rd ed.

Crystal, David, 1997, *The Cambridge Encyclopaedia of Language*, Cambridge University Press, Cambridge, 2nd ed.

Dykes, Barbara, 1992, *Grammar Made Easy: A Guide for Parents and*

Teachers, Hale & Iremonger, Alexandria, New South Wales

Gee, Robyn, 2004, *The Usborne Guide to Better English*, Usborne, London

Henderson, Elizabeth, 2003, *How to Have a Dyslexia Friendly School,* Beacon Office, Oldfield School, Maidenhead

Hyman, Peter, 2005, *1 Out of 10: From Downing Street Vision to Classroom Reality*, Vintage, London

McLoughlin, David, et al., 2001, *Adult Dyslexia: Assessment, Counselling and Training,* Whurr, London, 6th re-print

Miles, Tim, 1993, *Dyslexia: the Pattern of Difficulties,* Whurr, London, 2nd ed.

Morton, John and Frith, Uta, 1995, *Chapter 13 Causal Modelling: A Structural Approach to Developmental Psychopathology,* Developmental Psychopathology, Vol. 1 pp 357-390

Newby, Michael, 1995, *The Dyslexics Speak for Themselves,* in, Miles, Tim and Varma, Ved (eds), 1995, *Dyslexia and Stress,* Whurr, London

Stacey, Ginny, 2005, *A Taste of Dyslexia DVD,* Oxfordshire Dyslexia Association, Oxford

Stacey, Ginny, 2019, *Finding Your Voice with Dyslexia and other SpLDs,* Routledge, London

Stacey, Ginny, 2020a, *Organisation and Everyday Life with Dyslexia and other SpLDs,* Routledge, London

Stacey, Ginny, 2020b, *Development of Dyslexia and other SpLDs,* Routledge, London

Stein, John, Stoodley, Catherine, 2006, *Neuroscience, An Introduction,* Wiley, Chichester

Website information

OED Online, September 2020, Oxford University Press Accessed 24 October 2020

Series website: www.routledge.com/cw/stacey

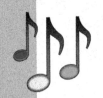

2 Foundations for Knowledge and Skills

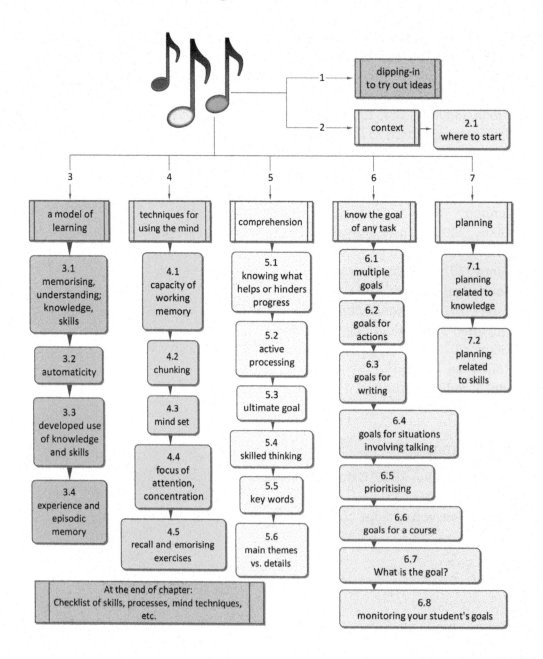

1 → dipping-in to try out ideas

2 → context → 2.1 where to start

3 — a model of learning
- 3.1 memorising, understanding; knowledge, skills
- 3.2 automaticity
- 3.3 developed use of knowledge and skills
- 3.4 experience and episodic memory

4 — techniques for using the mind
- 4.1 capacity of working memory
- 4.2 chunking
- 4.3 mind set
- 4.4 focus of attention, concentration
- 4.5 recall and emorising exercises

5 — comprehension
- 5.1 knowing what helps or hinders progress
- 5.2 active processing
- 5.3 ultimate goal
- 5.4 skilled thinking
- 5.5 key words
- 5.6 main themes vs. details

6 — know the goal of any task
- 6.1 multiple goals
- 6.2 goals for actions
- 6.3 goals for writing
- 6.4 goals for situations involving talking
- 6.5 prioritising
- 6.6 goals for a course
- 6.7 What is the goal?
- 6.8 monitoring your student's goals

7 — planning
- 7.1 planning related to knowledge
- 7.2 planning related to skills

At the end of chapter:
Checklist of skills, processes, mind techniques, etc.

Contents

≻, = Book 1, marks sections that are discussed in greater detail in Book 1 of this series. A brief summary is included here to support suggestions made in this book.

Thinking Preferences, p 72, are highlighted in orange in this chapter.

Examples of their use are listed in the *Index*: p 589

§8 is deliberately not on the map of the chapter.

Vital for dyslexic/ SpLDs, good practice for all

This chapter covers skills for dealing with information. The skills need to be specifically learnt by most dyslexic/ SpLD people since they are unlikely to pick them up subliminally – so these skills are VITAL for them to learn.

Learning the skills is also GOOD PRACTICE for everyone; being systematic about gaining the skills and making sure there are no gaps can be very beneficial for everyone.

Ⓖ p 575 subliminal

List of key points and summaries

Page		Box title
140	*K*	*Foundations of Knowledge and Skills and building an Individual, Personal Profile of Dyslexia/ SpLD and a Regime for Managing Dyslexia/ SpLD*
142	*K*	*Difficulties with Higher Order Skills*
143	*K*	*Check-list of Skills instead of Lesson Plans*
144	*K*	*It Has To Be Relevant to Your Student Now*
145	*K*	*A Model of Learning*
150	*K*	*Knowledge and skills*

K = key points
S = summaries

Working with the chapter: tutoring a student

The chapter covers some fundamental processes for working with information and ideas. Scan it so that you know what is covered and where, then find out from your student what her most pressing problems are, and which ones she would like to deal with first. Work with her to find her solutions. Record what is tried, how well any solution works, what doesn't work. Gradually, build a picture of how your student thinks well.

Remember to bear in mind the *MAJOR PRECAUTION* and help your student to avoid building any more dyslexic/ SpLD confusion into her brain.

MAJOR PRECAUTION: p 10

Some of the ideas in this chapter are here because they are worth discussing with your student or teaching her. Not all will be relevant to her, so you need to select those which will help her. I suspect many of these ideas will not be new to you, but you may not realise the significance of them as part of helping a dyslexic/ SpLD student.

The green line in the left-hand margin indicates those paragraphs that predominantly contain ideas to be discussed with or taught to your student. The meaning of the green line is also in the *GLOSSARY*.

Ⓖ p 572

Other ideas in the chapter are to help you understand more about the whys and hows of helping dyslexic/ SpLDs.

Some of the boxes are addressed to dyslexic/ SpLD people; it's the only way they make sense. They are marked with the green strip in the left-hand margin. The meaning of the green strip is in the GLOSSARY too.

Working with the chapter: for general understanding

The main themes are:

- that gaps in understanding happen despite all the right ideas being present
- how the capacity of working memory is reduced by the effects of dyslexia/ SpLD and what strategies can be used to increase the capacity
- the importance of identifying goals and prioritising effort
- that good planning can be very helpful even in minor tasks.

It is by having sympathetic enabling support that dyslexic/ SpLD people find out how to function well and to minimise the disrupting elements of their dyslexia/ SpLD. Your general understanding can make a lot of difference.

Working with the chapter:
for policies and public discussion

The main themes are:

- where to start: that work has to be known by the student to be relevant to her
- that gaps in knowledge can be undetected unless care is taken
- the need to deliberately teach skills that others learn subliminally
- lack of automaticity of skills means more time is needed for tasks
- how the capacity of working memory is affected by dyslexia/ SpLD and what techniques can be used to increase the capacity
- clear goals are needed, with help to decide priorities
- time set aside for planning, and help given
- the wide variation of the experiences even within a given SpLD syndrome means a flexible approach to issues needs to be adopted.

The policies that are put in place need to accommodate these various issues.

Public debate should include understanding of the difficulties and how they can be managed with flexible approaches to the needs of individuals.

Templates on the website

A1   *JOTTING DOWN AS YOU SCAN*
A2   *BOOKMARK – PURPOSE*
A4   *JOTTING DOWN AS YOU READ*
A5   *COLLECTING IDEAS THAT INTEREST YOU*
B1   *COLLECTING IDEAS THAT RELATE TO YOU* (specially for readers who are themselves dyslexic/ SpLD)

CHECK-LISTS FOR READERS describes a set of check-lists available on the website to help different reader groups engage with the ideas in the book. It also lists the most relevant sections of the book.

All the *TEMPLATES* suggested in this chapter are shown in the *LIST OF TEMPLATES*.

Appendix 1 Resources

This appendix will help you and your student collect information about the way she does anything, and how her dyslexia/ SpLD affects her.

The *APPENDIX* collects together some of the general skills she will need in order to make progress. They are skills you need to deliberately teach.

If you are dyslexic/ SpLD, this appendix will help you gather the information you want from this book.

TEMPLATES

CHECK-LISTS FOR READERS: p 21

LIST OF TEMPLATES: p 582

APPENDIX 1: p 524

Appendix 2 Individual, Personal Profile of Dyslexia/ SpLD and Regime for Managing Dyslexia/ SpLD

APPENDIX 2: p 538

Key point: *FOUNDATIONS OF KNOWLEDGE AND SKILLS* **and building an** *INDIVIDUAL, PERSONAL PROFILE OF DYSLEXIA/ SPLD* **and a** *REGIME FOR MANAGING DYSLEXIA/ SPLD*

Working on tasks, looking for the best ways to think about them is an opportunity for any dyslexic/ SpLD person to explore how her mind works well. Finding out what doesn't work is equally important, as is finding out the situations that increase the effects of the dyslexia/ SpLD.

As your student understands her dyslexia/ SpLD better and the way it varies, help her to be confident about herself. Help her to build the insights that emerge into her *PROFILE* and *REGIME*; these will allow her to become more autonomous.

Ⓖ p 575
autonomous

Appendix 3 Key Concepts

APPENDIX 3: p 554

This appendix has a summary of the key ideas I cover when doing an audit of skills and knowledge with a dyslexic/ SpLD student. They fall into the categories of

> *THINKING CLEARLY*
> *USING THE MIND WELL*
> *THINKING PREFERENCES*
> *USEFUL APPROACHES*
> *ASPECTS OF DYSLEXIA/ SPLD*

The appendix shows which of the 4 books in the series covers each idea in full.

1 Dipping-in to try out ideas

> Read the context and take note of where to start with any particular student.
> Read *WORKING WITH THE CHAPTER.*
> Read the stories, insights and examples.

Working with a student:
　　Brainstorm about your current student and decide which sections seem most relevant to her. If you work with more than one student, keep your brainstorming separate for each one.
　　Read the sections relevant to your student carefully; notice the other sections for future use.
　　Use the key points and summaries to prioritise the work you do with your student.

ⓖ p 575 brainstorm

LIST OF KEY POINTS AND SUMMARIES: p 136

For general understanding, policies and public discussion:
　　Brainstorm around your current interests in dyslexia/ SpLD and your questions.
　　Prioritise the interests and questions.
　　Read the sections relevant to your interests and questions.

2 Context

In *IMPARTING KNOWLEDGE AND SKILLS*, I discussed aspects that help or hinder the learning of dyslexic/ SpLD students. I also said that certain knowledge and skills have to be explicitly taught to dyslexic/ SpLD students, that they do not pick up some fundamental skills while learning another subject. This chapter includes knowledge and skills that need to be taught in their own right, which include:

IMPARTING KNOWLEDGE AND SKILLS: p 46

- comprehending
- fact-finding and gathering data
- following discussions
- questioning
- building theories or models
- evaluating, weighing up the relative merits of different perspectives
- presenting a line of argument
- knowing the goal of any task
- planning.

Key point: Difficulties with higher order skills

The above higher order skills involve organising thoughts. They are difficult for dyslexic/ SpLD teenagers and adults to gain, in much the same way that children have difficulty with:

- spelling and reading, dyslexia

- fine motor control, dyspraxia

- focusing attention and containing impulses, AD(H)D

- arithmetic and maths concepts, dyscalculia.

The processes involved relate to understanding anything:
> the daily news, banking procedures, travel options,
> day-release training courses, operating machinery,
> as well as academic courses.

A *MODEL OF LEARNING* is a framework for discussing all the stages where I have found dyslexic/ SpLD students lack appropriate skills and knowledge.

A *MODEL OF LEARNING:* p 145

COMPREHENSION is the mental grasp of something. It is important for all ways of gaining and understanding knowledge and skills.

COMPREHENSION: p 162

To *KNOW THE GOAL OF ANY TASK* gives a clear direction. It can be extremely helpful to clearly identify the goal early in any undertaking.

KNOW THE GOAL OF ANY TASK: p 181

Deliberate *PLANNING* can help

- to break down large tasks into manageable units
- a student to keep working in the right direction
- deadlines to be
  - seen well in advance
  - managed so that stress is kept at the level that suits an individual student.

PLANNING: p 200

Key point: Check-list of skills instead of lesson plans

Use a *CHECK-LIST OF SKILLS* to make sure you cover everything. Lesson plans are appropriate for children, but often not useful for adults and teenagers.

CHECK-LIST OF SKILLS, PROCESSES, MIND TECHNIQUES, ETC.: p 220

I use a check-list to make sure we cover all the skills needed. I used to have lesson plans, which meant I had decided between sessions which skills to cover next. However, working with my students taught me that sticking to the lesson plans was unhelpful to them, because when they came back for the next session, something else was more important; this is part of the *MENTAL ON/ OFF SWITCH*.

MENTAL ON/ OFF SWITCH: p 86

You have to convince students that they are the ones who have to make the effort and that they will enjoy the benefits of the new skills.

Story: Who eats the apple?

One school-teacher friend used to ask his children, "If you are hungry and there's an apple on the table, is it any good if I eat the apple?" "No, sir." "Learning is the same: it's your brain that has to do it."

I tell students that:

- I don't expect them to believe a technique is worth attention until they see it working for themselves

- they should try new techniques on some task that doesn't matter, otherwise their doubt and anxiety about the task will not give the new technique a fair trial

- it is just as useful to tell me about any techniques that don't work since it tells us more about the way their minds work.

Monitor the changes that happen as your student tries new techniques; see *MONITORING PROGRESS*. Observing what works for her is the best way to improve her understanding of how her mind works well. She will be able to see what works, under what circumstances, and how reliably. The confirmation she gets from using her skills in real-life situations is an essential part of honing her skills and building her confidence.

MONITORING PROGRESS: p 535

2.1 Where to start

Key point: It has to be relevant to your student now

Most of the time dyslexic/ SpLD people learn best when working on a subject or task that is important to them, interesting to them or currently needs their attention; all these personal connections help with *BEING ALERT*.

BEING ALERT: p 91

- You need to teach skills using material that keeps your student alert. You might be able to demonstrate that the skills are useful to her.

- Sometimes, the desire to gain new skills is a good way for your student to keep alert.

- When teaching skills, you have to draw attention to the skills she is using.

My (GS) practice is almost always:

- to work on something with high priority or interest to my student
- and, through the task chosen, cover:
    - the concepts covered in this book
    - issues about her dyslexia/ SpLD, using my knowledge from *Development of Dyslexia and other SpLDs* (Stacey, 2020b)
- I don't expect I will always know the answer and I back-track quickly if a suggestion doesn't seem right to the student.

My (SF) proactive approach is to ask:

- What do you do now?
- What do you want to be able to do?
- How shall we get there?

When deciding what topics to work on, it is worth bearing in mind the *MAJOR PRECAUTION* and asking your student to do the *EXERCISE FOR STUDENT: AVOID MORE PROBLEMS WHEN LEARNING NEW SKILLS*.

➤ 3 A model of learning

The way your student is processing her thoughts will have a significant impact on the progress she can make.

Key point: A model of learning

I have found that there are several stages at which you can help your student to make the best of her innate thinking strengths. The stages are underlined in *FIGURE 2.1*. They are important stages because when thinking is working well during them *NEURONS FIRING TOGETHER, WIRE TOGETHER* and progress is made.

The stages are listed in the *CHECK-LIST OF SKILLS, PROCESSES, MIND TECHNIQUES, ETC.*

GS: Ginny Stacey

Stacey (2020b)

SF: Sally Fowler

MAJOR PRECAUTION: p 10

EXERCISE FOR STUDENT: AVOID MORE PROBLEMS WHEN LEARNING NEW SKILLS: p 11

NEURONS FIRING TOGETHER, WIRE TOGETHER: p 88

CHECK-LIST OF SKILLS, PROCESSES, MIND TECHNIQUES, ETC.: p 220

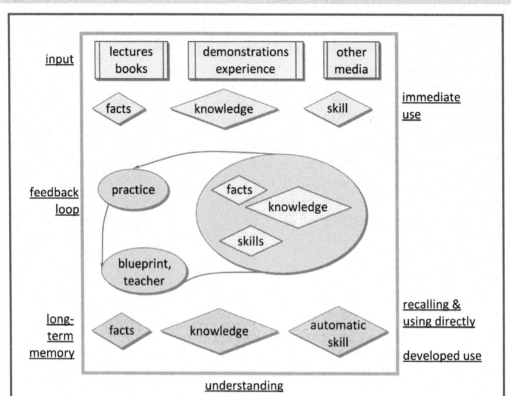

Figure 2. 1 A model of learning

Knowledge and understanding are often explained in terms of each other. In Figure 2.1 'knowledge' is used as part of the learning processes and 'understanding' is used as a different word to represent your student's deeper grasp of the issues involved.

Stage of model	Explanation
Input	any time new information is given.
Immediate use	very shortly after input.
Feedback loop	during this stage, knowledge is recalled or skills are practised repeatedly; regular repetition is used to learn both knowledge and skills; both are monitored to make sure they are correct and useful.
Recall	information is brought back from memory some time after input.

Direct use	information and skills are used exactly as they were input.
Developed use	knowledge and skills are modified in some way.
Long-term memory	knowledge and skills are established in long-term memory, and can be recalled.
Understanding	an appreciation of significant concepts has taken place.

Your student may find she uses different THINKING PREFERENCES for the different stages of this model. Focus on her progress with learning rather than looking for consistency of approach.

THINKING PREFERENCES:
p 72

You need to be aware that the feedback loop can look as if it is working when it isn't. The practice can be boring or too taxing. In either case, your student may, subconsciously or consciously, change the way she does it so that it looks as if she is practising well but the internal processes have not produced learning.

Insight: Learning to touch-type

Several touch-typing programmes are based on patterns of finger movements.

To learn the home keys: you might be asked to alternate left and right hands working out from 'f' and 'j'. You do this until you have reached a certain speed and then you move on to the next pattern.

If a dyslexic/ SpLD has been singing left-right-left-right to a tune to make the task more palatable, she will have lost any connection with the actual letters. Even repeating the letters can become a verbal task that gets disconnected from the finger movements.

So your student may achieve the desired, external result, but the internal learning hasn't happened.

When she works on another pattern involving the same keys, she will have to work out where they are again.

The solution is that the practice has to be random, not through patterns that can be predicted. As a result, the student has to think about every letter which then becomes connected to the movement. In the long run, this produces a more secure touch-typing skill.

Insight: Sight interfering with learning movements

Being able to watch while learning movements may interfere with establishing a reliable memory for the movement.

Elizabeth Henderson (2003), headmistress of two primary state schools, developed a method of teaching handwriting with the children not able to see their hands; she used eye patches. She realised that the signals from the eyes were causing problems for the children because they could see what they were doing and would be too critical too early. She taught them fine motor-control first in art work. Then, she taught them cursive writing and allowed them to practise as large as they needed to, on paper that was stuck to the table. This method resulted in better writing. She taught printing after cursive writing.

Henderson (2003)

The same principle can be used for learning to touch-type if a cardboard box, with one side removed, is placed over the keyboard and hands. Then, the eyes can't interfere with the movement, and the feedback is the letters on the screen.

It is worth considering whether a learner is focused too early on the result she can see, rather than learning the movement.

When *THINKING PREFERENCES* are an important part of your student's *PROFILE,* they can make a considerable difference to the way she manages any of the stages in the *MODEL OF LEARNING.*

THINKING PREFERENCES:
p 72
A MODEL OF LEARNING:
p 145

One pattern I have noticed about *THINKING PREFERENCES* relates to the input and feedback stages of a *MODEL OF LEARNING*. At these stages your student needs to be aware of her preference amongst the *SENSES* and her need for a *RATIONALE OR FRAMEWORK* of the material she is processing.

SENSES: p 74
RATIONALE OR FRAMEWORK: p 75

Some learning style theories are based on the sense that people use; sometimes only verbal and visual processing are included. Sometimes the kinaesthetic processing is also included. My work with dyslexic/ SpLD students has shown that the need for *RATIONALE OR FRAMEWORK* has to be considered at the same time and that the kinaesthetic sense should not be ignored.

Ⓖ p 575 kinaesthetic

Your student is looking for ways in which she can make progress; she should avoid a lot of effort that produces no results.

Story: Colour coding in applied maths

One student could not understand what she was being asked to do in working out the forces on a ladder leaning against a wall.

When we used different colours for the forces, she could immediately see the maths involved and could solve the problem[1] (visual), see *FIGURE 2.2*.

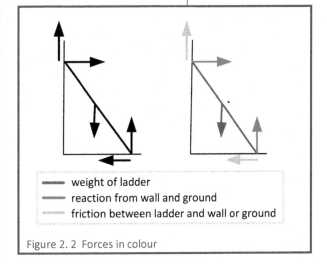

weight of ladder
reaction from wall and ground
friction between ladder and wall or ground

Figure 2. 2 Forces in colour

Your student may find she uses different *THINKING PREFERENCES* for different stages of working with information and ideas. You need to find out which ones are important for her and when. Build them into her *INDIVIDUAL, PERSONAL PROFILE OF DYSLEXIA/ SPLD* and help her to use them confidently.

INDIVIDUAL, PERSONAL PROFILE OF DYSLEXIA/ SPLD: p 540

---

[1] Problems are set in maths so that students work through them to gain understanding of the maths. For most of this book, problems are difficulties that impede progress rather promote it.

Insight: Using a variety of *Thinking Preferences* for the stages in *A Model of Learning*, p 145	
• I use mind maps to find the links between facts and ideas (holistic)	input and feedback
• I use all sorts of other visual devises to understand a topic: colour, symbols, analogies (visual)	understanding
• I will memorise a subject by the sense I make of it (rationale or framework)	feedback
• I will recall it again, using the logic of it (rationale or framework)	recall
• often I use the number of elements in it and sometimes the physical location of an idea on a piece of paper (it's the act of making the placement that I remember) (kinaesthetic, framework)	feedback
• when talking about an issue, I hold in mind the person involved when the issue first came to light. (MBPT – sensing)	developed use

Another person could use the same techniques but from different underlying *Thinking Preferences*. From many years' practice, I know these are the right *Thinking Preferences* for me. If they don't help with a future task, I will experiment with other styles of thinking.

3.1 Memorising and understanding; knowledge and skills

Key points: Knowledge and skills

It is important for your student to realise that:

• memorising and understanding are not the same thing

- competent use of knowledge includes appreciating the distinction between facts, discussion and evaluation
- there are significant differences between learning knowledge and learning skills.

3.1.1 Memorising

Memorising is the process of storing knowledge, skills and experience in memory. Being able to memorise and recall information is not the same thing as understanding it.

Many dyslexic/ SpLD students know they can read or listen to new ideas or information and that it gets lost somewhere in the mind and can't be recalled. It isn't available for any further processing. The situation can be significantly improved:

- by recalling relevant information from long-term memory by using *MIND SET*

  MIND SET: p 158

- the recalled information provides hooks that the new can link to
- these links are a way of *CHUNKING*

  CHUNKING: p 158

- the chunked new information can be stored in one storage chunk of working memory
- the *CAPACITY OF WORKING MEMORY* is increased and more information is available for the mind to work with

  CAPACITY OF WORKING MEMORY: p 157

- with the result that *COMPREHENSION* is much easier.

  COMPREHENSION: p 162

People can memorise information in their own particular way, and some do it very easily; for example, some people have a gift for remembering other people's names, and others seem to have the gift of forgetting names! It is worth finding out what kind of details your student memorises most easily.

3.1.2 Understanding

Understanding an idea or subject implies that your student has realised the links between the facts; how the information fits together; possibly what can be done with it; what is missing from it. There is a greater depth to her thinking about a topic or idea than being able to recall what she has memorised. It is useful to recognise the difference between memorising and understanding.

**Insight: A teacher's knowledge obscuring lack
in a student's knowledge**

You need to be particularly aware of this difference when helping
your student with written work. An essay can appear well
constructed, but be written from memory with either little
understanding or major gaps in understanding.

The gaps appear as you discuss the content. Someone, probably a
support tutor, who doesn't fully understand the topic can usefully
contribute a level of intelligent ignorance. As your student
explains her essay further, any gaps in her understanding will
probably emerge.

Tutors who know the subject will subconsciously use their own
understanding to fill in the gaps left by the student, which means
the gaps in the student's understanding go unnoticed.

3.1.3 Knowledge: facts, discussion and evaluation

A useful way to think about knowledge is to distinguish between facts,
arguments (or discussion) and evaluation.

Ⓖ p 575 argument

- Facts are statements about what is. They should be as close to
  objective statements as possible.

- Arguments are the discussions about the facts; they often include
  models that help to formulate the links between different facts,
  e.g. *A MODEL OF LEARNING* and *MODELS OF SPLD*. They may contain
  analogies to help understanding, for example, the comparison in
  PARK PATHS AND PRUNING NEURONS is based on an analogy. An
  argument will depend on the perspective of the person making it
  and quite often there are different arguments to be made from
  any given set of facts.

A MODEL OF LEARNING:
p 145

MODELS OF SPLD: p 57

*PARK PATHS AND
PRUNING NEURONS:* p 7

- Evaluation is the stage at which a judgement is made about the
  arguments and the facts. Your student should be able to show
  how she came to a particular evaluation, i.e. be able to present
  the facts and the arguments that led her to a particular
  evaluation.

Recognising the difference between facts, arguments and evaluations can be difficult for dyslexic/ SpLDs. Teaching these differences is used as an example in *Constant Content*.

Constant Content: p 92

Individual styles of thinking will alter the way facts, arguments and evaluations are presented, but this is a useful categorisation when it comes to appreciating some of the complexity of understanding.

3.1.4 Skills

Understanding something means your student has a body of knowledge about it. Having a skill means she can carry out a process in a competent way.

Skills can be physical or mental. They can range from automatic ones, which your student performs without conscious thought, to ones which are carried out with a good deal of conscious thought: no-one should use a chain saw without being fully conscious of their actions.

Driving is a physical skill that most adults learn, without understanding the mechanics of the car. In situations like this, learners need to repeat movements until they become automatic and can be performed without conscious effort while other things are done at the same time.

Examples of mental skills include maths and language skills, including *Comprehension*.

Comprehension: p 162

Some skills need to be practised until they can be used automatically.

➢ 3.2 Automaticity

Automaticity is the state of being automatic (OED Online, 2020). An automatic skill is performed without much conscious attention, if any. Spelling and reading are two skills that are expected to become automatic, but for many dyslexic/ SpLDs they remain skills that require active attention.

('automaticity, n' OED Online, 2020)

When working with ideas, it can be very disruptive if the mind has to pay attention to the spelling, pronunciation or meaning of any word. The switch of attention will break the links providing *Chunking*; it will mean a different chunk of working memory is used – so effectively, it will reduce the *Capacity of Working Memory*. A few suggestions for managing the disruptions can be found in *Spelling and Grammar* and *Talking Fluently*.

Chunking: p 158
Capacity of Working Memory: p 157

Spelling and Grammar: p 358
Talking Fluently: p 368

3.3 Developed use of knowledge and skills

There are some situations for which knowledge and skills are used exactly as they were memorised in the first place; there are other situations that require further processing before the knowledge or skills can be applied in the required manner. I think it is worth drawing attention to the fact that there are times when your student has to develop the knowledge and skills she already has in order to meet a particular circumstance.

Example: Knowledge used as learnt vs. developed use: 1

A very simple distinction could be made between a set of numbers that is only used as a single string of numbers, say for a bike lock, and a PIN number that is used for internet banking.

For the bike lock, your student learns and recalls the order of the numbers in a way that suits her; once the recall mechanism is reliable, she simply uses the numbers automatically.

For internet banking, your student has to select the numbers she uses every time depending on the questions on the login page. Often she will be asked for the number in a particular position in the PIN, so every time she has to think about her PIN number and decide on the correct answers.

Example: Knowledge used as learnt vs. developed use: 2

A more complex distinction between recall-and-use, and developed use might be: the recall of facts in order to answer questions in *Mastermind*[2] and the recall of events and discussions in order to develop environmental policies.

In the developed use of knowledge, your student is likely to understand issues more and more as she processes the information further.

Examples: Skills used as learnt vs. developed use

- Skills used as learnt:
Many medical practitioners learn the skills needed to measure a patient's blood pressure; they can become so familiar with using the equipment that they do it automatically with minimal attention to the procedure.

- Developed use of skills:
By contrast, sports people learn how to play their sport, but the conditions are always changing so they have to continually adapt how they use those skills.

---

[2] *Mastermind* is a TV programme for which participants need to recall information from memory.

Summary: Developed use of knowledge and skills

Much of successful learning involves developing knowledge and skills. Your student has to learn knowledge and skills in such a way that she can use them in sections and not just as single entities exactly as she first learnt them. She has to be able to adapt them and to add to them.

➤ 3.4 Experience and episodic memory

Experience is also stored in memory. Often, complete episodes are stored as complex networks, for example taking the dog out for a particular walk or singing the alphabet song.

Key point: Episodic memory remaining whole

This type of memory becomes a problem for dyslexic/ SpLD people if they cannot break the experience into smaller units, for example many dyslexic/ SpLD people can't break up the alphabet song to find out where a letter is. Some have to start at 'a' and sing the song until they get to the letter; some know roughly where the letter is and can start a little bit before, and then they sing the song until they get to the letter they want.

No amount of using the song this way allows them to learn where the individual letters are in the alphabet.

➤ 4 Techniques for using the mind

Finding Your Voice with Dyslexia and other SpLDs (Stacey, 2019) has 2 chapters, *About the Mind* and *Using the Mind*, which cover many aspects about the mind that I discuss with dyslexic/ SpLD students. The chapters have stories, background and references. The bullet points in this section contain sufficient information for the techniques

Stacey (2019)

to be used in the current book, however, they are not backed by stories, background and references. As you use the ideas in *INDIVIDUALS WITH DYSLEXIA/ SPLD* and these bullet points with your student, you will gain your own collection of stories and evidence.

INDIVIDUALS WITH DYSLEXIA/ SPLD: p 57

You should make sure the techniques are part of the work you do with your student and that she recognises when she is using them. Monitor her progress with them. Use the *CHECK-LIST OF SKILLS, PROCESSES, MIND TECHNIQUES, ETC.* to make sure you cover all the techniques she needs.

MONITORING PROGRESS: p 535

CHECK-LIST OF SKILLS, PROCESSES, MIND TECHNIQUES, ETC.: p 220

➢ 4.1 Capacity of working memory

- Working memory has 4 memory chunks (Stacey, 2019, 2020b; Baddeley, 2007).

Stacey (2019, 2020b) Baddeley (2007)

- Information is stored in each chunk providing there is a link between successive pieces of information.
- There isn't a limit to how much can be stored in each chunk.
- When there is a break in the links, the next chunk is used.
- When all four have been used, the first is used again by replacing what was already there, instead of adding to it.

- If a good reader is making connections between the ideas she is reading about they can all go into a single chunk.
- If a poor reader is not connecting the words together each word will occupy a single chunk, and the maximum words held in working memory will be 4.
- If the poor reader is still decoding at the single letter stage of reading, only 4 letters at a time will be available to working memory.

Using *THINKING PREFERENCES* well can improve the effectiveness of your student's working memory. It allows her mind to find links between pieces of information that she is processing, which amounts to using *CHUNKING* to increase the amount of information contained in working memory (Stacey, 2019).

THINKING PREFERENCES: p 72

Stacey (2019)

➤ 4.2 Chunking

- Chunking is the process whereby links are created between pieces of information so that they can be stored in the same chunk of working memory and thereby increase the *CAPACITY OF WORKING MEMORY*.

  CAPACITY OF WORKING MEMORY: above

- Chunking is achieved subliminally for most people.

- Chunking can be enhanced deliberately by using:

  THINKING PREFERENCES: p 72

  - *MIND SET*
  - *THINKING PREFERENCES*
  - various memorising techniques.

  RECALL AND MEMORISING EXERCISES: p 159

➤ 4.3 Mind set

- Mind set involves your student switching her mind on to the topic she is about to engage with.

- She can do mind set in a number of ways:

  - calling to mind what she already knows
  - remembering what she last did with this task or topic
  - building a mind map of what she knows
  - making a list of questions she has
  - drawing a picture or some other graphic
  - thinking about other people involved
  - anything that engages her mind with what is coming next
  - *MIND SET BEFORE READING* has other suggestions appropriate to reading.

  MIND SET BEFORE READING: p 244

- The process energises those neural networks that are already connected with the topic she is about to work with.

- These networks are then available to provide links for new information or repetition of a previous session.

  CAPACITY OF WORKING MEMORY: p 157

- The *CAPACITY OF WORKING MEMORY* is increased by more information being stored in the individual chunks.

- The firing together that leads to neurons wiring together has a better chance of happening.

  NEURONS FIRING TOGETHER, WIRE TOGETHER: p 88

➤ 4.4 Focus of attention, concentration

Being able to concentrate on the task in hand is often a problem for dyslexic/ SpLDs. Using *THINKING PREFERENCES* can give your student control of the focus of her attention.

THINKING PREFERENCES:
p 72

Whether she is learning knowledge or skills by *READING*, *LISTENING* or *DOING*, if she uses her *THINKING PREFERENCES* she is likely to stay engaged with the topic and not become bored.

If she is a holistic thinker, she needs to be aware of going off at a tangent or missing out links between ideas. Some of the characteristics listed for holistic thinkers in *DIFFERENCES IN THOUGHT PROCESSING* may also contribute to difficulty with focusing attention.

DIFFERENCES IN THOUGHT PROCESSING: p 114

➤ 4.5 Recall and memorising exercises

Anyone needs good recall from memory:

- to use information and skills already learnt
- to support new learning of information and skills
- to strengthen memories in long-term memory.

PREPARATION FOR DOING has some ideas for practical-based learning.

PREPARATION FOR DOING:
p 114

Key point: Use recall, not re-reading

Re-reading information does not strengthen memories in long-term memory.
Systematic recall does strengthen memory.

Exercise for student: Memorising exercises

This pattern can be used with any topic and any method for
capturing knowledge and creating a blueprint.

Ⓖ p 575
blueprint

- After a period of study or learning, create a blueprint that
  you will use to check future recall.

- One day later, recall as much of the knowledge as you
  can:
  - you can use words, mind maps, drawings, sound
    recordings: you just need the recall to be captured
  - compare your recall with the blueprint
  - notice what you remembered
  - notice how and why you remembered it (A)
  - notice what is missing
  - notice why you don't remember it (B)
  - use the how and why of (A) to link the missing
    information more securely to the rest of the
    information
  - repeat the same process
    - one week later
    - one month later
    - 6 months later
    - from time to time.

- The how and why at stage (A) tell you a lot about the way
  your mind thinks naturally

- Stage (B) tells you about the way your mind doesn't like
  to think and can be useful information as you work out
  how to manage your dyslexia/ SpLD.

- Build these insights into your *INDIVIDUAL, PERSONAL PROFILE
  OF DYSLEXIA/ SPLD* and your *REGIME FOR MANAGING DYSLEXIA/
  SPLD*.

*INDIVIDUAL, PERSONAL
PROFILE OF DYSLEXIA/
SPLD:* p 540

*REGIME FOR MANAGING
DYSLEXIA/ SPLD:* p 540

- Knowledge can be reviewed using the pattern of days, weeks and months for the review periods (adapted from Russell (1979)).

Russell (1979)

- Skills need to be practised little and often.

Information in the form of unrelated facts may be quite difficult for dyslexic/ SpLD people to learn. They may need to use an unrelated method of chunking the information together (Stacey, 2019). Once the right links have been found for the unrelated information, systematic review should enable the information to be stored in long-term memory (Stacey, 2019).

Ⓖ p 575 chunking

Stacey (2019)

Your student needs to find the right trigger that allows her to recall relevant information from her memory.

Story: Architecture in mind maps

One architecture student worked well with mind maps. During his final year at university, he put the whole of his course into mind maps on A3 paper and put them on his wall. He discovered that one key item on each mind map was all he needed in order to recall the whole of the map. He could select what he needed to answer the exam questions.

Russell (1979) calculates the efficiency of the repeat recall system set out above. If you spend an hour studying and do no reviewing, you will remember 10% of the material.

Russell (1979)

If you have a system of 1 hour study, and build in reviewing times:

      5 mins on work from the day before

      3 mins on work from each of

            1 week before, 1 month before and 6 months before

total review time 14 mins

which gives 1 hour 14 mins to gain 90% of the material, 'the overall gain in efficiency is 750%. *Thus a few minutes devoted to review makes the hours of studying effective and worthwhile.*' (Russell's italics.)

5 Comprehension

Comprehension is the 'act or faculty of understanding, especially of writing or speech' (OED, 1993). It is also described as 'mental grasp' of something. In order to have a mental grasp of something, your student's mind will have organised her experiences and thinking into some kind of pattern, or schema.

OED (1993)

ⓖ p 575 schema

Schemas, the organisation of thought, are fundamental to human thought processes. New knowledge and skills build on what has already been achieved; the building process involves re-enforcing what has been learnt before and schemas are extended by new experience.

Check that your student understands:

- the organisation of her subject
- how her discipline studies its subjects, in general
- how she has been asked to process a topic, in particular
- how to research around a topic or answer a set question.

She needs to have good working schemas for all these areas of study.

If you are helping someone deal with everyday life rather than a course, then the same principles apply but her schemas will relate to processes involved in the tasks of everyday living.

Key point: Creating schemas for comprehension

Most people do not have to be aware of the way their minds are organising experiences and thinking: it just happens and they use the result competently.

The same happens for dyslexic/ SpLD people when they are using their THINKING PREFERENCES in appropriate situations; for example many dyslexic/ SpLD people with good visual THINKING PREFERENCES will have no difficulty with map reading.

THINKING PREFERENCES: p 72

Most dyslexic/ SpLD people have to pay particular attention to creating schemas when the problems of the dyslexia/ SpLD cause confusion.

This section is a discussion of general issues that can assist dyslexic/ SpLD people to create the necessary schema.

5.1 Knowing what helps and what hinders progress

Gradually, as your student learns in a more conscious way, she will know what helps her to gain understanding and she will know what hinders her.

- She should learn her best rhythm for taking breaks and how to use her *THINKING PREFERENCES*.

- She may also learn how much she can process at any given time.

- It may be quite important to protect herself from being overloaded with new information. She is unlikely to function well when overloaded and she may need to negotiate the pace with managers and course leaders, as appropriate. Equally, she may function better under conditions that most people regard as too stressful.

Your student is the one who needs to know where her limits are and how to set about respecting them.

5.2 Active processing

Many dyslexic/ SpLD people find that words come into the mind and evaporate; they seem to leave no trace that can be accessed; they find listening in lectures or reading textbooks results in words leaving no impact.

Insight: A good sentence lost

I discuss phrasing of ideas with students. Many times one of us will say a sentence that captures an idea very well. We try to write it down straight away but neither of us can remember what it was.

But words do start to be retained when active processing is used i.e. when:

- your student is deliberately paying attention to what she is hearing or reading
- she is creating dynamic images
- she is supplying links to the information
- she is choosing to think well.

Several of the *TECHNIQUES IN USING THE MIND* will help your student to be active as she gains knowledge and skills.

TECHNIQUES FOR USING THE MIND: p 156

Summary: Active processing

Check how well your student is using the following techniques:

- *MIND SET* to switch her mind on
- *CHUNKING* to link pieces of information together
- *MEMORISING EXERCISES* to help retain previous work and check for consistency
- *FOCUS OF ATTENTION, CONCENTRATION* to improve effectiveness
- *METACOGNITION* to observe herself at the time of doing something and to make suitable choices
- *PRIORITISING* to separate the major themes from the minor ones.

MIND SET: p 158

CHUNKING: p 158

MEMORISING EXERCISES: p 160

FOCUS OF ATTENTION, CONCENTRATION: p 159

METACOGNITION: p 63

PRIORITISING: p 197

Observing others is often helpful, though she needs to remember that what works for others may not be suitable for her.

5.3 Ultimate goal

ⓖ p 575 goal

Knowing the goal of any work or task can be an aid to comprehension; it helps your student know how to organise and understand information.

1   Your student may be finding out about something because she wants the information for a specific reason and using that reason can provide guidance for the way she gathers the information. For example, if she needs information about a coach journey; the reason guides the way she searches.

2   She may be prompted by sheer curiosity and have no goal in mind.

3   She may be trying to assess whether she needs the information or not. For example, her car insurance renewal comes with 6 batches of information; she has to assess what is relevant to her choices in the renewal process.

4   If she is working on a skill, gaining the skill is a goal which could be used to direct the way she processes information about it. For example, as a musician, she could be working on a new piece for a performance or she could be working on her technique for general playing.

Story: Different goals in playing music

- To work on a new piece, I would avoid anything that would disturb the flow of the music from start to finish.

- To work on a new technique, I would make sure the practice was sufficiently disrupted so that I always had to focus on the technique, rather than the music.

Using goals is another area of working that varies greatly between dyslexic/ SpLD people.

Some find that they have no idea how a project will progress; if they put any structure in place too early, they have great difficulty in forgetting that structure, even when it has become quite clear that it is no longer suitable; see *First Learning Becomes Fixed*. Such people need to experiment to find out their best use of structure and goals, as outlined in *Exercise for Student: Avoid More Problems When Learning New Skills*.

First Learning Becomes Fixed: p 89

Exercise for Student: Avoid More Problems When Learning New Skills: p 11

Other dyslexic/ SpLDs find considerable benefit from using the goal:

- it gives a template for collecting the information
- it generates questions with which to assess priorities
- it makes achieving the goal much more direct at the end of the project.

When the ultimate goal is going to be useful, it is worth working with it from the outset of acquiring information.

Suggestions about using goals for the four possibilities listed at the beginning of this section are:

1   Given a specific goal[3]: look at *Know the Goal of Any Task*.

2   Sheer curiosity: use your student's curiosity to generate questions she would like answered.

3   Assessing whether she needs the information: *Mind Set* her need to be engaged with any of the content, or her interest in the topic, then look for key words (see *Exercise: Key Words*) and *Prioritise*, bearing in mind her time, energy and money.

4   To gain a skill: the *Major Precaution* is worth keeping in mind; sometimes the learning process is helped when your student is clear as to how different stages lead to the final skill.

Know the Goal of Any Task: p 181

Mind Set: p 158

Exercise: Key Words: p 176
Prioritising: p 528

Major Precaution: p 10

Generating Useful Questions: p 530

It can be very beneficial to create some 'research questions' or lines of thought which will help your student to assess the usefulness of the information, and its importance and relevance to her.

---

[3] In the academic world the word 'outcome' is often used instead of 'goal'.

5.4 Skilled thinking

Skilled thinking includes any series of thinking processes used in appropriate, efficient and effective ways to produce required results. Thinking processes include:

> discussing, assessing, recording, choosing, deciding, researching, questioning and many other ways of thinking.

To show the commonality of skilled thinking, I have described how thinking might be used in three situations:

- a plumber setting about a new job[4]
- a householder choosing an energy supplier
- an undergraduate doing a piece of coursework.

I have highlighted the thinking processes involved in the three situations, including 'to carry out' the plumbing job, as thinking will continue all the way through the work. In all three, when the thinking is organised into useful patterns, the outcome will be more satisfactory than if the thinking were confused. Sometimes our minds organise the thinking without conscious effort, sometimes conscious effort is needed. Dyslexic/ SpLD people are likely to need the conscious effort when others don't; *NOT REALISING WHAT YOU ARE DOING* is a good example of why conscious effort is needed.

NOT REALISING WHAT YOU ARE DOING: p 86

The following analysis is not intended to be complete; it is intended to promote awareness of this level of thinking. The *EXERCISE FOR STUDENT: THINKING PROCESSES* should also promote awareness. The processes have been highlighted in the following scenarios.

EXERCISE FOR STUDENT: THINKING PROCESSES: p 173

Example: Thinking processes for plumbing job

Plumber setting about a new job: 'What's needed to do a job?'
To describe the situation: The plumber is an operative within a small plumbing business which has office staff and a manager. The plumber will be given details of work, with client information.

---

[4] I've worked in the office of my husband's plumbing and heating business.

I am assuming the plumber has the skills and training for the job.
He needs to check the paperwork is complete, that he
understands what the client wants. He needs to organise
the paperwork so that he can find it when he needs it and
record information that the office will need for invoicing
purposes, or further discussion with the client.
He needs to assess how long the job will take, when he is likely to
get to the site and at what point (in time) he needs to tell
the client, or office, that he is likely to get there.
He should decide whether he needs to investigate the job first in
order to know what materials to use.
He will need to maintain his standard van stock as well as to order
and collect any materials specific to the job.
With everything to hand, he can carry out the job.

Example: Thinking processes for household decision

Householder choosing an energy supplier: 'Value for money'
It is usually assumed that consumers want the lowest possible
price for any goods. I am proposing some ideas for
consideration, namely that to make an informed choice, a
consumer needs to research a number of questions:
What are my values? Why are these my values? How much do I
know about the issues?
Areas to investigate: lowest costs; offers available; concern for
infrastructure maintenance; green issues; political concerns,
such as the company owner being foreign.
How reliable are the sources of information?
What do I know about the suppliers? What agendas do they
have?
What do I know about the different forms of fuel?
What do I know about different offers available?
Are there any opaque (non-transparent) practices to be aware
of?
What's in the small print of any offer? How does it change the
offer?

Having researched the information, the consumer can then compare and contrast the different sets of information, formulate an argument about pros and cons and decide on the best option.

Example: Thinking processes for coursework

Undergraduate starting a piece of coursework.
To describe the situation: An undergraduate has been set an essay title, given a reading list and is expected to write an essay of 2,000 words in 2 weeks.
The undergraduate has to understand the aims and outcomes of the course, know what the syllabus is and understand the themes in the essay title. She can also survey the reading list for further evidence about the themes of the essay.
She will need to organise her reading so that she has the books from a library and has down-loaded any online materials. She will need to take notes during her reading.
She will need to assess what is relevant to the question set, and recognise any other knowledge that will be important for other purposes, such as exams.
She will need to manage her timetable so that she does the reading early enough to write the essay, and proof-read it before handing in on time.

5.4.1 Elements of thinking

In each of these situations, facts are being gathered, arguments constructed and evaluations made, see *KNOWLEDGE: FACTS, DISCUSSION AND EVALUATION*. Each different job, course or hobby will have its own constructs and methods for building knowledge or skills. The set given here comes from work with undergraduates; it doesn't relate to any particular course and I hope it is general enough to be useful as a guide for producing the right set for any other situation, as shown in *EXAMPLE BOX: ELEMENTS OF THINKING IN GIVING A VOTE OF THANKS*.

KNOWLEDGE: FACTS, DISCUSSION AND EVALUATION: p 152

EXAMPLE BOX: ELEMENTS OF THINKING IN GIVING A VOTE OF THANKS: p 173

Skilled thinking involves:	Alternative words
framework	overview, plan, rationale, introduction; a model might be used as a framework
data	facts, statements, assumptions, examples, evidence, results, definition, description
practical work	experiments, investigation, doing, field-work, work experience, exercise for the reader, coursework
questions	conjectures, propositions, hypotheses, perspectives
analysis	connections, similarities, differences, alternatives, distinctions, agreements, disagreements, theory, model
discussion	explanation, argument, reasons, debate, presentation
quality	criteria, clarity, focused, self-correcting, self-reflection, degree of commitment, value, consistency
evaluation	critical assessment, appraisal, decision, judgement, priorities
outcome	result, conclusion, summary, implications, consequences, recommendations

Framework

A framework is a useful construct for holding knowledge together; it helps your student to understand the main points. She may be reading or listening or reflecting on her own or with others as she uses the framework.

Data

Data (facts) are the basis of any situation or body of knowledge. Your student also needs to be aware of assumptions made, because they will put boundaries on the facts she has. Examples, evidence and results also contain a considerable amount of data.

Practical work

Some knowledge is best gained through practical work. There are lab. experiments in most science subjects. Much of maths is learnt through practical worksheets. Many jobs entail practical skills as well as theoretical ones. Practical experience is fundamental to driving.

Questions

See *Generating Useful Questions:* p 530

Questions are very useful; they allow your student to clarify any thoughts that need further information. She can also generate a questioning attitude by stating perspectives, making conjectures or propositions, and proposing hypotheses. She can make questions based on the key words that she finds in her first approach to the work.

Sometimes a list of quite simple questions is useful, such as: Why? Who? What for? What conditions?

Analysis

Analysis is necessary to put information together and to weigh up the relationships that exist between different parts of the information. The relationships can be found by looking for connections, similarities, differences, alternatives, distinctions, agreements or disagreements. They are likely to be synthesised into a theory or model.

Discussion

Discussion provides a way of testing out the analysis by seeing how well ideas can be presented to others, and how robust they are when scrutinised by others.

Quality

In all of this thinking, the quality of data and analysis is important. Your student needs to know her criteria for assessing quality; she needs to know how consistent her information and thinking are and how clear. She needs to be focused, and not confuse issues by wandering off the topic. She needs to be able to self-reflect and self-correct to maintain quality. She probably needs a middling to high level of commitment, so that she doesn't reduce quality by stopping too early.

Evaluation

Evaluations involve weighing up the arguments that have been put forward about a collection of facts that have been gathered together. The judgement might be that more facts are needed; they might lead to a future course of action; they might be that something is good or bad; etc. Evaluations should not be presented without being backed by reasoned arguments based on facts.

Outcome

The final product of any thinking process varies depending on the scenario. For the plumber, it is the finished job; for the householder, a choice about energy supplier; for the student, an essay.

Many essays will end with a concluding section which will either be an evaluation of the arguments presented or a summary of them. It may contain the implications of the findings, the consequences of arguments or recommendations arising from them.

Some of these processes will also be relevant to the plumber: a summary of the work goes to the office; there may be implications or consequences from the work or even recommendations for future work.

The householder will make an evaluation; the outcome will be his final choice, even if that is to make no change of supplier. He may even find himself making recommendations to others as a result of his work and thinking.

Example: Elements of thinking in giving a vote of thanks

Applying the above *ELEMENTS OF THINKING* to 'Giving a vote of thanks at the end of a folk dance evening' produces the following:
You need a *framework:* who has to be thanked: caller, musicians, organisers.
Gather *data:* what has the occasion been like; how have dancers enjoyed the dances; were the dances new, easy, challenging?
Questions: probably unused.

ELEMENTS OF THINKING:
p 169

Practical work: probably unused.

Quality: Your comments should be made in a friendly manner, even if the evening was fraught with tension.

Outcome: You leave people happy at the end of the evening and everyone is thanked.

Exercise for student: Thinking processes

Reflect on a couple of situations you deal with regularly and decide what thinking processes are involved.

Use the patterns from *Example Boxes: Thinking Processes for Plumbing Job, for Household Decision, for Coursework*.

Write down what happens in the situations that you have chosen and then highlight all the thinking processes you are using.

Example Boxes:
Thinking Processes for
Plumbing Job: p 167

For Household
Decision: p 168

For Coursework: p 168

Reading to gain information and acquire knowledge involves a complex set of processes that is needed in everyday life, education and employment. The following example could apply to all three.

Example: Thinking processes applied to reading

Regular situation: reading, reviewing and evaluating the ideas

Framework: Gain an overview of the topic; assess the completeness of the material presented; review conclusions.

Questions: What is being discussed? Why? How? What are the significant issues?

Practical: Discussion with peers.

Quality: Reasonable overview needed; deep understanding of underlying issues to be gained.

Analysis: Weighing up reliability of facts; any assumptions made or missing; soundness of arguments put forward.

As a result of applying these thinking processes in a deliberate way:

Outcome: Good understanding of the topic read and a clear assessment of the quality of the work.

5.4.2 Patterns of thinking processes

Different groups of thinking processes are useful for particular types of tasks, as you can see from the plumbing, householder and student examples. One person could be involved in several different situations and regularly use various patterns of thinking processes.

When your student frequently needs to repeat a set of thinking processes:

- she may decide to settle for a particular pattern so that she makes sure she covers all the areas with minimum effort to manage her thinking

- she may decide that what's necessary is so obvious that the task drives itself

- somewhere between these two extremes: for some parts she follows a particular pattern; and for other parts she lets the task dictate the processes.

Insight: Remembering the system

If she needs to use a specific pattern, encourage her to record it in some way and some place so that she doesn't forget her decision. It is quite easy to design a system one day, forget what it was and design another the next day and end up confused between the two systems.

5.4.3 Results of skilled thinking

It is satisfying to think with skill. In many circumstances, skilled thinking saves time and energy and produces the required result of any task. It can enable people to make appropriate, informed choices.

In academic work, skilled thinking can lead to good quality, critical thinking in which:

- the fine details of a topic are known
- credibility of evidence is assessed
- arguments identified and analysed
- models and theories are discussed with insight
- evaluations are well grounded.

Summary: Skilled thinking

Dyslexic/ SpLD people need to learn the advanced processes of skilled thinking as skills in their own right.

Skilled thinking applies to many different situations and subjects.

Skilled thinking is necessary to gain a good understanding of any issue.

The elements of skilled thinking are included in the *CHECK-LIST OF SKILLS, PROCESSES, MIND TECHNIQUES, ETC.*

CHECK-LIST OF SKILLS, PROCESSES, MIND TECHNIQUES, ETC.: p 220

5.5 Key words

Exercise to do with your student[5]: Key words

The following passage from *The Brain Book* by Peter Russell (1979) can be photocopied before doing the exercise. It is useful to have clear space down one side of the passage for writing on.
Read the next four paragraphs and then follow the instructions below.
Key Words
(From *The Brain Book* by Peter Russell)

'We saw earlier that words that had greater significance, had greater meaning, were more outstanding, and generated stronger images were very much easier to remember. When we read, we automatically pick out these more memorable words from the text, and the rest of the material is generally forgotten within a second or two. Thus, take the following sentence: "Astronomers are now suggesting that black holes may not, after all, be entirely black, but may in fact be capable of radiating energy." The key ideas in this sentence, the words that are most memorable and contain the essence of the sentence, are *astronomers, black holes, not black, radiating energy*. The rest of the words are merely grammatical constructions and emphasis; they are not necessary for recall.

'Key words tend to be the nouns and verbs in a sentence—though sometimes adjectives and adverbs may be significant enough to become key words. Key words are generally concrete rather than abstract. It has been found that concrete words generate images faster than abstract words—one and a half seconds faster on the average— and that the images they generate are richer and have more associations [(Gregg, 1975)]. For this reason they are better remembered.

'In a study by Michael Howe [(1977)] at Exeter University students' notes were examined and the ratio of key words to non-key words measured. It was found that the higher the percentage of key words present in the notes, the better was the recall. Because of their greater

Russell (1979)

Ⓖ p 575 concrete

Gregg (1975)

Howe (1977)

---

[5] When doing this exercise with anyone, I read the passage first, then I read out each sentence as we work on it.

meaningful content key words "lock up" more information in memory and are "keys" to recalling the ideas. In the foregoing case you have only to recall the two keys *black holes* and *radiating energy* to unlock the memory of the main idea contained in the sentence.

'So that you can get a feel of key words, go back and count how many words in the above three paragraphs of this chapter are actually key words.[6]'

Comment

One instinct that many dyslexic/ SpLD students have is that all the words in a passage are so important that none of them can be left out. So, reading the very last paragraph of that passage, the usual answer is "No way can I miss out any of those words".

Instructions:

Discuss the comment above.

Work on the passage sentence by sentence.

For each sentence:

1 select key words that contain the essence of the sentence and highlight them

2 decide what the purpose of the sentence is; use the ELEMENTS OF THINKING to help your student with this second step.

Discuss METACOGNITION as you do step 2 with the first sentence together.

ELEMENTS OF THINKING:
p 169

META-COGNITION:
p 63

Typical results of working with a group of people are shown in *DISCUSSION OF KEY WORDS EXERCISE*.

DISCUSSION OF KEY WORDS EXERCISE:
p 216

Both parts of this exercise are very valuable. Being able to assess the essence of a sentence and select its key words helps your student's understanding of the detail of the sentence. Deciding on the purpose of the sentence helps her comprehension of the whole topic; being aware of that purpose helps to develop METACOGNITION.

META-COGNITION:
p 63

Unravelling the sentences can lead fruitfully to discussion about *SENTENCE STRUCTURE*.

SENTENCE STRUCTURE:
p 97

---

[6] "About thirty." Footnote from *The Brain Book* (Russell, 1979)

5.6 Main themes vs. details

The importance of main themes is that they show your student how the information fits together; therefore, they help comprehension. Without them it is almost like doing a jigsaw without a picture, she has nothing to guide her. Using key words and the purpose of sentences and paragraphs will help her pick out the main themes from the detail.

Insight: Difficulty in assessing importance

Dyslexic/ SpLD people often find it hard to see the different levels of importance within a topic, subject or situation. If your student is unsure of the way her mind is processing information it is a very scary action to relegate any part of it to the 'minor detail' box. Once she has mentally put it there, she may find it difficult to reassign it to a major idea category; it's as if the initial tag never gets removed. She can't work with the length of words either because words like 'not', 'or', 'and' are small, but they significantly alter the meaning of the text.

Tip: Calligraphy pen to distinguish importance

One practical tip for distinguishing main themes from detail while taking notes is to find a calligraphy pen, a fibre tip one which has two different thicknesses. Important points are written with the thick side, the others are written with the narrower side. Your student is actively assessing the importance of information as she writes, which helps her to make the decision.

My practice is to teach the value of finding main themes through demonstrations. In this book, the SUMMARY OF THE CHAPTERS gives the main themes of each chapter. The CONTENTS of each chapter gives the section headings. The DIPPING-IN TO TRY OUT IDEAS sections indicate the major sections in the chapter.

THE SUMMARY OF THE CHAPTERS: p X

Instructions of any kind are useful places to practise finding the main themes; your student could practise using the publicity that comes by post.

Example: A Water Company leaflet on changes of ownership of sewers

This was an eight-paged A5 leaflet about changes in legislation. It's the type of document that takes me ages to read in the standard way and it's one I felt I ought to read.

Dealing with it by way of comprehension means
　　looking for key words:

1st page: Legal changes   ownership
　　　　your sewers   property owner

2nd page: dates involved   types of drains involved

3rd page: note that says I don't need to do anything; note that
　　　　new costs to Water Company may get passed on to their
　　　　customers → US, the customers

4th 5th pages: diagrams that show the changes → I can see how
　　　　we're affected

6th page where to get extra info → tells me to store the leaflet
　　　　for future use

7th 8th pages: reaching people in 21 languages.

Fairly quickly, I have everything I need to know, and I know where
　　　　to keep the leaflet for future use.

Summary:
The main theme is that the law has changed, and the position
　　　　along the sewer at which ownership switches from public to
　　　　private changed on Oct 1st 2011.
We didn't need to do anything, except pay up when prices go up!
　　　　I could file the leaflet in such a way that I could find it if
　　　　needed for a year, and then ditch it without further reading.

Summarising is a skill that often needs lots of practice. You have to choose the material to summarise carefully:

- if your student is not remotely interested in the topic, she probably will find it very hard to practise summarising, even if she really wants the skill
- if she is very interested, she may know too much already and have difficulty staying with practising the skill
- she needs to acquire the skill before applying it to something
  - very interesting to her
  - that she is studying or that is work-related.

Crook (2010)

Example: Finding the important ideas in a paragraph.

The following paragraph was part of the instructions for a piece of coursework and was rather incomprehensible to the student I was working with.

Course aims and objectives from a module on Historical Writing and Research Skills: An Introduction to Independent Study (Crook, 2010):
'This is a level 2, single module, and as such it will enable students to build on ideas and skills developed during their first year. In particular, the module is designed to give students the practical skills with which to approach their dissertations. It will prepare undergraduate students for advanced independent study in History, both in terms of the acquisition of key research skills and in the development of a critical, reflective engagement with questions of method and interpretation. It will cover the structure and development of an argument, supporting the use of primary sources, debating historical questions and reviewing literature.'

The flow chart we made of the paragraph is given in FIGURE 2.3. The space used to separate out the ideas is also important. The student was able to understand the major themes of the coursework.

Aims of
Historical Research & Writing:
An Intro to Independent Study

acquisition of key research skills

critical reflective engagement
with

method

interpretation

structure & development of an argument

supporting use of primary sources
debating historical questions
reviewing literature

Figure 2. 3 Important ideas in a paragraph

Essay titles and exam questions, meeting notes and agendas can be worked on in the same way. Your student can reduce them to a map or flow diagram much like *FIGURE 2.3*. She can highlight the main issues; she can add margin notes summarising the main points. Your student can draw pictures and diagrams that will help her to bring to mind the topic under discussion. She can survey long reading lists to pick out the main themes. Further discussion of essay titles and exam questions can be found in *GOALS FOR WRITTEN WORK*.

MARGIN NOTE:
examples of visual
strategies

GOALS FOR WRITTEN WORK: p 195

6 Know the goal of any task

Key point: Knowing the goal

The final element in your student's *REGIME FOR MANAGING DYSLEXIA/ SpLD* is to know her goal in any task. In using knowledge and skills your student is aiming to achieve a particular result, or several results. If she is very clear about what she wants to achieve, she is more likely to stay on task and be able to minimise the effects of her dyslexia/ SpLD.

REGIME FOR MANAGING DYSLEXIA/ SpLD: p 540

Knowing her goal will also help your student to *PRIORITISE*. She will be able to relate different aspects to the main goal and decide how important they are.

PRIORITISING: p 197

Example: Main goal and details

Suppose you have been asked about buses that run from A to B and suppose you have lived in the town for many years through several bus company changes. You know the history of the buses over several years. If you have been asked by a history researcher, everything you know is going to be relevant. But if the person needs to get from A to B, the current bus is all the person is asking about.

Your goal is determined by the need of the questioner, so is the amount of detail to include.

It is really important for HOLISTIC thinkers to be aware of the goal, in order to avoid going into too much detail. They have minds that produce a wealth of information given an initial thought. They are likely to touch on many different ideas in response to the first one and other people can become quite lost.

HOLISTIC VS. LINEAR: p 75

MULTIPLE GOALS, §6.1, is about the need to identify all possible goals.

GOALS FOR ACTIONS, §6.2, has three examples from everyday life and two relating more to education and employment.

GOALS FOR WRITING, §6.3, uses three different types of written work to look at the purpose, the recipient and the motivation for writing.

GOALS FOR SITUATIONS INVOLVING TALKING, §6.4, looks at issues specific to talking; it builds on the previous two sections.

PRIORITISING, §6.5, is about the need to do so.

GOALS FOR A COURSE, §6.6, summarises the sections within the book that will help your student to sort out course goals; it is usually very useful, if not essential, to identify them.

§6.1: p 183

§6.2: p 184

§6.3: p 187

§6.4: p 196

§6.5: p 197
§6.6: p 198

WHAT IS THE GOAL?, §6.7, includes an exercise to help your student indentify her goal.

§6.7: p 199

MONITORING YOUR STUDENT'S GOALS, §6.8, includes an exercise to help your student assess how she is meeting her goals.

§6.8: p 200

6.1 Multiple goals

Any action or piece of work might have two different types of goal. You dig your garden or allotment. One goal is to maintain the garden and allotment. Quite often, another goal is to get rid of tension caused by other situations in life. Separating these two goals from each other could influence the choices you make about what to do in the garden; you could end with a more satisfactory outcome as a result of your informed choices.

Example: Two different goals

A report about a new medical drug:
The report describes the drug, the trials, its benefits, any side effects; the report makes recommendations about the drug's use.
1st goal: to give medical evidence
2nd goal: to persuade people to use the drug.

Both types of goal are important and need to be identified, and both will affect the planning of the report. They can be identified by the same means.

Essay writing also involves two goals. The first is to write well about the subject matter; the second is to demonstrate knowledge to a teacher. Sometimes, it can hamper your student's writing style to think that the reader (the teacher) already knows more than she (the student) does. It can be important for her to be clear about the different goals in order to maintain her best level of fluency.

If there is a goal that is not being met and which your student is only subconsciously aware of, it can interfere with her progress and increase the problems from dyslexia/ SpLD. If she brainstorms around the task she is doing, she should be able to identify all the goals.

The goal of a task may also determine the best way of acquiring information and knowledge in the first place. In the research *EXAMPLE: TWO DIFFERENT GOALS*, knowing both goals in advance should be part of the research programme that initially undertook the work: the research needs to cover all the likely concerns of the eventual users of the medical drug.

EXAMPLE: TWO DIFFERENT GOALS: p 183

6.2   Goals for actions

Anyone could be helped by knowing the goal of an action. The important concepts for helping dyslexic/ SpLD people are:

- actually realising what the goal is
- recording it, i.e. doing more than thinking about it and leaving it inside the head
- putting it in a prominent position so that it can't be forgotten.

Discuss these concepts with your student, using any of the ideas in this section.

'Going away for a weekend' is an action that could have many different goals.

Example: Goals for going away for a weekend

Reasons for going away could include:

- to attend a conference
- to go fishing
- to see relations
- to go on a course
- to see a show
- etc.

If you are going to see a show, it is unlikely to take up all the time, so you may add secondary goals that will determine how you spend your time.

Suppose you have the primary goal of seeing the show and 5 secondary goals of seeing people or exhibitions; you could mentally think of 6 'things' to see.

As you plan, you might find that not everything is possible, so you start seeing what to miss out. You could find that you can do 5 things if you miss out the show, or you can do the show and one other.

If you put more importance on doing as many as possible you could rule out the show, which was the reason for the weekend excursion in the first place.

If you remember that your primary goal is the show, you won't miss it.

How many times have you gone up stairs to fetch object A, come back with several other things, but not A? So the equivalent of missing the show is quite a common occurrence, and not just for dyslexic/ SpLD people.

Example: Goal for family gathering

Clearly identifying the primary aim helps in many situations. The purpose of a family gathering is more likely to be for people to talk to each other than for the kitchen to be tidy all the time.

Example: Goal for shopping

You may decide to go shopping on the way to a meeting. You can't determine how long the shopping will take, so you need to bear in mind that getting to the meeting is your goal, and you need to be able to abandon the shopping when you run out of time.

Example: Goal for engaging with practical work

You might be someone who likes thinking about concepts and ideas and who is not motivated to do practical work.

You could have some far-reaching policies or theories that you might want to put into practice. The effectiveness of your ideas will be increased if they match reality well. Practical work can be seen as a way of testing how well ideas match the real world: the goal of the practical work is to investigate the ideas. Thus, practical work supports the work on ideas and every part of the practical work is seen in terms of the policies or theories. Then, the person whose thinking preference is for ideas (possibly, Myers-Briggs intuiting) has a more satisfactory goal for engaging with practical work.

MYERS-BRIGGS PERSONALITY TYPE: p 76

Key point: *THINKING PREFERENCES* and managing dyslexia/ SpLD

In the above example, the innate *THINKING PREFERENCES* of a person are engaged with the work. For many dyslexic/ SpLD people using their innate *THINKING PREFERENCES* is key to managing dyslexia/ SpLD because the effects of dyslexia/ SpLD get worse when thinking processes are not right for the individual concerned.

THINKING PREFERENCES: p 72

Example: Goal for practical demonstration

The goal for a practical demonstration is usually to illustrate knowledge, or a skill; the people watching will have a variety of *THINKING PREFERENCES*. The goal of good communication will be achieved when both these factors are kept in mind and the demonstration is tested against them while it is developed.

6.3 Goals for writing

One often has to produce written work for some particular purpose. Your student's writing will be better focused if she can keep the goal in mind as she writes.

In the discussion below, I have taken three types of written work, colour-coded for ease of recognition:

- CVs and job applications (these are discussed in more detail in *Job Application*)

Ⓖ p 574: CV
Job Application: p 504

- essays and exam questions
- reports and articles.

To draw out the differences between them, I have dealt with all three together in terms of:

1   the purpose
2   who your student is writing for, and what motivation is prompting the written work
3   ideas to help her know her goal in writing the piece.

The last but one subtopic of this section has some brief ideas about *Other Types Of Written Work*. The final subtopic gives examples of *Goals For Written Work*.

Other Types Of Written Work: p 194

Goals For Written Work: p 195

Sometimes a lot of preparation is too restrictive and your student may need to let her ideas flow in her writing without being too conscious of her goal. Usually, she will then need to edit her work so that it does achieve the purpose she has for it.

6.3.1 The purpose

A CV is written to give the facts about your student's experience to an employer or a tutor or an institution. Her goal is to convey the facts clearly and in a way that is going to tell the reader the sort of information they need to know. The same is true when dealing with a job application.

Your student may have been given an essay title or an exam question. Then, her goal is to show her understanding of the material through addressing the title or the question. In order to do so, she has to understand the essay title or exam question, see *Process And Content Words*.

Process And Content Words: p 189

Reports and articles are often about ideas your student wants to make available to others. Her goal is defined when she decides exactly what she wants others to gain.

6.3.2 Who is your student writing for and why?

In all these situations, your student is aiming to share her knowledge with someone else, for a specific reason, and by writing.

- CVs and job applications are an example of specific information requested by the reader.

- In an essay or exam question, she is demonstrating to the reader that she has a sound grasp of the material and she is using a specific pattern of writing in order to do so. The reader often knows more than your student, which can hinder writing. She needs to focus on the goal of demonstrating her knowledge and not confuse herself by thinking she is imparting new knowledge to this reader. This is an example of the two types of goal mentioned in *EXAMPLE: TWO DIFFERENT GOALS*, and it is a situation in which it is useful to be clear about them both.

EXAMPLE: TWO DIFFERENT GOALS: p 183

- In a report or article your student is presenting information, some of which may be new; she may be making the case for a certain action, or she may be drawing conclusions towards some future aim. The work may have been requested or it may come out of her interest.

6.3.3 Knowing the goal

Knowing what others have included is often a good way for your student to start being clear about her goal. It is often helpful to see an example, or several examples, of how others have set out their writing. Your student can assess how easy she found the material to read. You can help her analyse the way others have written by using the *ELEMENTS OF THINKING* together with the *EXERCISE TO DO WITH YOUR STUDENT: KEY WORDS*. Your student should allow her own style to develop; however, knowing that she is including all the necessary elements can be very reassuring, and it can help her confidence and writing fluency.

ELEMENTS OF THINKING: p 169

EXERCISE TO DO WITH YOUR STUDENT: KEY WORDS: p 176

For CVs it is helpful to use *Mind Set* and apply it to why your student is writing the CV.

For other information that has been requested, for example in a job application, use *Mind Set* to think about the job: What is the job? Why does your student want it? What does the employer want to know about her? What can she bring to the job? There are other ideas in *Planning*.

Mind Set: p 158

Planning: p 200

Knowing the goal for an essay or exam question[7] depends on reading the title or question accurately, see *Process and Content Words*.

Process and Content Words: p 189

Some reports and formal writing are also determined by other people, and your student can define her goals in much the same way as the *Example: An Exam Question about Atmospheric Management*. It may be useful to write a sentence that states the purpose of the report, rather like creating an essay title.

Example: An Exam Question about Atmospheric Management: p 191

For reports and articles that stem from your student's own interest, she needs to clarify her goal in similar ways; the difference is that she, and not someone else, is the source of the ideas and processes.

6.3.4 Process and content words

Essay titles and exam questions will have two different types of word: process words and content words.
This classification of words is also relevant in:

everyday life: instruction manuals; online forms; holiday-booking processes; self-service checkouts; etc.

education: maths problems and exams questions; science practical work, problem sheets and exam questions; etc.

employment: job descriptions, task instructions, filling in forms; etc.

An exam question is used as an example and analysed in detail to show the value of identifying process words and breaking content words into component parts.

---

[7] There is little difference between essay titles and exam questions. For the former, students are expected to find out information before they write, for the latter they are expected to know everything necessary already.

The process words tell your student what to do; the content ones tell her what to apply the process to. In 'Explain and evaluate the Keynesian argument for increases in government spending as a cure for economic crises', 'explain' and 'evaluate' are the processes which your student has to apply; the rest of the words are the content that she is being asked to explain and evaluate.

It is useful for your student to practise identifying process words in exam questions of a subject she is not studying. Then she will not be distracted by the content but will be more able to focus on the process words and what they are telling her to do. It is also useful to decide whether the process words relate to *FACTS, DISCUSSION* or *EVALUATION*.

KNOWLEDGE:
FACTS, DISCUSSION AND EVALUATION: p 152

Process words		
Facts	*Discussion or argument*	*Evaluation*
Analyse	Examine the argument that ...	Assess
Describe	How far ...	Compare
Outline	Show how ...	Consider
State	What arguments can be made for and against	Criticise
Summarise	...	Discuss
		Evaluate

The exact process can depend on the subject studied. It is worth your student finding out how to interpret the words most used for her subject.

If your student is studying maths or a science subject, make a list of appropriate process words and what they mean.

If your student is not in education, then she can practise on material that is similar to information she needs to understand; again if it is not familiar, she will not get distracted by the content. Make a list of process words she is likely to encounter.

Question:
Outline what points need to be considered when creating an operational urban air pollution alert system capable of predicting, detecting and reacting to a pollution episode within a time scale of days or hours. Wherever possible, illustrate your discussion with existing urban air pollution alert systems.

Comments:
One difficulty with this question is that students start to write about urban air pollution alert systems because they don't see the question is about the points to consider when constructing one.

Question re-written:
Comprehension is helped a little if the question is re-written with just 2 new words and 4 hyphens, as shown by the underlining:
Outline <u>the</u> points <u>that</u> need to be considered when creating an operational urban <u>air-pollution</u> <u>alert-system</u> capable of predicting, detecting and reacting to a pollution episode within a time scale of days or hours. Wherever possible, illustrate your discussion with existing urban <u>air-pollution</u> <u>alert-systems</u>.

The two process words are 'outline' and 'illustrate'.

I am cautious about the way I re-write exam questions. I don't stray very far from the original, otherwise my students become uncertain that everything is included.

 Example continued:

1) The question can be re-arranged as in *Figure 2.4*, with all the component parts in separate boxes; rounded corners of two boxes show the characteristics of the alert-system. The words on the arrows help to show the relationships between the boxes.

The diagram highlights the goals of the answer. It can also be used for planning the answer.

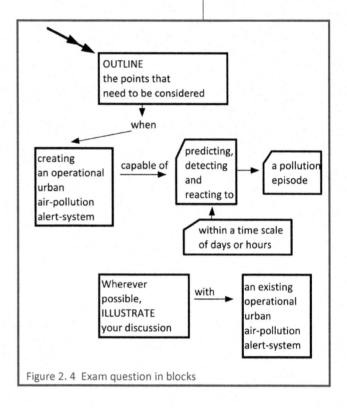

Figure 2. 4 Exam question in blocks

The diagram is likely to help visual and holistic thinkers because it is spread out and uses visual symbols and details. Logical thinkers could be helped because the flow diagram shows relationships.

The diagram can be further enhanced by using colour, as in *Figure 2.5*. The two figures have slightly different layouts: *Figure 2.4* has the process words in a vertical line and *Figure 2.5* has them in a horizontal line. Which one will be suitable depends on whether a student needs to focus on each stage separately or needs to keep the second stage in mind while processing the first.

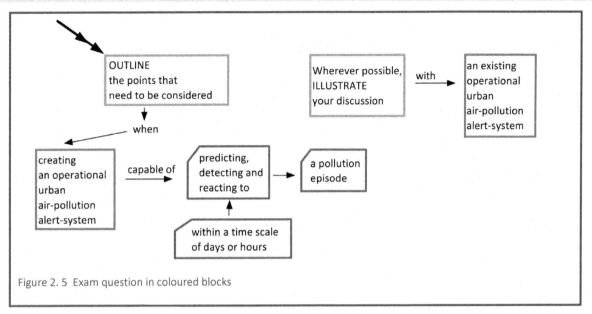

Figure 2. 5 Exam question in coloured blocks

   Example continued:

2) For list makers, the question can be spaced out with the component parts on separate lines.

The list is likely to help verbal and linear thinkers.

Outline the points that need to be considered when

- creating an operational urban air-pollution alert-system
- capable of predicting, detecting and reacting to
- a pollution episode
- within a time scale of days or hours.

Wherever possible[8],
illustrate your discussion with

- existing urban air-pollution alert-systems.

Exam question as a list

---

[8] 'Wherever possible' has been indented so that the two process words, 'outline' and 'illustrate', are in the same vertical line and are against the margin. 'Wherever possible' is not so important; it could have been moved, but it is good to demonstrate techniques that don't alter the order of the words.

3) The question can be colour coded or highlighted:

Outline the points that need to be considered when creating an operational urban air pollution alert system capable of predicting, detecting and reacting to a pollution episode within a time scale of days or hours. Wherever possible, illustrate your discussion with existing urban air pollution alert systems.

Visual thinkers would use the colours and verbal thinkers the words.

In all three suggestions, kinaesthetic thinkers will gain through the actions involved.

In none of these options has the question been reduced to key words; your student should keep the precise instructions and the relationships between the components, so using only key words could be unhelpful at this point. Later in the planning stage, key words could well be all she needs.

6.3.5 Other types of written work

The writing tasks discussed above are not the only ones your student may have to do: knowing the goal can facilitate many types of writing.

- Your student can treat formal letters as short reports in order to define her goals.

- If she finds informal letters difficult, she can use MIND SET as a way of deciding what her goal for the letter is.

  MIND SET: p 158

- For emails and text messages she will often need to be quite clear about her purpose because they are so succinct that they are often open to misinterpretation.

- Filling in forms online, especially boxes that require continuous prose, is often difficult for dyslexic/ SpLD people (and others!). It can be useful to have a text document open alongside. Your student can then construct her answer in the text document and copy and paste into the online form. The techniques above should help her be clear about the ideas or information she needs to convey. Having the text document also stops her losing her typing when something happens to the form and it disappears.

- Filling in paper forms involves several difficulties for dyslexic/ SpLD people; it is almost always a good idea to make a copy of the form before she starts writing anything.
    - She can't erase once she starts writing using a pen.
    - The boxes don't expand, so she has to make sure that what she wants to write will fit.
    - As she progresses through the form, she may realise that she didn't identify what the form-writer requires, so her first answer is off the point.
    - As with proof-reading, if possible she should leave time between entering the answers on the copy of the form and transferring them to the form to be sent; she may find she has a better understanding of what she was being asked.
- Creative writing is altogether a different genre. Often the first stage is to write as the ideas flow into her head. She will probably then have to reflect on her writing in order to communicate her ideas to another person.

This list is not comprehensive. For any other type of writing, your student can choose the ideas that suit her work best, and experiment to find the approaches that help her to maintain her best fluency in writing.

6.3.6 Goals for written work

e.g.	Examples: Goals for written work
Letter to a friend	Keep in contact; share your news; enquire about your friend.
Letter to local councillor	Put a point of view: state a situation; present facts; put a consistent, telling argument; summarise with point of view.
Answer exam question	Demonstrate your ability and knowledge of the subject.
Undergraduate dissertation	Demonstrate your ability to carry out research: present the background, your methods, your findings, any relevant further research. The findings are not the main point; to show that you can do research is the main purpose.

Research thesis	The findings are the main point and any conclusions that can be drawn from them. The evidence, analysis, methods all contribute, as does the background.
Newspaper article	To catch attention: should be to inform with accuracy.
Report	Set out a problem, research the causes or possible solutions and consequences, make recommendations. Good cover of facts will be needed, and well-argued discussion giving a full discussion of different points of views.

6.4 Goals for situations involving talking

Meetings, seminars, debates, presentations, one-to-one conversations are all situations when it can be useful for your student to know what her goals are.   In this section, ideas specific to these situations are added to the ideas in GOALS FOR WRITING.

A meeting could be a one-off event for a particular purpose. It could be part of a series of meetings. Formal meetings tend to have an agenda, minutes are kept and approved. Your student can decide about the goals involved from the overall purpose of the meeting and from the agenda. It can also help to think about her interests and motivations in relation to the meeting and those of the other members.

Seminars tend to be for exchange of ideas and knowledge about a specific topic; this exchange is the goal, together with an increased understanding of the topic.

At a seminar, it's important to think about the different levels of experience of the participants. All should feel confident enough to contribute. If your student is one of the more experienced, it is good to make sure the less experienced aren't intimidated by her knowledge. If she is one of the less experienced, she needs to recognise her goal of gaining a deeper understanding, possibly by asking questions.

To debate is 'to engage in discussion or argument; esp. in a public assembly' (OED Online, 2020). A debate is not an exchange of ideas

See also GROUP WORK: MEETINGS, SEMINARS AND DEBATES: p 446

GOALS FOR WRITING: p 187

('debate, v.1.4.b' OED Online,2020)

or a examination of possibilities. Teams in a debate have already made up their minds. They listen to the points made by opponents in order to disprove them. The outcome of a debate is that one side wins the argument.

Making a presentation is also a time when your student will find it useful to be clear about her goal. While she is presenting, her focus of attention is on herself; she needs to know what helps her keep her thoughts together while she talks. It is unlikely she will achieve any goal if she loses her fluency when talking, see *TALKING* for further discussion.

TALKING: p 362

One-to-one conversations range from informal chats to formal discussions. Goals tend not to be relevant to informal chats, except for two points. Dyslexic/ SpLD people aren't always in tune with the other person and don't let go of an idea or goal early enough; we tend to pursue a thought long after others have switched to something else. Sometimes an important idea will occur to your student while someone else is talking, and the challenge is how to keep hold of it long enough to be able to mention it, without being rude and abruptly interrupting another speaker, see *INSIGHT: CAPTURING THOUGHTS IN MEETINGS*.

INSIGHT: CAPTURING THOUGHTS IN MEETINGS: p 473

For a formal one-to-one conversation, e.g. work-based appraisal or viva examination, your student can use the ideas in *EXERCISE FOR STUDENT: WHAT IS YOUR GOAL?*

EXERCISE FOR STUDENT: WHAT IS YOUR GOAL?: p 199

6.5 Prioritising

There are usually several tasks for your student to do in order to achieve her goal. Some will be vital, so that if they are not done her goal will not be fulfilled. Others will be less important; if they are not done, her goal will still be achieved, though not quite as well as might be. Others will be relatively unimportant and hardly impact on achieving her goal.

Example: Going away for the weekend to see a show

Vital task: booking the tickets or have some money to buy them
Important, but not vital: packing a wash bag
Unimportant task: packing a good book to read.

Prioritising includes assessing how important the individual tasks are, and in what order to do them. Your student will need to know how long each of them takes, whether doing some together will make them easier to do, whether each one can be done or not. She needs to consider how she will feel if any of them are not done.

Making a plan can help her prioritise, or she could use the ideas in *PRIORITISING*. Once she has sorted out her priorities, she can experiment and find out to what extent following the plan helps her. For some things, like writing an article, the plan may be a major tool for achieving her goal. For other things, like going away for a weekend, it may be too restrictive if followed rigorously.   In our household, plans are not binding, they are 'something to hang modifications on' and as such they are very useful.

PRIORITISING: p 528

6.6 Goals for a course

In undertaking any course, it is very useful for your student to know her goals, which should be the knowledge and skills that the course is designed to teach her. She should be able to find this information in the course materials.

To find the goals from the course materials your student can apply similar approaches to those shown in *EXAMPLE: FINDING THE IMPORTANT IDEAS IN A PARAGRAPH* and in *EXAMPLE: PREPARATION FOR A LECTURE*. A good set of goals for a course can be very useful material when it comes to revision.

EXAMPLE: FINDING THE IMPORTANT IDEAS IN A PARAGRAPH: p 180

EXAMPLE: PREPARATION FOR A LECTURE: p 271

6.7 What is the goal?

In many different situations having a clear goal in mind helps a dyslexic/ SpLD person avoid some of the effects of their dyslexia/ SpLD. Knowing the goal is the fourth element in the *REGIME FOR MANAGING DYSLEXIA/ SPLD*.

REGIME FOR MANAGING DYSLEXIA/ SPLD: p 540

Exercise for student: What is your goal?

- Use the *MATERIALS AND METHODS* that suit you best for collecting your thoughts together.

MATERIALS AND METHODS: p 565

- Look at *FIGURE 2.6*. It uses a mind map to put questions to help you identify your goal.

- Do you want to change the questions to suit your situation better?

- Answer the questions in an order that suits you.

- Can you identify your goal?

- If not, what else do you need to know in order to identify it?

- Carry on collecting information until you know what your goal is.

What is the task?

What is the reason for doing the task?
Is it the same as the goal of the task?

Are there any dyslexia/ SpLD pitfalls to take into account?

What is your goal?

What is the main goal of the task?

What are the priorities in achieving the goal(s)?

Are there any secondary goals?

Figure 2. 6 What is your goal?

6.8 Monitoring your student's goals

How will your student know that her goals are being met?
What does she expect to be the result of achieving her goals?

Exercise for student: How well am I doing?

Use a list or a mind map or a table. You could also use any suitable electronic device.
Write down your goals and note any priorities you have established.
Include any minor goals that need to be reached along the way to achieving the main one.

For each goal, write out the results of that goal being realised. Include any relevant time information.

From time to time come back to these expectations and decide how well you are doing and whether you need to adjust your expectations.

Monitoring your student's goals can help her to see whether she is approaching a task in the right way or whether she needs to change the way she does things.

7 Planning

Good planning can assist learning knowledge and skills, and using them.

Key point: Planning

- Planning can be undertaken before your student has all the necessary knowledge or skills; the planning allows her to be clear about any work still to be done.

- Knowing what she wants to achieve (i.e. *KNOW THE GOAL OF ANY TASK*) before she does any research can make the research processes much more effective.

- Knowing what she wants to achieve can also help her to be clear about any skills she needs to acquire.

KNOW THE GOAL OF ANY TASK: p 181

The summary of *MATERIALS AND METHODS* will help your student reflect on ones that she can use easily. She may find she varies the materials depending on the task or situation. Using separate sheets of paper or cards, or working on a computer may help her to re-order her ideas once she has collected them all; this technique is especially useful for big projects.

MATERIALS AND METHODS: p 565

Formats to use for planning include:
1   brainstorming, see *MIND SET*
2   tabular formation to show relationships
3   flow diagram
4   separate sheets or cards that can be shuffled around, either using previous sheets of notes or making them as part of the planning process – Post-it notes can be used in this way too
5   adapt any note form, see *TAKING AND MAKING NOTES,* to suit your present purposes.
Using a *TABULAR FORM* can be particularly helpful when comparing different collections of information or ideas.

MIND SET: p 158

TAKING AND MAKING NOTES: p 300

TABULAR NOTES: p 321

While planning, it can be useful to look at influences that assist or prevent progress. Any of the formats listed above could be used. *FIGURE2.7* uses the brainstorming format. You need to bring to mind:

    the task
    your goal(s)
    what needs to be planned
    your strengths
    any difficulties you might expect
and then you can plan with some confidence.

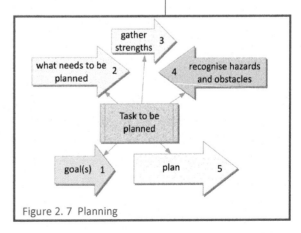

Figure 2. 7 Planning

Her strengths, hazards and obstacles can come from her *Individual, Personal Profile of Dyslexia/ SpLD*. It is important to include them and be realistic about them; doing so should enable her to minimise the effects of her dyslexia/ SpLD and maximise her potential.

Ⓖ p 575 hazard, obstacle

Individual, Personal Profile of Dyslexia/ SpLD: p 540

7.1 Planning related to knowledge

Writing or talking

To keep the language simple *Prompts for Planning* and *Three Examples of Planning* are worded as if your student is writing for at least two *readers*; but the words like 'writing' and 'readers' are in italics as a reminder that she may be talking to listeners. The suggestions that follow are appropriate to writing or talking to either a single person or many people and to preparing for meetings.

7.1.1 Prompts for planning

The following prompts take the form of questions to guide your student's thinking about planning:

- the first four relate to how she is going to *write* (purpose goal[9]);
- prompts 5, 6 and 7 relate to the subject matter (content goal[10]);
- prompts 8 and 9 relate to both goals and how she is working to achieve both.

How she is going to *write* often alters the selection of what she will *write*, so it is worth starting with the first four prompts.

Any constraints on her work should emerge from the prompts, or be considered with the answers to the prompts. She needs to scrutinise the instructions for her work, to see whether there are limits on its *length*, and details of its *layout* or *style*.

Prompt 1   Why is your student undertaking this piece of *writing*?

Did she establish an overall goal, or purpose, as in *Know the Goal of Any Task*? As she uses the next three prompts, she should keep considering how she will achieve this goal. If she doesn't have a purpose, one may emerge during planning or *writing*.

Know the Goal of Any Task: p 181

---

[9] Purpose goal – dealing with the purpose of the task
[10] Content goal – dealing with the content; see *Example: Two Different Goals:* p 183

Prompt 2   Who are her *readers*?

Tutors, other students (peers[11]), particular people – real or imaginary

Employer, line manager, fellow employees (peers), clients

Friends, others who share her interests (peers)

Official people: bank manager, local councillor

If there are no special people, your student can choose some to give herself *readers* to *write* for. It is much easier to *write* with people in mind than not; it helps to keep the mind focused.

Prompt 3   Consider the *readers*:

What do they know?

What might they want to know?

What does your student want to tell them?

What is their life-style?

What are their entrenched views?

Is your student trying to persuade them about some idea?

Does her material cater for a wide range of THINKING PREFERENCES?

THINKING PREFERENCES:
p 72

Prompt 4   Is your student *writing*:

as herself

on behalf of another person, e.g. a client, a relative

on behalf of a group?

If she is not *writing* as herself, who are the authors and what are their views?

Prompt 5   Look at the question or title or statement about the topic:

What is the subject?

How has your student been asked to process it? or How has your student decided to process it?

Prompt 6   What does your student know? What does she need to find out?

Your student can use any form of notes, see TAKING AND MAKING NOTES, to collect ideas so that she recalls what she knows about the subject.

TAKING AND MAKING NOTES: p 300

---

[11] 'Peers' are her equals and in many situations they will be invaluable as *readers*.

As she researches for *writing*, she should notice the way others have treated the subject, especially within her field or company[12]. Your student can use the *Exercise To Do with Your Student: Key Words* to analyse some of the sources that she uses.

Exercise To Do with Your Student: Key Words: p 176

She can *Generate Useful Questions* for which she needs answers, and use these for further research.

Generating Useful Questions: p 530

Prompt 7   What other information does your student need?

Your student can use the *Elements of Thinking* to check whether she has included everything needed to achieve her goals and to ensure she is making a good argument.

Elements of Thinking: p 169

Prompt 8   Having gathered the information, arrange it in a suitable way:

Does it achieve your student's goals?
What are the important ideas? Maybe number them.
What conclusion does your student want to put across?

Prompt 9   Is your student on target?

Your student should keep checking that what she is doing satisfies the purpose of the *piece of writing* and is processing the subject matter in the desired way, see *Multiple Goals*. Has a *word* or *page limit* been set? Has she got too much or too little material, or about right? See *Length (Writing), Duration (Talking)*.

Multiple Goals: p 183

Length (Writing), Duration (Talking): p 206

7.1.2 Examples of planning

Examples: Three examples of planning:

First example
A geographer was asked to *write* on behalf of an environmentalist group about environmental issues in reply to an anti-environmental letter-writer.

---

[12] There is often a house style; for example, companies will want reports written in particular ways; educational fields have specific ways of discussing subjects.

He needed to assess three collections of information:

1 the environmentalist group's viewpoint

2 the anti-environmentalist letter-writer's viewpoint

3 the current 'scientific' evidence relating to environmental issues.

He put the three sets of ideas side-by-side in a table.

He needed to take the anti-environmentalist's points and use the scientific evidence to present the group's answers in a *written reply.*

Second example

A scientist had to *write an essay* to show tutors that she understood a topic.

She was *writing* as herself; her *readers* were knowledgeable; her preparation was to sort out her ideas about the topic, to appreciate their order of importance and how they relate to each other.

Third example

A student of politics had to *write* about different policies of conservatism. The lecturer had discussed the policies from three or four different perspectives.

A table was drawn up. Each perspective was made into a column; each policy was made into a row. The features of each policy were written in a horizontal line across the columns. This form gave the student an overview of the similarities and differences, which was then used to plan and write the essay.

7.1.3 If your student is stuck

1 If your student cannot carry on because of physical fatigue, she needs to take a break and *RELAX.*

RELAXATION: p 558

2 If progress is not happening, compare what she is doing to what she was intending to do, or has been asked to do, i.e. her goals. Sometimes, there is a conflict of ideas that prevents progress.

3   Her *THINKING PREFERENCES* may not be engaged; especially her main
     MOTIVATION. See *EXAMPLE: GOAL FOR ENGAGING WITH PRACTICAL WORK*
     for an example of changing perspective so that a main *THINKING
     PREFERENCE* is engaged.

THINKING PREFERENCES:
p 72

*INPUT, OUTPUT AND
MOTIVATION:* p 73

4   Her environment may not be helping her: one student needed
     yellow around her; another needed to see the outside world;
     another needed to spread her resources over a wide surface.

*EXAMPLE: GOAL FOR
ENGAGING WITH
PRACTICAL WORK:* p 186

5   Something completely unrelated to her work may be
     undermining her progress and she will struggle to continue until
     it is acknowledged, and possibly solved, see second insight in
     SOME UNOBVIOUS PROBLEMS.

*SOME UNOBVIOUS
PROBLEMS:* p 64

The processes of *MIND SET* can be useful to see why she is stuck and to
see if there is any way she can change the use of her *THINKING
PREFERENCES* to help her continue.

MIND SET: p 158

7.1.4 Length (writing), duration (talking)

It is often useful for your student to think about the length of her final
work before she starts work on it. There is no point in doing the
research for a major report, if she is writing an article for a magazine
and she is only allowed 300 words. She might be given 2 minutes to
deliver a notice at a meeting, which she hopes will produce an
enthusiastic response from the audience.

The following examples cover a long report, a short essay, and talks of
varying duration. In each case there is a given length for the work.
The first is a table with a fairly detailed breakdown of the word count,
which can be adapted to apply to the other examples.

The purpose of tables such as this is as a guide: your student should
not feel that she has to keep rigidly to the division of words or
minutes. Her aim is to achieve a balance between the subtopics
bearing in mind their relative importance to the overall theme of the
work and the length, or duration, in which she can develop her
arguments.

10,000 words for a report may be broken-down into an introduction, 4 major sections and a conclusion. Usually the introduction and conclusion are half the length of a major section, giving the equivalent of 5 sections of 2,000 words each. Each major section could well have a similar pattern of an introduction, 5 themes and a conclusion, giving the word count pattern in the table. Taking each theme at a time then becomes less daunting.

To get a balance of ideas, probably 5 themes are needed to make a good argument for each main section.

Total words : 10,000			
	Words	Section	Words divided between themes
	1,000	Introduction	
	2,000	Section 1	165 Introduction 334 Theme 1 334 Theme 2 334 Theme 3 334 Theme 4 334 Theme 5 165 Conclusion
	2,000	Section 2	ditto
	2,000	Section 3	ditto
	2,000	Section 4	ditto
	1,000	Conclusion	

Example: Word count for an essay divided between subtopics

1,000 words (with short paragraphs) is about 2 typed pages. Half a page is about 334 words. Often when your student breaks-down a large piece of work into components and sees how little she has for each topic, the whole doesn't seem so enormous and she may start to worry that she has too much to write!

1,000 words would probably be suitable for an introduction, three themes and a conclusion. With this structure, each theme would be about 500 words, and the introduction and conclusion about 250 each. Your student doesn't have to start writing at the beginning, she could start with theme 3.

Example: Minutes for talks divided between subtopics

A similar analysis for different lengths of talks would be:

15 minutes:	3 mins. each for introduction, 3 main ideas and conclusion.
half-an-hour:	5 mins. each for introduction, 4 main ideas and conclusion.
1 hour:	introduction and conclusion 5 - 10 mins. each, with either 5 main ideas or 3 main sections equally spaced in the rest of the time.

7.2 Planning related to skills

A skill is an 'ability to do something, acquired through practice and learning' (OED, 1993). Skills are likely to have both physical components and mental ones. They can be developed for a mainly physical, practical task, or for a mainly mental task. 'Practical' means 'relating to practice or action as opposed to speculation or theory' (OED Online, 2020).

OED (1993)

('practical, adj.1.a.' OED Online, 2020)

PLANNING TO USE PRACTICAL SKILLS is primarily about skills with a practical purpose. *PLANNING TO USE MENTAL SKILLS* is about those with a mental purpose.

PLANNING TO USE MENTAL SKILLS: p 212

7.2.1 Planning to use practical skills

There are many jobs that are practical and in which kinaesthetic skills are used.
For instance:

operating farm machinery	electrical work	scientific research
making clothes	using a computer	playing musical instruments
sculpture	painting	carrying out medical procedures
playing sports	building	cooking
and more.		

Within these jobs, many different skills will be used. The job as a whole will probably need planning. How your student sets about planning to use the individual skills is the subject of this section.

There are skills that your student will learn primarily by watching others, or being with them and doing, or by doing and experimenting on her own; such skills can be used in a kinaesthetic way.

People who are good at these skills are using the body-kinaesthetic intelligence from the theory of *Multiple Intelligences* (Stacey, 2019). Different *THINKING PREFERENCES* can also be used to learn practical skills, but the body-kinaesthetic intelligence will have to be involved in using them.

Stacey (2019)

THINKING PREFERENCES: p 72

Your student may know the skills in a practical, kinaesthetic way, and they may not be held in her mind in a verbal way, so communicating her knowledge of them via language may be difficult when others don't share her way of thinking.

Many practical jobs and skills also have theoretical knowledge that needs to be known and used alongside the practical skills.   Practical people sometimes have difficulty with the theories. The practical and theoretical sides of work and study can be related using the ideas in *MYERS-BRIGGS PERSONALITY TYPE AND NOTE MAKING*. Making these connections helps the theory to become relevant.

MYERS-BRIGGS PERSONALITY TYPE AND NOTE MAKING: p 332

Some dyslexic/ SpLD people are very sensitive to their environment, to the extent that their ability to execute actions can be seriously disturbed by the wrong environment (Stacey, 2020a). Use the ideas in *ACTION, RESULT, NEXT STEP* to help your student understand how the environment affects her. The headings for information could be:

Task   Environment   Reflection   Adaptation

'*Adaptation*' would include her constructive way forward and anything that she needs to negotiate with others.

Stacey (2020a)

ACTION, RESULT, NEXT STEP: p 527

Summary: Suggestions for planning to use practical skills

- As ever, your student should use her *THINKING PREFERENCES* so that any thinking involved is as reliable and as easy as possible.

- She can mentally rehearse actions, or sequences of actions, to reinforce the mental patterns involved and make them active; this is mind set for action, see *MENTAL REHEARSAL OF MOVEMENTS*.

- Identify reliable mental triggers so that she knows how to get into an action and maintain it well, see *INSIGHT: MENTAL TRIGGERS*.

- Use *PROMPTS FOR PLANNING*, with appropriate adaptations:

  Prompt 1: Why is your student doing this action?

  Prompt 2: Who benefits from this action?

  Prompt 3: What do they want?

  Prompt 4: What is her purpose for the action?

  Prompt 5: Are there any instructions? Has she understood them?

  Prompts 6 & 7: Is there anything else she needs?

  Alter the questions and text under the prompts to fit her skill.

- Assess the environment in which the action takes place.

THINKING PREFERENCES: p 72

MENTAL REHEARSAL OF MOVEMENTS: p 292

INSIGHT: MENTAL TRIGGERS: p 211

PROMPTS FOR PLANNING: p 202

Insight: Mental triggers

Your student may need to create a reminder that she sees just before she goes into action.

Many pieces of music have repeated sections; I only know where I am when I have woven a story for a piece and I relate the story to myself as I play. I have a note to myself on the music to remind me to think through the story.

Your student's motivation for taking-action can have an important influence on how well she will do the action. She should identify any strong influences at the planning stage.

Ⓖ p 575
taking-action

Is she taking this action:

>   for joy and to share with others, e.g. music

>   to give a good performance, e.g. job interview or exam

>   to win, e.g. at sport

>   to impress others, e.g. cook a meal

>   other?

She should choose the motive that she wants to use, or that suits her best, and build it into the way she prepares for taking-action. Make sure it is part of the way she keeps her mind focused during the action.

Often a collection of practical skills are used together and the planning for each skill may be slightly different. In the *Story: Medical Examination (OSCE)*, we had to think through all the skills being examined.

Story: Medical Examination (OSCE[13])

An OSCE is a practical exam in which students have to demonstrate expertise in about 12 different situations that they will meet in practice. Actors take the part of patients; there is equipment and the students have to record their observations.

For one student, we assessed the difficulties she would face because of dyslexia and dyspraxia; we devised strategies when we could; then we negotiated with the examiners, explaining how her dyslexia/ SpLD impacted on her performance, and how any accommodation would allow her to show her ability. We also had to argue how the adjustments would not give her an unfair advantage.

Many experts in the building trade have to renew their qualifications on a regular basis; the exam situation can be very similar to the one described for the OSCE exam, e.g. gas fitting qualifications.

7.2.2 Planning to use mental skills

There are mental skills involved in dealing with everyday life and using knowledge, including:

understanding	imagining	skilled thinking
planning	reading	listening
assessing situations	writing	talking
and more.		

Some of these skills are discussed in this book. In general education, some of these skills are taught deliberately, at least to begin with. Many are assumed to be picked up subliminally.

Ⓖ p 575 subliminal learning

---

[13] OSCE: Objective Structured Clinical Exam

Key point: Being deliberate

It is often assumed these mental skills will be learnt subliminally, i.e. without conscious effort, through dealing with knowledge.

Dyslexic/ SpLD people need to learn them and practise applying them in very deliberate ways.

Several skills will probably be used together to achieve a specific outcome:

> read an email; understand the message and any implications; decide on the response; write the reply.

When your student is using a skill at a level that is easy for her, she may not need to do any planning.

When the overall task becomes more difficult, she may need to be deliberate in the way she uses the skill.

Summary: Suggestions for planning to use a mental skill

- As ever, your student should use her *THINKING PREFERENCES* so that her thinking is as reliable and as easy as possible.

  THINKING PREFERENCES: p 72

- She can use *MIND SET* to switch her mind on to the skill and the topic she will be working on, and gather her thoughts together.

  MIND SET: p 158

- She needs to think how she uses the skill; again she can use the processes in *MIND SET*.

- She should assess the *ENVIRONMENT* in which she is working.

  ENVIRONMENT: p 70

In the following example, the elements in *FIGURE 2.7* are applied to the mental skill *recall*. The ideas could have been gathered in a mind map, a list or a table.

Time was a more important 'environmental' factor than place.

FIGURE 2.7: p 201

Example: Planning to create a reliable recall system – part 1

Task to be planned	to develop a recall and memorising system
1 goal	to have a system that works for me and that I want to use
2 what needs to be planned	a card system to check recall notes, or other source, to check how complete and accurate the recall is time to use the recall system
3 strengths	logic, visual patterns, use of colour motivation increases when a project is for others in some way
4 hazards	too busy getting over-enthusiastic, then disappointed, then giving up
4 obstacles: ideas that won't work	recall in spontaneous ways, or at need, may not happen if the system is too rigid
5 develop ways forward	set up basic card system, and full backup notes decide on a few things to commit to memory and some skills to learn monitor how good the recall is, how well the system is working and adjust accordingly

A few examples that could benefit from a good recall system:

> using a stopwatch for a sports activity
>
> names of people in a new group
>
> a technique for teaching English
>
> practice and knowledge for a music exam.

Monitoring the recall system

Your student should monitor any system she develops:

- to make sure it is working for her
- to notice anything that needs changing
- to continue to develop her skill in planning.

Example: Planning to create a reliable recall system – part 2

Comments on part 1:

time: just noticing how easy it is to let other things take up the time sharpened up the attention given to the recall system

over enthusiasm → giving up: make sure each part works before using the system on anything else

ideas that won't work: completely acceptable that some won't work; change to ideas that will work; this is all a useful part of developing dyslexia/ SpLD management.

other: do any other factors seem to affect recall? Some of the material needs to be remembered out of sequence. Triggers for recall need to be set up so that they can be used in a random order.

Proof of the pudding:

Recognising the problem with time meant the system was given a high priority; it got used and was not consigned to oblivion. The growing sense of satisfaction, achievement and joy helps to maintain the discipline to use the system.

---

8 Discussion of *KEY WORDS EXERCISE*

The following table summarises a typical discussion prompted by doing the *EXERCISE TO DO WITH YOUR STUDENT: KEY WORDS*. The left-hand column gives the number of key words in the text written out in the middle column. The right-hand column has the discussion points. The exercise can teach *METACOGNITION* as well as key words. A valuable reading tool is to understand and use the relationships between sentences, in particular how they give your student the information. The same tool can be used while writing and talking.

EXERCISE TO DO WITH YOUR STUDENT: KEY WORDS: p 176

METACOGNITION: p 63

No. of key words	Text from the *EXERCISE: KEY WORDS*	Discussion points
•2•	Key Words	
•8•	'We saw earlier that words that [1]had greater significance, [2]had greater meaning, [3]were more outstanding, and [4]generated stronger images were very much easier to remember.	[1, 2, 3, 4] This sentence contains a list of four characteristics, as indicated by the numbers. It is often important in reading to realise where an author has created a list of equivalent ideas. Discussion about the difference between 'greater significance' and 'greater meaning' is useful; as is the discussion about 'were more outstanding' and 'generated stronger images'. People need to consider how important the differences are and whether noting all four characteristics improves their use of key words. This sentence is generally recognised as being an opening to the topic; almost a definition of 'key words'.
•0•	'When we read, we automatically pick out these more memorable words from the text, and the rest of the material is generally forgotten within a second or two.	This sentence expands the idea of key words, but none of the words are seen as key to remembering or understanding.

(9)	'Thus, take the following sentence: "Astronomers are now suggesting that black holes may not, after all, be entirely black, but may in fact be capable of radiating energy."	This sentence is an example. Some people prefer to note and remember examples rather than principles. The discussion as to who needs which type of information is a useful one as it validates differences in THINKING PREFERENCES.
•0•	'The key ideas in this sentence, the words that are most memorable and contain the essence of the sentence, are *astronomers, black holes, not black, radiating energy.*	Explains the example. No words usually seen as key words.
•0•	'The rest of the words are merely grammatical constructions and emphasis; they are not necessary for recall.'	Explains the example further. Again no words seen as key words.
	The first paragraph gives information about key words and how they work in a context. The second paragraph tells the reader what kind of words to look for and what is particularly useful about concrete words. It is useful to discuss the difference types of information in the two paragraphs and that these differences warrant two separate paragraphs.	
•4•	'Key words tend to be the nouns and verbs in a sentence—though sometimes adjectives and adverbs may be significant enough to become key words.	Instructions: The sentence tells the reader what to look out for as key words. Often students tell me they don't know what nouns, verbs, adjectives and adverbs are; they feel this information is a little wasted on them.

•1•	'Key words are generally concrete rather than abstract.	Again tells the reader what to look for. Discussion about concrete versus abstract is useful; concrete is a quality readers want to look for, whereas abstract is not going to be very useful, so why would they treat the word as a key word? My students and I usually have a useful discussion about ignoring any material that they don't need.
•10•	'It has been found that concrete words generate images faster than abstract words—one and a half seconds faster on the average—and that the images they generate are richer and have more associations [(Gregg, 1975)].	Tells the reader why the concrete quality of key words is so important.
•0•	'For this reason they are better remembered.'	Restates the main theme of the passage. No new key words.
	The next paragraph contains evidence. We usually discuss the role of evidence. If a reader is learning about key words to gain the skill of using them, she only needs to use the information about the percentage of key words. She doesn't need any of the rest of the paragraph as key words, though it may be reassuring to read. If the reader is an education or psychology student, she might be writing an assignment about the use of key words; in this case key words from this section would be important. The change of colour indicates the change of purpose of the key words. It is instructive to pause and think that the purpose for which a student is reading material alters its importance for her.	

-13-	'In a study by Michael Howe [(1977)] at Exeter University students' notes were examined and the ratio of key words to non-key words measured.	Introduces the research carried out and tells the reader what was measured.
•8•	'It was found that the higher the percentage of key words present in the notes, the better was the recall.	Gives the results.
-0-	'Because of their greater meaningful content key words 'lock up' more information in memory and are 'keys' to recalling the ideas.	Repeats the purpose of key words.
-0-	'In the foregoing case you have only to recall the two keys *black holes* and *radiating energy* to unlock the memory of the main idea contained in the sentence.'	Recalls the example in the first paragraph.
	•25• key words to learn about them (9) key words in the example •8• key words in the evidence that are useful in learning about key words -13- key words only relevant to the evidence	The selection of key words is not always the same. The phrasing for the use of the sentences also varies. The visual impact of key words highlighted is probably more telling than a count of the key words. The use of different colours for the different purposes also makes greater impact. The exercise is probably better done as a discussion.

9 Summary: check-list of skills, processes, mind techniques, etc.

Summary: Check-list of skills, processes, mind techniques, etc.

Appendix 2 p 538
Individual, Personal Profile of Dyslexia/ SpLD
 	
    Thinking preferences
    Pausing (Thinking clearly)
    Pitfalls
    Accommodation
	Regime for Managing Dyslexia/ SpLD
	    Pitfalls
	    Pausing (Thinking clearly)
	    Thinking preferences
	    Goals

Thinking Preferences p 72
    Visual, verbal and kinaesthetic
    Rationale or framework
    Holistic vs. linear
    Motivation
    Myers-Briggs Personality Type
    Multiple Intelligences
	Techniques for Using the Mind p 156
	    Chunking
	    Mind set
	    Concentration
	    Recall and memorising exercises
	Useful Abilities of the Mind p 63
	    Metacognition
	    Objective observation
	    Reflection

Model of Learning stages p 145
    Input
    Immediate use
    Feedback loop
    Recall
    Direct use
    Developed use
    Long-term memory
    Understanding
	Appendix 1 processes p 524
	    Collecting information together
	    Prioritising
	    Generating useful questions
	    Surveying
	    Recording and scanning
	    Monitoring progress
	also
	    Materials and methods p 565

Foundations of Knowledge and Skills	Skilled Thinking p 167	
Comprehension p 162	Framework	Data
Key words p 176	Practical work	Questions
Main themes vs. details p 178	Analysis	Discussion
Know the goal of any task p 181	Quality	Evaluating
Planning p 200	Outcome	

References

Baddeley, Alan, 2007, *Working Memory, Thought, and Action,* Oxford University Press, Oxford

Crook, Tom, 2010, *U67923: Historical Writing,* Oxford Brookes University, Unpublished

Gregg, Vernon, 1975, *Human Memory,* Methuen, London

Henderson, Elizabeth, 2003, *How to Have a Dyslexia Friendly School,* Beacon Office, Oldfield School, Maidenhead

Howe, M. J. A. and Godfrey, J., 1977, *Student Note Taking as an Aid to Learning,* Exeter University Teaching Services, Exeter

OED[14], Brown, Lesley Ed in Chief, 1993, *The New Shorter Oxford English Dictionary on Historical Principles*, Clarendon Press, Oxford

Russell, Peter, 1979, *The Brain Book: Know Your Own Mind and How to Use It,* Routledge, London

Stacey, Ginny, 2019, *Finding Your Voice with Dyslexia and other SpLDs,* Routledge, London

Stacey, Ginny, 2020a, *Organisation and Everyday Life with Dyslexia and other SpLDs,* Routledge, London

Stacey, Ginny, 2020b, *Development of Dyslexia and other SpLDs,* Routledge, London

Website information

OED Online, September 2020, Oxford University Press Accessed 24 October 2020

Series website: www.routledge.com/cw/stacey

---

[14] The online OED has been consulted every time, and the meanings are consistent. Sometimes the words used in the hard copy of OED (1993) are clearer, or more to the point in the context of this book, in which case, the reference is to the hard-copy edition.

3 Guidance for Non-Linear Readers

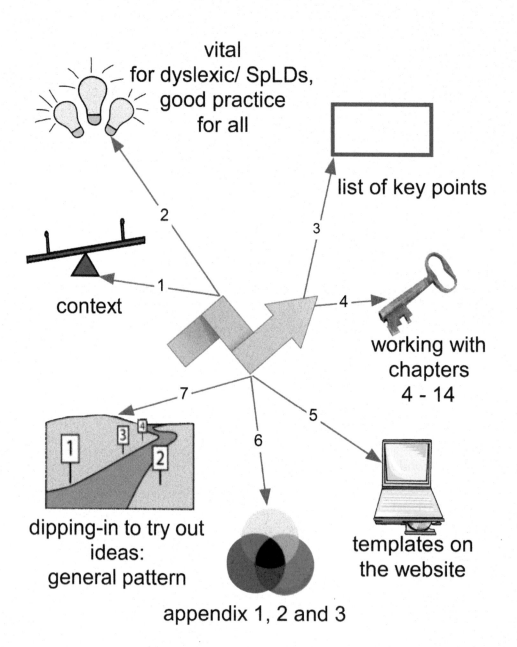

vital for dyslexic/ SpLDs, good practice for all

list of key points

context

working with chapters 4 - 14

dipping-in to try out ideas: general pattern

templates on the website

appendix 1, 2 and 3

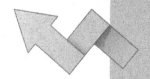

Contents

THINKING PREFERENCES, p 72, are highlighted in orange in chapters 4 – 14.

Examples of their use are listed in the *INDEX*: p 589

1 Context

I have put information at the beginning of every chapter in this series to help non-linear readers find the sections most useful to them. Chapters 4 – 14 are each about a specific topic you might be working on with your student, and the information for non-linear readers is the same except for the lists of sections to scan or read. It has been put into this chapter rather than repeat it in every chapter.

'He/ she' is used in this chapter because the pronoun used for your student could be either in chapters 4 – 14.

Some of the boxes and paragraphs are addressed to dyslexic/ SpLD people; it's the only way they make sense. They are marked with the green strip in the left hand margin. The meaning of the green strip is also in the *GLOSSARY*.

Ⓖ p 572

The green line in the left-hand margin indicates those paragraphs that predominantly contain ideas to be discussed with or taught to your student. The meaning of the green line is also in the *GLOSSARY*.

Ⓖ p 572

2 Vital for dyslexic/ SpLDs, good practice for all

Vital for dyslexic/ SpLDs, good practice for all

The techniques and skills discussed in these chapters are ones that are VITAL for most dyslexic/ SpLD people to learn deliberately and not picked up alongside other learning. They are also good practice for anyone.

With any student who has no specific condition that is causing difficulty you can use the ideas and techniques and probably ignore all reference to anything that is causing a hindrance.

With a student who has a different condition that is causing difficulties you should use the symptoms of his/ her own condition instead of the dyslexia/SpLDs insights and find which of the general ideas and techniques will help him/ her.

3 List of key points

K = key points

4 Working with chapters 4 – 14

4.1 Working with chapters 4 – 14: tutoring a student

These chapters are about finding solutions that allow your student to solve his/ her difficulties. You both will need to explore the difficulties to make sure the solution is addressing the heart of the problem, see *Some Unobvious Problems*. Solutions need to be monitored; they can be developed as necessary to apply to new situations.

Some Unobvious Problems: p 64

As your student engages with the exploration, monitoring and developing, he/ she will gain control over his/ her dyslexia/ SpLD and so become an autonomous person, see *Appendix 2*, below. Even knowing when to ask for accommodation is part of having control. It

Ⓖ p 575 autonomous

Appendix 2: p 226

is important for your student to realise most people have problems of some kind; his/ hers just happen to have a label.

For each chapter, select from the *Check-list of Skills, Processes and Mind Techniques etc.* those that are appropriate for your student. Use the *Check-lists for Exploring Behind the Obvious* to find the best tools and insights to use. Check that your student is gaining skills and knowledge as he/ she works. He/ she can:

- make a list of them
- observe his/ her use of them and record it
- develop his/ her own list for future use.

Check-list of Skills, Processes and Mind Techniques etc.: p 220

Check-lists for Exploring Behind the Obvious: p 67

4.2 Working with chapters 4 – 14: general understanding

These chapters work through the tasks that dyslexic/ SpLD people need to approach in their own way. As a general reader, the chapters will give you deeper insights into the complexities of managing dyslexia/ SpLD. They will show you ways you can help to avoid the difficulties in communication.

4.3 Working with chapters 4 – 14: policies and public discussion

As policy-makers, these chapters will help you to understand how dyslexia/ SpLD people can be enabled to fulfil their potential with minimum disruption from their dyslexia/ SpLD.

These chapters will help campaigners and media personnel to understand the issues that affect the lives of dyslexic/ SpLD people. Public dialogue based on a wider appreciation should bring faster progress to diminishing the problems.

5 Templates on the website

Templates that are generally useful:

A1   *Jotting Down as You Scan*

A2   *Bookmark – Purpose*

A4   *Jotting Down as You Read*

A5   *Collecting Ideas That Interest You*

B1   *Collecting Ideas That Relate to You* (specially for readers who are themselves dyslexic/ SpLD)

B7   *Recording Template - 3*

Templates

TEMPLATES are also recommended in some of chapters 4 – 14. All the TEMPLATES suggested are listed by chapter in the LIST OF TEMPLATES.

LIST OF TEMPLATES: p 582

CHECK-LISTS FOR READERS describes a set of check-lists available on the website to help different reader groups engage with the ideas in the book. It also lists the most relevant sections of the book.

CHECK-LISTS FOR READERS: p 21

6 Appendices

6.1 Appendix 1 Resources

APPENDIX 1: p 524

This appendix will help you and your student collect information about the way he/ she does anything and how his/ her dyslexia/ SpLD affects him/ her. It collects together some of the general skills he/ she will need in order to make progress.

> If you are dyslexic/ SpLD, this appendix will help you gather the information you want from this book.

6.2 Appendix 2 Individual, Personal Profile of Dyslexia/ SpLD and Regime for Managing Dyslexia/ SpLD

APPENDIX 2: p 538

The heart of this book is teaching your student skills that will enable him/ her to become as autonomous as possible. He/ she will be able to study more effectively, and will be able to make his/ her best contribution to everyday life and employment.

G p 575 autonomous

It is important to benefit from tasks, including trying new ideas, that don't work. The ways and reasons they don't work can tell you both a lot about the workings of your student's mind.

As he/ she learns these skills you will be able to COLLECT INFORMATION TOGETHER and MONITOR his/ her PROGRESS. The insights you both gain can be build into a PROFILE OF DYSLEXIA/ SPLD and a REGIME FOR MANAGING DYSLEXIA/ SPLD. The desired autonomy comes when your student has ownership of his/ her PROFILE and REGIME, and uses them on a daily basis.

COLLECTING INFORMATION TOGETHER: p 526

MONITORING PROGRESS: p 535

The *PROFILE* is not a fixed set of characteristics about your student. He/ she needs to know how to keep exploring and developing other ways to do and think. He/ she can build the new insights into his/ her *PROFILE* and *REGIME*.

Key points: Your student's *INDIVIDUAL, PERSONAL PROFILE OF DYSLEXIA/ SPLD* and *REGIME FOR MANAGING DYSLEXIA/ SPLD*

Working with this book provides opportunities for your student to discover where his/ her strengths lie and how to use them.

As your student understands his/ her dyslexia/ SpLD better and the way it varies, help him/ her to be confident about him/ herself.

Help him/ her to build the insights that emerge into his/ her *PROFILE* and *REGIME*; these will allow him/ her to become more autonomous.

6.3 Appendix 3 Key Concepts

APPENDIX 3: p 554

This appendix has a summary of the key ideas I cover when doing an audit of skills and knowledge with a dyslexic/ SpLD student.
They fall into the categories of:

> *THINKING CLEARLY*
>
> *USING THE MIND WELL*
>
> *THINKING PREFERENCES*
>
> *USEFUL APPROACHES*
>
> *ASPECTS OF DYSLEXIA/ SPLD.*

The appendix shows which of the 4 books in the series covers each idea in full.

7 Dipping-in to try out ideas: general pattern

The ideas here give a pattern that is essentially good practice for finding the material you are most interested in when reading any non-fiction. You should teach the pattern to your student, including how to modify it to suit other material and topics, see *Adapting Dipping-in to Try Out Ideas: General Pattern*.

Adapting Dipping-in to Try Out Ideas: General Pattern: p 400

Step 1: are you interested in:

    a   teaching

    b   dialogue

    c   indirect communication

    d   general understanding

    e   policy implications?

Key point: Avoid generating more difficulties

Read *Major Precaution*, if you are interested in helping a dyslexic/ SpLD person to gain knowledge and skills, whether by teaching or by sharing strategies.

Major Precaution: p 10

Step 2: It may help to brainstorm about one or two students, or people you know. Use: *B7 - Recording Template - 3* with headings:

Templates

A = date

B = situation

C = what happened

D = comment. Your comments can be anything that helps to clarify what you want to find out more about

E = key issue for each entry.

If you work well with mind maps, you could build a mind map instead of using the template or you could summarise your entries from *B7 - Recording Template - 3* onto a mind map.

Can you formulate some questions to which you would like to find answers?

Step 3: decide how the key issues in column E relate to chapters 4 – 14. Use the book mind map, the contents list or the mind maps and contents of each chapter. Use *TEMPLATE: A1 - JOTTING DOWN AS YOU SCAN* to record the page numbers of any material of interest.

Step 4: prioritise: decide which issues are most important, which have middling importance and which are least important. Include the time factor: something that is not a really important issue may be relevant to the present time and therefore have a higher priority.

Step 5: decide what you want to start with. It might be better to start with something that is of middling priority than to start with the highest priority.

Step 6: for each issue:
Go to the relevant chapter. The dipping-in to try out ideas section of each chapter has a list of the sections to read and a list of the sections to scan.
Read the sections listed for reading.
Scan those listed for scanning.
As you read and scan, jot down anything you want to come back to, with where it is in the chapter.
Read those parts that are relevant to your students, or to your current interest.
Go back to your brainstorming: what answers can you find to the questions you had?
What further questions do you have?
How do you want to use what you have found?

Website information

Series website: www.routledge.com/cw/stacey

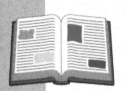

4 Reading

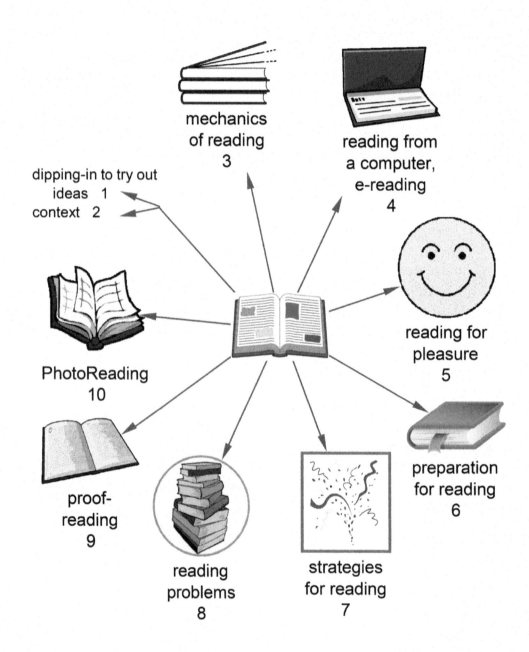

mechanics
of reading
3

reading from
a computer,
e-reading
4

dipping-in to try out
ideas   1
context   2

PhotoReading
10

reading for
pleasure
5

proof-
reading
9

reading
problems
8

strategies
for reading
7

preparation
for reading
6

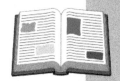

Contents

Thinking Preferences, p 72, are highlighted in orange in this chapter.
Examples of their use are listed in the *Index*: p 589

List of key points and summaries

K = key points
S = summaries

Templates on the website

TEMPLATES

Information for non-linear readers

Before the context of the *USEFUL PREFACE* and *CHAPTERS 1* and *2*, there is information that I hope will help non-linear readers as they approach the chapters. For chapters 4 – 14, this information would be identical except for which parts to scan and read. I have put all the information together into *GUIDANCE FOR NON-LINEAR READERS, CHAPTER 3*. It is worth reading *CHAPTER 3* at some stage of working with this book.

GUIDANCE FOR NON-LINEAR READERS: p 222

1 Dipping-in to try out ideas: reading and scanning lists

Start with *DIPPING-IN TO TRY OUT IDEAS: GENERAL PATTERN*.

DIPPING-IN TO TRY OUT IDEAS: GENERAL PATTERN: p 228

Read:

    MECHANISMS OF READING (VISUAL STRATEGIES): p 234

    PREPARATION FOR READING: p 243

Scan:

    STRATEGIES FOR READING: p 246

    READING PROBLEMS: p 252

    READING FROM A COMPUTER, E-READING: p 240

    KEY POINTS AND SUMMARY BOXES: the list is on p 231

1.1 Key points: for policy-makers and general readers

Key points: For policy-makers and general readers

- For dyslexic/ SpLDs, reading is a vulnerable skill that can easily be disrupted.

- Accommodation that helps dyslexic/ SpLDs to read more easily:
  - o need not be expensive
  - o will be good practice for many others
  - o will be cost-effective.

- Read *READING PROBLEMS* and *STRATEGIES FOR READING*.

- If you are in charge of producing reading material:
  - o check whether the material supports the reading strategies of dyslexic/ SpLD people
  - o consult several dyslexic/ SpLD readers for their comments.

READING PROBLEMS:
p 252

STRATEGIES FOR READING:
p 246

2 Context

Your student is reading to understand. As you help him, use other relevant ideas in this book from:

This chapter covers other information and insights about reading, including the MECHANICS OF READING. I have found these insights can make significant improvements. Again, what works for one student doesn't work for another, so your student needs to experiment with the ideas and use those that help him.

MECHANICS OF READING (VISUAL STRATEGIES): this page

3 Mechanics of reading (visual strategies)

**Insight: An instinct to change:
To begin reading AT The Beginning**

Many dyslexic/ SpLDs are strongly programmed to start at the beginning of a book or article, to read every word in a linear fashion until they get to the end. They move their eyes smoothly over the words. Often they have difficulty finding the next line. They find they don't make much sense of what they have read.

Understanding and working with the mechanics of reading has helped many dyslexic/ SpLDs to change this programming so that reading works better.

- They don't start at the beginning.
- They start by searching for what they want to know.
- They feel free to move around the text.

3.1 Eye movement

There are two sets of neural pathways that take signals from the eyes: 1) operates when there is movement of the eyes and 2) the other when the eyes are stationary, i.e. zero movement.

When the eyes are moving, the mind is using one set of neural pathways and looking for the gross position of a potential enemy or food (going back to the time of our ancestors); it is not processing colour or fine detail; it is using the signals from the peripheral area of the retina. By contrast when the eyes are still, the mind is using the other set of neural pathways; it is looking for fine detail, relative positions and it processes colour; it uses the centre of the retina, an area called the forvea. The mind switches between the two sets of neural pathways depending on the movement or not of the eyes; there's a toggle switch: either one or the other is operating, not both together (Russell, 1979; Buzan, 2010).

Russell (1979)
Buzan (2010)

It is possible to show the difference between peripheral vision and central vision by making two transparencies of the same text and rotating them in relation to each other, as in *FIGURE 4.1*. The clear writing at the centre represents the fine detail seen by the stationary eyes. The blurred text represents the peripheral vision, which is mostly used by the moving eyes. The point being looked at by the stationary eyes is known as the fixation point.

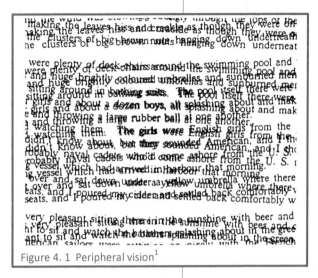
Figure 4. 1 Peripheral vision[1]

For reading, your student needs to be able to process the fine detail; he needs to see 'rubber', as at the centre of *FIGURE 4.1*; any random order of the letters will not be helpful for reading!

The eyes should move in saccades[2] during reading. That is they stop momentarily to take in the information and then move on to the next fixation point. It is thought that peripheral vision is used to guide the distance between fixation points. The mind stores the information during saccades in order to integrate it all together. Thus, *FIGURE 4.1* represents one fixation point with the centre clear and the peripheral not so clear. Central vision gives 'a large rubber ball'; peripheral vision is hinting at 'another', 'English' and 'American' which help to make the jump to the next fixation point. The integration over several fixations is what we expect to happen in the process of reading.

Skilled readers don't pay attention to the movement of their eyes. Their eyes don't fixate on every word; their eyes probably fixate 2 or 3 times across a line of text, depending on the length; they will go back and check a word, if there is something they don't understand.

---

[1] The text in *FIGURE 4.1* is from *Man from the South* (Dahl, 1979)
[2] Saccades, from the French for jerks, so named by Professor Javel in 1879, the first person to realise the eyes moved this way. (Russell, 1979)

Over many years, interest in eye movement during reading led to my interest in eye-span and the use of exercises to explore this part of the mechanisms of reading.

Using some eye exercises from *Harrap's Swift Readers, Book 5* (Elder and Wood, 1975), I found many dyslexic/ SpLD students' eyes don't fixate but keep moving smoothly; the students only take in a few letters at a time. They really struggle to understand what they are reading.

Elder and Wood (1975)

The two exercises on *TEMPLATE : G6 - EYE-SPAN EXERCISES 1 AND 2* are adapted from those by Elder and Wood.

TEMPLATES

For the first, the eyes are trained to move down the page focusing on the cross, while attention is paid to seeing group of letterset increasingly further apart, as shown in *FIGURE 4.2*. For the second, the eyes are still moving straight down the line, while sentences of different widths are read, see *FIGURE 4.3*.

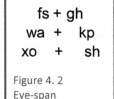

Figure 4. 2
Eye-span
exercise 1

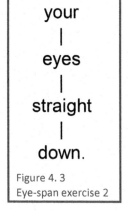

Figure 4. 3
Eye-span exercise 2

I've given these exercises to many dyslexic/ SpLD students and most struggle to keep their eyes from moving from side to side as they read. I suggest that they practise for a while. Enough students have reported improvement in their reading to make these exercises worth considering; others don't find any benefit.

Give your student the *EYE-SPAN* exercises from the website and let him see how his eyes move while reading. If he has difficulty in keeping his eyes from moving from side to side, suggest that he does the exercises regularly until his eyes track downwards more easily. He needs to check for any responses that override the purpose of the exercise: for example, some people get so engrossed in the movement of their eyes, they fail to look at the letters or the words. When the eye-span has increased, more of the text is processed together and reading improves.

TEMPLATES

3.2 Meaning-related groups of words

The *TEMPLATE: G7 - EYE-SPAN EXERCISE 3* uses meaning-related groups of words. The extra spacing highlights relationships. As your student's eye-span increases he will get used to looking for groups of words. If you teach him the building blocks of language, he will learn to work with meaning to decide which words to process together; see *TEACHING LANGUAGE* and *TEMPLATE: G8 - THE STORY PAPER SPLIT TO SHOW WORD GROUPS.*

TEMPLATES

TEACHING LANGUAGE: p 94

3.3 De-coding

While reading, dyslexic/ SpLD people can be decoding letter by letter, syllable by syllable (and missing a few as they go), word at a time, or phrase at a time. When the initial capture of letters and words is too slow, the links between the parts will not allow chunking to expand the *CAPACITY OF WORKING MEMORY*. An analogy I've used is that of going to an art gallery and looking at one of Rembrandt's large pictures. If your student stands close to the picture he can see the fine detail of the brush strokes and colour, but he won't appreciate the picture as a whole; to do that he needs to stand at the other side of the room. In slow decoding he can't grasp enough to be able to understand what he is reading; he needs to read faster to take in more at a time.

Ⓖ p 575 chunking

CAPACITY OF WORKING MEMORY: p 157

To stop slow de-coding, I suggest that people force themselves to read slightly faster than is comfortable. Your student can do this by moving a piece of paper, or a ruler, down the page or by spreading his fingers out so that they form a line across the page and then he can move his hand down the page to increase the speed of his reading. Gradually, as his reading improves, he will find he uses different speeds depending on how well he knows the information or on how complex it is.

3.4 Colour

Colour makes a difference to the reading skills of many dyslexic/ SpLD people.

Those who find that reading makes their eyes tired or who experience visual disturbances when they read, such as text moving around or striped effects on the page, are those who are most likely to be helped by colour. It is important to ensure that eyesight has been tested because the person might just require glasses. The optimum colour can vary from person to person.

We all tend to think that what happens for us is what happens for everyone. Dyslexic/ SpLD people are no exception in this respect: they may be unaware that others don't experience the same visual effect during reading. It is worth everyone experimenting with coloured filters and backgrounds to see if the colour helps.

There are two approaches to determining the most appropriate colour. One approach involves an individual's response to yellow and blue filters being investigated and glasses of the appropriate colour being given to those whose reading improves (Stein, 2014). Many people have been helped by these glasses. The other approach investigates an individual's response to a wide range of colours (Singleton, 2008). When a colour is found to help, the person can either have glasses of that colour or can opt to use coloured sheets covering the text. I've known people really delighted with their coloured glasses: "At last the world stays still!" Your student can buy coloured reading rulers (Crossbow Education) which can then be used, as described above, to increase the speed of processing. I have known many people to be helped by the use of coloured filters.

Stein (2014)

Singleton (2008)

Crossbow Education
Accessed 1 Sep 2020

There can be a stigma attached to dyslexia/ SpLD and I've known people refuse to use a colour just to avoid comment from others. Personally, I use coloured filters when reading is not working and nothing else seems to help; it just gets me over the moment of difficulty and I usually don't use one for very long.

Those who find colour helps their reading will often print onto coloured paper. Many find reading on computer screens can be helped by changing the colour scheme, the colour of the major working area of each window and the colour of the font.

There are frequently questions about the best colour to use when producing paperwork for many different readers. The general advice is to use pastel colours and to avoid harsh contrast. Black on white is about the worst combination.

3.5 Font[3]

Many dyslexic/ SpLD people find that not all fonts are equally easy to read. To a certain extent it is a question of what your student is used to and familiar with.

Fonts with serifs[4] are usually not recommended. Full justification[5] increases difficulties for some, as the words change shape or the spacing between words alters, so left justification is recommended. The difficulty with the spaces between words changing is that some people's minds focus on the spaces and not the words and 'rivers of white' stand out better than the words. Some people find italics difficult. Fonts which don't have much space between the words are difficult for some people.

The size of the text is also an important issue. Too small and the reader may struggle to see the words clearly; too large and the dyslexic/ SpLD reader can feel as if he is being treated as a child. Your student needs to find the size that works best for him.

Find the font that your student finds easiest. If he has his own computer, he can alter the settings to his best font.

Many of my students have felt they mustn't 'give in' to the problems; they will struggle with an unsuitable font, colour, etc. rather than make life easier. I suspect this is the wrong way round the problems. Rather than continuing to struggle, if your student eases the difficulty (in this case, reading a font he doesn't like) his mind can build up comprehension skills. Then, when the comprehension skills are firm, they will help him de-code the less easy fonts and help him with other reading problems. From my own experience, I find that I can read text so much more easily in general now; when I'm struggling, I find taking my own advice improves my reading.

---

[3] Font: A complete set or assortment of type of a particular face and size; ('font, n.2' OED Online, 2017)
[4] A serif is a small line attached to the end of a stroke in a letter or symbol. Fonts without serifs are called 'sans serif'.
[5] Justification refers to the alignment of text either against the left or the right margin or both margins of the page, which is called 'full justification'.

Summary: Mechanics of reading

- Choose best place to start reading, not necessarily the beginning
- Eye movements
- Meaning-related groups of words
- De-coding
- Colour
- Font, typeface, size, characteristics such as bold, italic, etc.

4 Reading from a computer, e-reading

Many alterations or strategies are available when reading from a computer or other electronic device.

Colour and font

Your student can change the general settings of his computer so that he is working with the *Colour* and *Font* that suit him. He can change the page size, which will increase the size of words without altering the relative position of anything.

Colour: p 237
Font: p 239

Web browsing

He can alter the settings on his web browser to suit his own requirements; there are packages that allow him to change the look of web pages.

Screen ruler

Using a screen ruler could help him to keep his place when reading on a computer; it can also be used to make sure he keeps his speed faster so that he avoids slow *De-coding*.

De-coding: p 237

Scrolling

Scrolling can interrupt comprehension if your student has to switch from reading to working out how far down to scroll. Your student could experiment with the highlighting tool to see if that will help him. Two suggestions are:

- read the text that is visible; highlight a word in the last line; scroll until that word is at the top of the screen; and then continue reading

- switch the highlighter tool on; select text as he reads; when he gets to the end of the screen allow the text to be coloured; then scroll until only one line of coloured text is visible at the top of the screen. He can select word by word or line by line; either way might help him to keep his place.

Text-to-speech

Many people find a text-to-speech program really helps them to understand when they are reading electronic material. It is very important to make sure the package allows your student to choose a voice that he can understand easily. Seeing the text while it is read can be extremely helpful. For some, the best programs are those which highlight the text as it is read.

Comfort

Your student needs to avoid physical discomfort while reading from, or working on, a computer, including visual discomfort. Stress at any level (physical, mental, psychological) is going to make the processes of reading and understanding much more difficult.

Summary: E-reading

- Default screen colour
- Default font: style, colour, justification
- Thesaurus or dictionary to look up unfamiliar words
- Customise web browsing
- Scrolling strategy
- Assistive technology:
  - screen ruler
  - text-to-speech
  - choice of voice
- Comfort

5 Reading for pleasure

Reading for pleasure can be quite different from reading for study or work. Your student will have his own interest to follow; his imagination might be sparked by the story or material; he is likely to be curious about the book. It also doesn't usually matter whether he remembers what he has read or not.

Story: Reading for pleasure vs. study reading

One student was describing her reading over a vacation. There was a difference in her tone of voice when discussing the 'academic' reading and that done for 'pleasure'. She told me the titles of the books and they all came from the same reading list given by a tutor.

The 'academic' books were needed for an essay; understanding the material would make a difference to the work load; the tutor would be expected to see the fruits of the work.

The books read for 'pleasure' she chose to satisfy her interest; there was no immediate purpose in reading them; they weren't going to be useful during the term.

However, she was quite happy to do the extra reading because she'd had the experience in previous exams that material read for pleasure was remembered better than that read for an essay; consequently the answers to questions on the pleasure reading were better than those on material read for an essay.

It is worth finding out how your student's mind responds and helping him to change his perspective, if necessary, to give him most satisfaction from his reading.

With several students, a difficulty has arisen because interest in the subject has evaporated during the course. The lack of interest, and of pleasure, creates an extra difficulty in reading; we usually work quite hard to find some way for the student to re-gain positive motivations, either through thinking preferences to re-engage with the course, or by changing the motivation from learning the subject to the deliberate development of skills.

6 Preparation for reading

Key points: Preparation for reading

- Mind set
  - o   Survey
  - o   Know the goal
- Thinking clearly
- Avoiding distractions

Reading is hard for most dyslexic/ SpLDs, so your student might as well do everything he can to make it easier, including wearing his coloured glasses, even if they provoke a lot of comments! I told one student he was a 'Wally' for not using the coloured glasses because he didn't like the comments; he was quite clear that they improved his reading.

The *ENVIRONMENT* in which your student reads may be important. Some need a quiet place; some find noise a way of keeping themselves focused. Many need to be able to spread out as they read; they need to see everything on the top surface; it is no good building up piles of books or papers as anything below the top becomes lost to the mind for these individuals. If your student is 1) working from a book, 2) making notes on a laptop, and 3) using other sources of information, he may need to see everything at the same time.

ENVIRONMENT: p 70

6.1 Mind set before reading

MIND SET is the process of switching the mind on to a topic before reading about it. There are two aspects worth reinforcing here with respect to reading: *SURVEYING* and to *KNOW THE GOAL OF ANY TASK.*

MIND SET: p 158

SURVEYING the book or article is a combination of searching for *KEY WORDS* and sorting out *MAIN THEMES VS. DETAILS.* Your student is aiming to build a schema for the topic which will help his subsequent reading to make sense. The back cover often gives a summary of the content. The contents page can also be useful.

SURVEYING: p 533
KEY WORDS: p 176
MAIN THEMES VS. DETAILS: p 178

- Your student can look at:
    - the structure of the book
    - the way the book is laid out
    - any visual devices that are used
    - boxes for key ideas
    - the use of colour, bold or other font changes to show important words
    - photos and diagrams.
- He can move his pencil or fingers over diagrams so that he notices the full curve of a graph, for example.
- He can inspect tables and headings.
- He can analyse the abstract or preface in the same way as used in *EXAMPLE: FINDING THE IMPORTANT IDEAS IN A PARAGRAPH.*

EXAMPLE: FINDING THE IMPORTANT IDEAS IN A PARAGRAPH: p 180

- He can notice and look up *Unfamiliar Words* before he starts reading the book.

Unfamiliar Words: p 246

Time spent this way will yield results.

Knowing his purpose before he starts reading will also help, see *Know the Goal of Any Task*. Don't let him be vague and think "I need to know this stuff." What does he need to know? Why? ... He must be as clear as possible about the topic he is engaged with and the level of detail he wants. Deliberately thinking about the goal will also switch on the neural networks already engaged with the topic.

Know the Goal of Any Task: p 181

Some people find it is useful to survey the material the night before, then, after a night's sleep, do a brief brainstorm before settling down to read.

Ⓖ p 575: brainstorm

He could make a list of those strategies that he finds helpful on the template *A3 - Bookmark – Profile and Techniques* and then use the bookmark to remind himself to use them.

Templates

Selecting from course book lists or processing documents for a meeting, for example, can be simplified using mind set, surveying and knowing the goal. Your student can identify the most important topics and know where to find the information.

6.2 Thinking clearly

Take your student through the 2 suggestions in *Thinking Clearly*, and see which one helps him to engage with his reading and stay alert. Discuss the issues in *Reading Problems* to uncover any that may hamper his reading.

Thinking Clearly: p 79
Reading Problems: p 252

6.3 Distractions

Distractions from the environment are outlined in *Environment*. Your student may also experience distractions from his own mind. *Objective Observation* should help your student to recognise the root of them; he can use the *Recording Templates, B5-8,* on the website to capture his observations and to make sense of them. If underlying thoughts are trying to attract his attention, they may well interfere with his reading until he pays attention to them. Having a note-pad for them and knowing how and when he will deal with them should mean that he can put them on hold while he reads.

Environment: p 70

Objective Observation: p 63

Templates

6.4 Unfamiliar words

Fluency in reading can be disrupted if there are unfamiliar words. Your student might stop and look up those words; this approach will break his focus on the topic. He may hope the meaning will become clear; this approach leaves an undermining thought, "You don't really know what's meant." Either way his understanding of the topic will be affected.

It can be much better to scan the text for unfamiliar words; look them up; create a list that can be used quickly as the words are read in the context of the material he is reading.

7 Strategies for reading

General

Using the CHECK-LIST OF SKILLS, PROCESSES, MIND TECHNIQUES, ETC., your student can make his own check-list of those strategies and ideas that particularly help him. He can make the list into a bookmark.

CHECK-LIST OF SKILLS, PROCESSES, MIND TECHNIQUES, ETC.: p 220

It may help him to work through a set of questions as he starts to read.

Key points: List of questions to guide reading:

- Why am I reading this?
- How much time do I have?
- What is this about?
- What are the themes?
- What are the aims?
- What's the structure of the material?
- What layout devices are used to help understanding?
- Is there any small print? Have I scanned it for key issues?

- Have I looked at:
  - back cover
  - front cover
  - contents
  - index
  - abstract (for an academic paper)
  - beginning and end of chapters?
- Have I looked up unfamiliar words?

Story: Systematic reading

One student used an early draft of these books while on a break from university. He used the *TEMPLATE: A4 - JOTTING DOWN AS YOU READ* with a set of general guiding questions at the top. When asked if the template helped, he said that it had because he'd never been that systematic with his reading before.

TEMPLATES

COMPANION @ WEBSITE

In reading this part of the draft:

- he was motivated because he had a large number of books to read for a piece of work
- he used the following ideas from the draft
  - there are strategies for reading and retaining information
  - focusing on the main themes keeps comprehension high
  - using note-taking skills while reading helps retention
  - reorganising words into points helps memory.

In reading his text books:

- he skimmed over the text looking for useful ideas
- he took notes
- he used the abstracts
- he used the beginning and end sections of chapters.

He finished his reading in 2 days, a much shorter time than usual; his reading was efficient and effective.

7.1 Pay attention to small print

In surveying and looking for main ideas, it is important to remember that the small print holds information that could be very important:

- deadlines for action
- clauses that significantly affect the context of the main document
- costs that might be incurred
- etc.

You need to process the small print as well as the larger text. Using surveying techniques is likely to be more satisfactory than trying to understand the detail of every point.

7.2 List of strategies involving *THINKING PREFERENCES*

The visual strategies are listed here so that the list is complete; the discussion about them is in *MECHANICS OF READING*.

MECHANICS OF READING
(VISUAL STRATEGIES):
p 234

Summary: Strategies involving *THINKING PREFERENCES*

THINKING PREFERENCES:
p 72

Visual

DE-CODING: p 237

- Move your eyes fast enough to avoid inefficient, slow *DE-CODING*.

COLOUR: p 237

- Use a *COLOUR* filter, as suits you.

MEANING RELATED
GROUPS OF WORDS:
p 237

- Look for *MEANING-RELATED GROUPS OF WORDS*.

Verbal

VERBAL STRATEGIES:
p 249

- Read aloud into a recording device.
- Scan the text into a computer and use text-to-speech software.

Searching for meaning (Rationale or Framework)

SEARCHING FOR
MEANING: p 249

- Look for the main idea in a paragraph, and the second
- Read the first and last sentences in a paragraph
- Read the introduction and the conclusion first.

Kinaesthetic

- Re-organise the words in the author's sentence(s)
- Taking notes: helps comprehension, stops important ideas being lost
- Use Post-it notes
- Have a template to gather ideas from different sources.

KINAESTHETIC STRATEGIES: p 251

Work through these different strategies with your student so that he knows about them all and can select those that help him.
DIFFERENT WAYS TO READ in the USEFUL PREFACE sets out different practices that have been used in the book to support the needs of different readers. Discuss the section with your student and ask him to do the EXERCISE: READING STYLE.

DIFFERENT WAYS TO READ: p 12

EXERCISE: READING STYLE: p 13

7.3 Verbal strategies

1   Read aloud into a recording device
2   Scan text into a computer and use text-to-speech software

Many people process what they hear better than what they read; some of these find they can record themselves reading out loud; they use the punctuation to help them read, see STORY: USING PUNCTUATION TO READ.

STORY: USING PUNCTUATION TO READ: p 256

Your student might be able to scan text into a computer and then use text-to-speech software, see READING FROM A COMPUTER, E-READING.

READING FROM A COMPUTER, E-READING: p 240

7.4 Searching for meaning

1   Look for the main idea in a paragraph, and the second
2   Read the first and last sentences in a paragraph
3   Read the introduction and the conclusion first

The third suggestion can be applied to a chapter or to a whole book. In the case of a whole book, the suggestion includes reading any introductory and concluding chapters.

These are all strategies for actively working with the text and searching it for the ideas. Having a pattern for working with text helps those who need a framework.

Using the third suggestion often allows your student to realise what the book is all about, to find the rationale of the book.

Exercise for students: Main and second idea in a paragraph

Read *G9 - THE SHORT STORY: PAPER* on the template section of the website.

It has 4 paragraphs:
1) the first group of sentences
2) the next pair of sentences
3) and 4)   the last two are obvious paragraphs.

What is the main theme of each paragraph?
What is the second theme?

TEMPLATES

This exercise is adapted from Buzan (2010).

Buzan (2010)

You could use any short story where the main theme is not obvious and needs to be thought about. It is good to work with a group, because the discussion shows how different people are reacting to the text. It is useful for students to realise that different people react in different ways.

A paragraph, especially one giving information with discussion, should have a shape as shown in Figure 4.4. Surveying the first and last sentences of paragraphs can give your student a good understanding of the text.

The introduction and conclusion of a chapter often give summaries of the chapter. Sometimes one is better than the other; your student has to keep questioning as he searches for information.

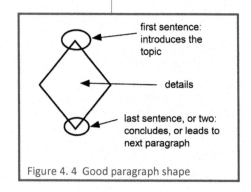

Figure 4. 4 Good paragraph shape

7.5 Kinaesthetic strategies

1   Re-organise the words in the author's sentence(s)
2   Making notes: helps comprehension, stops important ideas being lost
3   Use Post-it notes
4   Have a template to gather ideas from different sources.

These four strategies involve doing, which probably brings in the kinaesthetic sense.

KINAESTHETIC: p 74

Ⓖ p 575
kinaesthetic

In re-organising an author's sentence(s), your student is re-constructing the language. He might:

- change passive sentences into active ones
- change negatives into positive statements
- make long sentences into several shorter ones, or into bullet points
- make the lists in a sentence more obvious
- find and use other possibilities that work for him.

As he makes the changes, he will be thinking actively about the sentence and that will help him make sense of it.

TAKING AND MAKING NOTES as he reads can help your student to be doing something relating to reading. If he needs to make marks on the text, he should either get his own copy or work on a photocopy.

TAKING AND MAKING NOTES: p 300

Using Post-it notes is either
1   a way of marking where important points are
2   a way of making notes in the book while reading.

People can go back over the Post-it notes and decide which ones contain the most important ideas and then transfer the selected notes into their computer or into their paper-based notes system.

Scanning material into a computer or getting it from a website allows your student to adapt it into useful notes for himself. Ordinary text can be copied and pasted into a word processed document; text in a pdf document can sometimes be copied. Maths or material with a lot of symbols is usually put on a website as a pdf file, since not everyone will have the software to reproduce the content correctly; this material can be captured as screen shots and pasted as a box in your student's notes file. He can then use highlighting or other means to make the material into notes that work for him. These procedures can help a student with his reading because he is actively engaged with the material through the way he is making the notes.

Having a template to collect information is particularly useful when your student is comparing several different sources, as the householder would have done in the *EXAMPLE: THINKING PROCESSES FOR A HOUSEHOLD DECISION*. He is then able to search for the same type of information in all his sources and he can see where he has got information and where there are gaps; he is well placed to make the comparison required at the end of his reading.

EXAMPLE: THINKING PROCESSES FOR A HOUSEHOLD DECISION: p 168

8 Reading problems

Many dyslexic/ SpLDs say they struggle to stay awake when reading. They can be doing all the right things:

- using strategies they know work

- be in a comfortable environment

- be really keen to get the information

- be sleeping and eating well.

Yet with some books, reading is the quickest way to sleep.

Key point: Fighting against sleep while reading

I have learnt to recognise that fighting against sleep while trying to read means that I am not processing properly the material that I am reading; I have to look for something that is not being solved by the above list of approaches:

- the author's style may be wrong for me

- the grammar may be ambiguous

- negatives can be used in a complicated way

- there may be unfamiliar words, or unfamiliar use of words

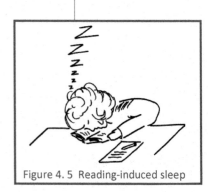

Figure 4. 5 Reading-induced sleep

- I may have questions about the background
- my mind can be engaged on another topic
- other.

I find the problem has to be identified and the underlying problem addressed. Otherwise a lurking sense that all is not quite right undermines my reading ability and nothing else I do will get it working again.

8.1 Author's style

The author may be putting a point of view that your student doesn't agree with:

He needs to recognise the disagreement.

He probably needs to mentally note which ideas he disagrees with, and which he can accept.

The active processing allows him to continue reading.

The author may have a hidden agenda: the words may have an obvious meaning, but the underlying message is quite different, see *STORY: AN UNDERLYING MESSAGE MISSED*.

STORY: AN UNDERLYING MESSAGE MISSED: p 266

The author may have a different paragraph shape. *FIGURE 4.6* is equivalent to leaving out the way one paragraph links to another; *FIGURE 4.7* is equivalent to the main idea being placed somewhere inside the paragraph. With either style, recognising how the ideas are presented allows your student to adapt it to the logic that makes sense to him.

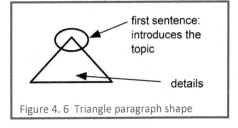

Figure 4. 6 Triangle paragraph shape

The book may be written as dialogue with very little punctuation. While dyslexic/ SpLDs may not know how punctuation works, we can still find it useful in reading. It helps to show which words combine to make meaningful phrases.

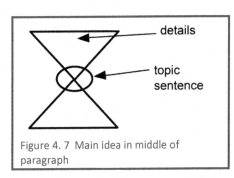

Figure 4. 7 Main idea in middle of paragraph

8.2 Comments about grammar

Sometimes a word can have several meanings and it isn't completely clear which one to choose:

> 'As the lens on a camera focuses an image onto the sensitive screen, the lens of our eyes focuses a scene on to the sensitive cells of the retina that curves round the back of the eyeball.' (Gilling and Brightwell, 1982)

'As' can mean 'at the same time', or 'in the same way', or 'because'; unless your student already knows about cameras or eyes, he won't know which meaning to choose.

The grammar may not be correct. In the above passage, 'eyes' is plural while 'lens', 'retina' and 'eyeball' are all singular. Your student could form a mental picture of the lens going between the two eyes.

A book sometimes doesn't have just one or two complications or errors like these; it can have many of them. Eventually your student may find he is not making sense of the material.

Long, involved sentences are often hard to read.

The subject can be separated by several lines of words from the verb it relates to; if your student's mind is not storing words effectively in working memory, he won't hold onto the subject for long enough to make sense of the sentence, see *CAPACITY OF WORKING MEMORY*.

For example in:

> The weather which is not following the usual patterns that have persisted over many decades, though some say they haven't changed for several centuries, is a good topic to start a conversation with a stranger.

'weather' is the subject and 'is', the verb, follows 2½ lines later.

Gilling and Brightwell (1982)

CAPACITY OF WORKING MEMORY: p 157

'This', 'that', 'these' and 'those' can be difficult to relate to the idea they refer to. In the following, 'that' could refer to 4 different ideas .

Example: This, that, these, those

In the following instructions, the underlined 'that' is not clearly used.

Always put the source, page number and date of working on every page of your notes, then you can organise them quickly to put them away, or to move them so that you have space to work. If you don't do that, you

- either have notes without an order and you then don't use them

- or you have to take too much valuable time just working out how the pages fit together.

What does 'that' refer to?

- Moving the pages?

- Putting them away?

- Organising them to put away?

- Putting source, page number and date on them?

If your mind takes it to be the last idea you have read, you won't make sense of the sentence. You have to refer 'that' back to the first idea in the sentence, namely putting source, page number and date on the pages.

8.3 Punctuation

Punctuation should be used to show the structure of text. It should be an aid that helps your student read fluently, even if he is not aware of the rules of punctuation. The lack of good punctuation may be part of your student's problems reading certain texts. It is worth recognising when this happens. Your student could treat putting in the punctuation as a puzzle that helps him understand the meaning. Recognising the lack of useful punctuation should be helpful in limiting the demoralising effects of struggling to read.

Story: Using punctuation to read

One student used the punctuation to help her read aloud while recording herself. She didn't try to understand what she was reading. She used the punctuation to modulate her voice, so that it became softer at the end of phrases and sentences.

She then listened to her recording. The rise and fall of her voice helped her to understand what she was listening to. For her, this was much more satisfactory than re-reading a passage several times and still not understanding. It was better than reading aloud on its own because she could go back over any passage if necessary.

8.4 Negatives can be complex

There are times when text has several negatives together or when a strong image is given but in a negative, complex way. The EXAMPLE: COMPLEX NEGATIVE, below, leads to contradictions that can go unnoticed and when they do, they can disrupt reading.

It is usually possible to write more directly.
For example, the double negative 'not infrequently' could be written as 'frequently' in many circumstances.

As a further example, at some stage I wrote:
> Besides not getting something right, the dyslexic/ SpLD person can get it wrong in different ways, randomly. The lack of a consistent set of brain connections means that dyslexia/ SpLD cannot be corrected in the same way that short- or long-sight can be corrected with glasses whereby one optical correction deals with all the problems and nothing more needs to be done. (Word count 62)

On proof-reading, I decided it was difficult to read these two sentences and that they contained a double negative.

Example: Double negative

The double negative in the text above is effectively:
'not only do you not get something right, but you can get it wrong in different ways, randomly'.

The paragraph would be understood better re-written as:

You often hear an analogy made between glasses used to correct short-sightedness and teaching strategies to dyslexic/ SpLD people. The analogy breaks down because of the random nature of dyslexia/ SpLD. Most short-sightedness changes slowly over time, so that glasses need changing every other year. The lack of a consistent set of brain connections means that dyslexia/ SpLD doesn't respond to a set strategy programme that will remedy the effects.   (Word count 70)

On re-writing, I decided an example would help:
I have a strategy for telling that 'practice with c' is a noun, and 'practise with s' is a verb. The strategy is not present in my mind as I write; randomly I spell them right, and randomly wrong.

Example: Complex negative

Two statements from a questionnaire demonstrate complex negatives:

1
I have been fascinated with the dancing of flames in a fireplace.   TRUE / FALSE
You picture the flames in your favourite fireplace and give the answer: TRUE

2
The warmth of an open fireplace hasn't especially calmed me.   TRUE / FALSE
You see yourself by a fireplace, relaxed, at ease with the world and answer: TRUE

BUT there's a negative in there (The warmth... hasn't ...calmed me.'), so the picture you've imagined is contrary to the statement. The answer for you is: FALSE.

8.5 Background to the material

Your student may be very familiar with the subject he is reading about and know more of the background to it than the author. The author may have stated one detail incorrectly, but it isn't important to the ideas he is really writing about. Your student may be very interested in what he has to say, but the incorrect detail keeps coming into your student's mind in such a way as to interfere with his reading. He may need to go and think about what is wrong and be sure that it has no impact on the other arguments, before he can continue reading effectively.

Your student may have found one chapter in a book that he is particularly interested in and he doesn't want to spend time reading the earlier chapters. His mind may keep telling him that he doesn't know the earlier discussion and it may eventually destroy his confidence in his ability to read the interesting chapter.

8.6 Mind engaged on another topic

There may be something else that is demanding your student's mental attention. However hard he tries to ignore it and remind himself that he has it under control, he may find that he is not convinced and again his reading will gradually deteriorate.

He may only make progress if he gets his thoughts down in a way that he will remember. Sometimes it is enough just to make a note and jot down some details; sometimes he may have to go and do something. If the latter happens too often, your student probably needs to look at the way he is organising his life and make some changes; he may find useful ideas in *Organisation and Everyday Life with Dyslexia and other SpLDs* (Stacey, 2020).

Stacey (2020)

There may be some completely different problem that your student is subconsciously worrying about; he hasn't recognised what it is, but it is disrupting his reading processes and until he finds out what is worrying him, your student will struggle to make any progress; the second bullet point in SOME UNOBVIOUS PROBLEMS is an example of such a situation.

SOME UNOBVIOUS PROBLEMS: p 64

8.7 Other reading problems

The problems listed here are just a few of those that I've come across while helping dyslexic/ SpLDs. They have become visible by discussion with careful listening; by using the *OBJECTIVE OBSERVATION*. Each time your student is not reading at his most effective rate, he would do well to stop and try to find out why.

OBJECTIVE OBSERVATION: p 63

Summary: Other reading problems

Sleepiness

Author's style

Poor use of grammar

Dealing with negatives

Knowing too much or too little of the background of the topic

Identifying other distractions

9 Proof-reading

Insight: Reading your own work

It is a fairly common, if disheartening, experience to write some work, proof-read it, be pleased that it expresses your ideas so well and expect a good grade, and to hand it in confident of a good mark, only to get it back with a much lower mark than you expected. Then when you read it, you struggle to remember what you wanted to say and you wonder how you thought it was good.

What I think is happening here is that while your student is writing, his ideas can be pretty clear and good and they are strongly present in his mind as he works. When he proof-reads, the words on the page prompt his mind to be conscious of his ideas; the ideas dominate and your student doesn't see that the words on the page are not clearly expressing his ideas; the beautiful essay stays in his head.   Until the memory of his ideas is not so strong and immediate he is unlikely to proof-read well. He needs to find out how long to wait after writing until his ideas have faded from his mind. He will actually read the words and assess how well they give his meaning. The delay can be more than a day.

One strategy that works for proof-reading is to read the text out loud; doing so should make your student pay attention to each word. Another is getting the computer to read it to him. Both of these methods combine audio with visual. They can help your student to notice:

- repeated words, e.g. 'the' followed by 'the'

- some confusions, e.g. 'through' and 'thorough'

- subject and verb not agreeing, e.g. 'he have the paper'.

Summary: Proof-reading

- Leave sufficient time after you finish writing and before you start proof-reading.

- Find the software that will help you best.

- Read the text aloud, or use text-to-speech.

- Ask someone to check your work. (This is GOOD PRACTICE for all.)

10 PhotoReading

PhotoReading (Scheele, 1999) is a system for reading that has been used successfully by many people I have taught, again not by all. There is considerable overlap of techniques with those in this chapter. It is worth trying the system to see if your student can use it. I have found that there are several ways it can be adapted to the different needs of dyslexic/ SpLD people. Discussing the system in depth is beyond the scope of this book.

Scheele (1999)

References

Buzan, Tony, 2010, *Use Your Head*, BBC Active, Harlow

Dahl, Roald, 1979, *Tales of the Unexpected,* Penguin Books, London

Elder, T., Wood, R., 1975, *Harrap's Swift Readers, Book 5 with Teacher's Book,* Harrap, London

Gilling, Dick and Brightwell, Robin, 1982, *The Human Brain,* Orbis, London

Russell, Peter, 1979, *The Brain Book: Know Your Own Mind and How to Use It,* Routledge, London

Scheele, Paul, 1999, *PhotoReading* 3rd ed., Learning Strategies Corp., Minnetonka, MN

Singleton, C.H., 2008, , Educational & Child Psychology, vol. 25 (3), pp 8-20

Stacey, Ginny, 2020, *Organisation and Everyday Life with Dyslexia and other SpLDs,* Routledge, London

Stein, J., 2014, *Dyslexia: the Role of Vision and Visual Attention,* Current Developmental Disorders Reports, vol. 1, pp 267-280

Website information

Crossbow Education, Reading rulers, http://www.crossboweducation.com/visual-stress-software/reading-rulers   Accessed 1 September 2020

OED Online, June 2017, Oxford University Press. Accessed 2 Nov 2017

Series website: www.routledge.com/cw/stacey

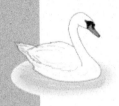

5   Listening

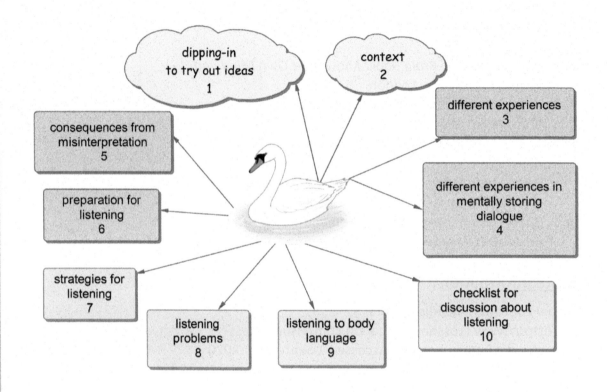

Contents

THINKING PREFERENCES, p 72, are highlighted in orange in this chapter.
Examples of their use are listed in the INDEX: p 589

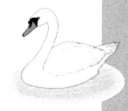

List of key points and summaries

K = key points
S = summaries

Templates on the website

TEMPLATES

COMPANION @ WEBSITE

Information for non-linear readers

Before the context of the USEFUL PREFACE and CHAPTERS 1 and 2, there is information that I hope will help non-linear readers as they approach the chapters. For chapters 4 – 14, this information would be identical except for which parts to scan and read. I have put all the information together into GUIDANCE FOR NON-LINEAR READERS, CHAPTER 3. It is worth reading CHAPTER 3 at some stage of working with this book.

GUIDANCE FOR
NON-LINEAR READERS:
p 222

1 Dipping-in to try out ideas: reading and scanning lists

Start with DIPPING-IN TO TRY OUT IDEAS: GENERAL PATTERN.

Read:
   KEY POINT: A RANGE OF LISTENING EXPERIENCES: p 267
   THE STORY BOXES: p 265, p 266, p 268, p 270, p 276
   LISTENING CHECK-LIST: p 265

Scan:
   CHECK-LIST FOR DISCUSSION ABOUT LISTENING: p 279
   PREPARATION FOR LISTENING: p 271

DIPPING-IN TO TRY OUT
IDEAS: GENERAL PATTERN:
p 228

1.1 Key points: for policy-makers and general readers

Key points: For policy-makers and general readers

- Listening can be the best way for some dyslexic/ SpLD people to absorb information.

- Listening, interpreting the spoken word, can be a difficult skill for dyslexic/ SpLD people.

- Subsequent actions may not be in line with a speaker's intentions.

- If you need to be clearly understood:

    read   ○ *KEY POINT: A RANGE OF LISTENING EXPERIENCES*

    ○ *PREPARATION FOR LISTENING*

    ○ *STRATEGIES FOR LISTENING*

- Check that your material and delivery assist dyslexic/ SpLDs to listen well.

KEY POINT: A RANGE OF LISTENING EXPERIENCES: p 267

PREPARATION FOR LISTENING: p 271

STRATEGIES FOR LISTENING: p 275

2 Context

The spoken word is another way in which ideas are passed from one person to another. For some dyslexic/ SpLD people, listening is very much easier than reading; while for others, it presents a range of problems.

Your student is listening to understand, so the ideas in *COMPREHENSION* are relevant to listening. Good *PREPARATION FOR LISTENING*, when possible, can make listening very much easier.

COMPREHENSION: p 162

PREPARATION FOR LISTENING: p 271

Your student may need to use her *THINKING PREFERENCES* in a very deliberate way. Sometimes, she may find that her mind is not retaining information, even when it is well within her capabilities.

THINKING PREFERENCES: p 72

Such a situation can happen when the information has no obvious links to her *THINKING PREFERENCES*. You can work with her to establish links and explore how they can help her to understand.

Swans glide with seeming ease on the water, but their feet are putting in effort; the swan image for this chapter reflects the apparent calm and passivity of listening and the effort that dyslexic/ SpLD listeners often make in order to understand while listening.

Story: Listening requires effort

Normally I engage my motor skills to aid listening, by taking notes. When listening to synthesised voices, the added strain of decoding the strange sounds increases my spelling difficulties. To help me follow, I try visual techniques, such as knowing what picture could be associated with the ideas.

Both methods are better than hoping I will remember what's been said, but both require effort.

Key point: Listening check-list

What am I interested in?

What's important to me?

What is the topic under discussion?

Is this main theme or detail?

Do I need to take notes?

Can I take notes?

Do I need to jot down my own thoughts briefly?

It is worth noticing a difference between listening and reading in respect to going back over material. What you read usually stays still while you read it and you can go back to it to check you have understood it correctly (not that you can always do that on the web, if you can't remember how you got to a particular page!). The spoken word is not always stored in a way that allows for repeated access, even over a very short space of time, see *Story: A Good Sentence Lost*. Recording devices can be used to allow repeated access to the spoken word.

Story: A Good Sentence Lost: p 164

One of the difficulties mentioned in *Author's Style*, is that the author may have an underlying message. In a similar way, speakers do not always say exactly what they mean. The words may have an obvious, surface meaning but as your student listens she may feel there is something that the speaker is not saying; for example, two people may be trying to organise their time together and one of them can be so polite and considerate that she is not thinking of what she would really like to do, although it is lurking in her subconscious, and it can be hard work to listen for her needs.

Author's Style: p 253

Story: An underlying message missed

One social work student was very pleased when his placement report was returned. As she handed it back, his tutor said, "I can see you haven't written many placement reports."

The student thought the tutor meant, "From reading your report, I understand this was your first placement." He took the comment as one of interest and encouragement.

About a week later, he told me he'd realised that the tutor meant, "Your report is not at all good."

3 Different experiences

Key point: A range of listening experiences

As always there's a wide range of experience:

- some dyslexic/ SpLDs find the hearing sense much easier to use than the visual

- some can't recall what they hear immediately, but it will be remembered when it is needed

- some listen by watching (visual preference) a speaker's mouth and, if they can't see the mouth, listening is very difficult which makes using a phone hard

- others find that what they see interferes with listening; they need to look away to listen properly

- a different accent may be really difficult to understand, as can the mechanical voice of some disabled people and the near robotic voice on some text-to-speech software

- holistic thinkers may have problems because what they hear triggers too many ideas and their minds start to think about these other ideas; then, without a mind that holds the words for later processing, they have no record of what's been said and they lose the thread of the conversation or lecture

- words may not connect to the right meaning fast enough for your student to understand; so the conversation or lecture moves on and she gets lost, see *MEANINGS OF WORDS*.

MEANINGS OF WORDS: p 98

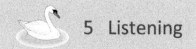

The following are some of the stories behind these experiences.

Story: A word losing its context

I was part of a group of parents talking about the new ways of teaching maths. Someone started talking about multiplication. As a physicist, I know about multiplication, but suddenly the word seemed strange and I had to work out that it was related to maths. While I was doing so, the conversation carried on. I don't have a mind that stores words, so I lost the thread of what was being said and it was some time before I could make sense of what others were saying.

Story: A gardener remembering instructions

One dyslexic gardener found he could listen to the instructions for the coming week; he would never be able to repeat them back to the head gardener; but as the week went by, the instructions came back to him as he needed them.

Story: Can listening and seeing work together?

I described to one group of students how I discovered that my senses of seeing and listening don't work together: I can't hear Handel's *Music for the Royal Fireworks* and see a fireworks display. I can listen or see but not both. My story made sense of one student's childhood experiences.

As quite a young child, he had realised that he heard better if he looked away from the person speaking to him. He was frequently told by exasperated adults, "Will you look at me while I speak to you."

4 Mentally storing dialogue

Some people can store a lot of dialogue without any effort[1], and recall it to process it and use it; I haven't yet met a dyslexic/ SpLD person who can do this, but it is worth knowing that it can be done and that it is part of the differences that exist between the ways different minds work with sound.

5 Consequences from misinterpretation

When I taught a module to a class of 20 students who were all dyslexic, I knew my words were being internalised in many different ways. You could tell some of the differences by the words they used in the conversation:

- some used words about
    - seeing
    - action, their own or someone else's
    - hearing
- some were looking for links and rationale.

The words used indicated different views of what I had said; they weren't exactly what I had said.

With the range of different interpretations dyslexic/ SpLD can have, there is a strong possibility for misinterpretation, which then leads to unexpected, unrequested actions.

---

[1] The mind is probably using one memory store and making the necessary links without a person's conscious effort, see CAPACITY OF WORKING MEMORY, p 157. One of the best known examples of a phenomenal memory was written about by Luria (Baddeley, 1982).

The emphasis put on words can also lead to misinterpretation.

Story: I want to be there early for once

2 friends went to a birthday party together. They arranged to go in one car.

The driver emphasised that she wanted to be early and to arrive before 6pm. She said she'd pick her dyslexic friend up an hour earlier, at 5.

When she arrived at 5pm, the dyslexic wasn't remotely ready, thinking there was still an hour left before the car owner would arrive.

So they were unhappy and late.

The emphasis on arriving early made 6pm the important time.

When it comes to getting ready, the important time is when to start getting ready, so 6pm had become the time to start getting ready.

Very often the misinterpretations are not recognised until later action is not what is expected. Gradually, your student needs to recognise where there is a difference in how she interprets what she hears. You need to work with her so that she can:

- find strategies to check she's got the right information
- gain co-operation from those around her to deal with any results of misinterpretation.

6 Preparation for listening

Make sure your student has the right pronunciation for words.

- It is disheartening to work on a set of words in preparation and then find a lecturer, or other speaker, uses a different pronunciation which she doesn't recognise as being the word she worked on.

- She can ask someone to record the words for her, or find them spoken by a natural voice on the internet, not a digital one.

The many different ways of doing *MIND SET* can be used in preparation for lectures or meetings. This is so important there are two exercises below for your student: *PREPARATION FOR A LECTURE* and *PREPARATION FOR A MEETING*.

MIND SET: p 158

The first exercise involves course aims and objectives, the syllabus and lecture notes. The information about courses is often in the course handbook, whether online or in hard copy.

Exercise for student: Preparation for a lecture

You need: the course aims and objectives, the syllabus, course handbook, the summaries of the lectures.

1 The course aims and objectives usually tell you the skills you will be developing and some very general ideas that will be covered, see *EXAMPLE: FINDING THE IMPORTANT IDEAS IN A PARAGRAPH*.

EXAMPLE: FINDING THE IMPORTANT IDEAS IN A PARAGRAPH: p 180

2 The syllabus will usually be more specific about the subject matter that you will be studying. If you get an electronic version, you can reduce it to the key words and phrases; probably with one idea per line. You can space out the material, so that closely related themes are together; you can indent to show subtopics.

You can work with the aims and objectives, and the syllabus at the beginning of a course.

3   You can then use the lecture summaries before each lecture[2].

   o   You should find the best time, possibly the night before or in the hour before.

   o   You can use key words with a spatial layout if that helps you.

   o   You can relate the topics in the lecture to the skills and general ideas from the course aims and objectives, and to the subject matter from the syllabus.

Select any way of using *MIND SET* that suits you. Use suggestions from *SURVEYING* and look for *KEY WORDS*.

MIND SET: p 158

SURVEYING: p 533

KEY WORDS: p 176

Verbally: you are using the key words.

Visually: you can use space to emphasise relationships; any other visual method can be used.

Kinaesthetically: you are doing the work and the design.

Rationale or framework: you can make sure you understand the relationships, or you can formulate questions you want answered.

---

[2] Lecture notes aren't always available in time; this way of using them is a good point to use to encourage lecturers to make them available early.

Example: Preparation using a lecture summary

Lecture synopsis (Crook, 2010):

Crook (2010)

> The aim of this lecture is to introduce students to the practice of historical writing and what makes it distinctive. The lecture will review the various genres which make up the discipline (social history, economic history, imperial history, and so on). Much of the lecture will consider whether historical writing should be concerned with telling (good) stories and will discuss the genre of 'micro-history'.

Synopsis keywords, separated out for clarity:

Historical writing

- distinctive
- genres:
  o social history
  o economic history
  o imperial history
  o micro-history
  o other

- telling stories   (good ones)

If this list is written on an A4 page and space left between the lines, the main ideas in the lecture can be added, or questions that the student wants answered by the lecture can be written on the sheet.

The initial purpose of creating the list is to prepare for the lecture.

In a lecture your student is a passive listener, in a meeting she will be expected to take part. She has to listen, hold on to her own ideas and talk. The problems and solutions for talking in meetings are discussed in *TALKING*, *STORY: TOO MANY IDEAS SPARKED BY OTHER PEOPLE TALKING* and *INSIGHT: CAPTURING THOUGHTS IN MEETINGS*.

TALKING: p 362

STORY: TOO MANY IDEAS SPARKED BY OTHER PEOPLE TALKING: p 472

INSIGHT: CAPTURING THOUGHTS IN MEETINGS: p 473

The second exercise involves meeting notes, agenda, circulated papers and other sources.

Exercise for student: Preparation for a meeting

You need: the agenda, the minutes of the last meeting, any papers circulated, any other sources of information, e.g. internet pages you've found, newspaper cuttings.

If there are a lot of materials, put them in a ring binder with an index showing the order. The index could also have a brief summary that tells you what you need to know about each section of information.

You process the material in much the same way as is explained in the *EXERCISE* and *EXAMPLE* above.

Highlight the key words and important passages, if this helps you.

Brainstorm your particular interests in the subjects under discussion.

Ⓖ p 575: brainstorm

line spacing adjustment here

This type of preparation helps your listening because:

- you have organised the material in a way that suits you
- you have given yourself aids to find things when you need them
- you can concentrate on listening.

MIND SET: p 158

When there is a lot of reading to do, do it in advance of the meeting, and then use *MIND SET* a little before the meeting. If papers are presented only at the beginning of the meeting, you may need to move yourself to a quiet place to read; trying to read while listening may mean you do neither.

As you listen, you may find ideas are generated in your mind by what others say, a strong tendency for holistic thinkers. You want to come back to these ideas, but it may be rude to interrupt another person talking. In the preparation for a meeting, I make sure the first page for taking general notes has the area marked out for capturing ideas I want to return to.   During a meeting, I reserve a particular space on my notes pages for such ideas, see *INSIGHT: CAPTURING THOUGHTS IN MEETINGS*; once an idea has been captured I can return to attentive listening.

INSIGHT: CAPTURING THOUGHTS IN MEETINGS: p 473

7 Strategies for listening

- If the preparation is done quite close to the meeting, it will act as *MIND SET*, otherwise doing *MIND SET* in the hour before a meeting will be helpful. Your student will be able to keep focused on the points of the meeting, even when other members go off task.

MIND SET: p 158

- As with reading, if I'm going to sleep while listening, it is a sure sign I am not processing the words well.

- *TAKING AND MAKING NOTES* helps some kinaesthetic people deal with listening problems. The notes may never be used again; their purpose was to help the writer to be an active listener. *TAKING AND MAKING NOTES* during ordinary everyday events strikes some people as odd but it may be the only way to keep listening well.

TAKING AND MAKING NOTES: p 300

- Some people just doodle while listening; the action of the hand is all that's needed (kinaesthetic).

- Your student could record discussions, meetings or lectures. Many smart phones have a recording facility that allows markers to be inserted at important points. Using markers should help your student to organise using playback to regain the information. She needs to ask permission to record anything.

- Your student's listening skills can improve if she uses her *THINKING PREFERENCES* to enhance her interpretation; she will be actively

THINKING PREFERENCES: p 72

understanding what she is listening to. She is likely to be using chunking to increase her *CAPACITY OF WORKING MEMORY*. For example:

(G) p 575: chunking

CAPACITY OF WORKING MEMORY: p 157

- o   visual sense: to make pictures, to see the story (and even abstract academic material often has a story)
- o   practical knowledge (kinaesthetic): to think of the practical application of the material.

- Your student can use the lecturer's anecdotes, with her *THINKING PREFERENCES:*

- o   to process her thoughts and check her understanding
- o   as stories to act as tags for the main ideas.

Story: *THINKING PREFERENCES* assisting listening

One social work student was finding it very hard to listen to the lectures about the more theoretical side of her course.

She was a kinaesthetic, visual thinker who loved being out on practice as part of her course.

During the theoretical lectures, she thought of her clients and chose the one most appropriate to the lecture. She imagined herself working with this client and she related the theories and policies to the client. She was able to use both her visual and kinaesthetic senses as she listened. The lectures made very much more sense to her.

It's really a question of knowing what your student's capabilities are now and experimenting to see what skills she could develop.

It will also help if she notices when she stops listening. What is it that stopped her listening? Once she knows that, she can start to find the solution; or she can give herself permission to not listen.

8 Listening problems

It's important for your student to realise that some problems with listening can't be solved and that some of them don't originate with her. She may not be able to listen because:

- the speaker doesn't speak clearly or is too disorganised for her to follow
- there are extra noises around
- there are people moving about
- there is very little oxygen in the room
- other reasons.

Work with your student to find out what her particular problems are and then let her explore solutions.

Summary: Listening problems

Among the problems are:

- the effort required
- the need to see something related to the ideas
- in contrast the previous need: sight may interfere
- seeing and hearing don't work together.

Words:

- pronunciation not known or not recognised
- unfamiliar accent of a speaker
- lose their meaning
- trigger different internal representations
- the wrong word is emphasised.

Thoughts:

- too many new ideas to be remembered
- too many ideas triggering other ideas
- limited working-memory capacity for words
- underlying message missed
- no framework
- no goal
- losing own ideas.

9 Listening to body language

A major part of communication when people are together is body language.

The way a person moves

- can be in harmony with what is being said
- can be contrary
- could be totally irrelevant.

This book isn't the place for a full discussion of body language.

The important aspect is whether your student's listening is aided or impaired by another person's body language.

For example: a person might:

- pace the floor while talking
- stand with hands on hips while discussing what to eat that evening
- have their head on one side while listening or talking
- use a lot of energy while talking
- look straight at your student
- not look at her at all.

The list of ways we use our bodies is long and the significance of any gesture depends on the context.

Using *OBJECTIVE OBSERVATION* and recording the observations using one of *TEMPLATES: B5-8 - RECORDING TEMPLATES - 1-4* will allow your student to observe what is happening, how she is affected by it and to decide whether any changes need to be made. If she decides changes are necessary, she might know what to do now she has seen what is happening. It may be the changes relate to something in this book, in which case use the relevant parts. It may be she needs other resources to make the changes, so she needs to make sure she finds those that she can use well.

OBJECTIVE OBSERVATION: p 63

TEMPLATES

10 Summary: check-list for discussion about listening

Summary: Check-list for discussion about listening

Discuss the various listening experiences and strategies with your student.

- How does her experience compare with what has been discussed?
- What's the same? What is different?
- What preparation does she make for formal and informal occasions?
- What does she feel is a problem?
- What strategies can she explore?
- How will she monitor changes in the way she listens?
- Does she feel good about her listening capabilities, or does she need to feel more competent?

Use the *TEMPLATES: B3 - COMPARE EXPECTATION AND REALITY* and *B4 - ACTION, RESULT, NEXT STEP* to collate your discussion and her progress.

MONITORING PROGRESS: p 535

TEMPLATES

References

Baddeley, Alan, 1982, *Your Memory: A User's Guide,* Penguin Books, London

Crook, Tom, 2010, *U67923: Historical Writing,* Oxford Brookes University, Unpublished

Website information

Series website: www.routledge.com/cw/stacey

6 Doing

summary: learning-by-doing 9

problems relating to doing 8

strategies for doing 7

preparation for doing 6

knowledge learnt-by-doing 5

learning a skill 4

doing and thinking preferences 3

context 2

dipping-in to try out ideas 1

Contents

THINKING PREFERENCES, p 72, are highlighted in orange in this chapter.

Examples of their use are listed in the *INDEX*: p 589

List of key points and summaries

K = key points
S = summaries

Templates on the website

TEMPLATES

Information for non-linear readers

Before the context of the *USEFUL PREFACE* and *CHAPTERS 1* and *2*, there is information that I hope will help non-linear readers as they approach the chapters. For chapters 4 – 14, this information would be identical except for which parts to scan and read. I have put all the information together into *GUIDANCE FOR NON-LINEAR READERS, CHAPTER 3*. It is worth reading *CHAPTER 3* at some stage of working with this book.

GUIDANCE FOR NON-LINEAR READERS: p 222

1 Dipping-in to try out ideas: reading and scanning lists

Start with *DIPPING-IN TO TRY OUT IDEAS: GENERAL PATTERN*.

DIPPING-IN TO TRY OUT IDEAS: GENERAL PATTERN: p 228

Read:

KEY POINT: PROCESSES FOR ACQUIRING AND APPLYING KNOWLEDGE AND SKILLS, p 283

INSIGHT: IMPORTANCE OF INITIAL STAGES OF LEARNING, p 287

SUMMARY: LEARNING-BY-DOING, p 299

Scan:

CONTEXT, p 282

1.1 Key points: for policy-makers and general readers

Key points: For policy-makers and general readers

- Learning-by-doing engages the kinaesthetic sense.
- A significant number of dyslexic/ SpLD people learn through their kinaesthetic sense.
- If this sense is left out of educational situations, these learners may have no way to engage with the material that society wants them to learn.
- Dyslexic/ SpLDs' practical skills would be very valuable to society if only they could learn in their right way.
- Policies for education should include the kinaesthetic sense.
- Those who don't find practical tasks naturally easy need a flexible approach that allows them to use other ways of thinking to help with practical tasks.
- The same approaches need to be adopted in the work place.

G p 575: kinaesthetic

2 Context

By communicating with others, people acquire knowledge and skills by reading and listening, and people pass on knowledge and skills by writing and speaking. These are language-based systems and clearly verbal processing is involved but visual and kinaesthetic processing are also involved in reading, writing, listening and talking. Moreover, visual aids use spatial awareness to enhance the verbal processing and they are well developed in communication and teaching.

Additional kinaesthetic processing is not well developed and is often given no attention. It can be a key element in the way dyslexic/ SpLDs learn and then communicate their learning. In order to keep my thinking clear while discussing kinaesthetic processing, I have chosen 'doing' to represent acquiring knowledge and skills and 'taking-action' for applying knowledge and skills. I have also emphasised the learning

G p 575: taking-action

aspect in this chapter by using learning-by-doing and learning-through-doing (and other variations of the verb to learn). I can't define a difference between the two but sometimes 'by' seems a better word to use and sometimes 'through'.

Key point: Processes for acquiring and applying knowledge and skills

acquiring	vs.	*applying*
reading	vs.	writing
listening	vs.	speaking
doing	vs.	taking-action

Doing and taking-action are not just about communication; they are involved in many other situations that use the kinaesthetic sense, in particular, practical work and physical experiences. It is not always so easy to separate kinaesthetic processing into doing and taking-action because the same physical action can be involved in both.

For some situations and people, the kinaesthetic sense is used to 'read' the situation more effectively than listening to words, and communication using gestures can be faster than speaking words. The situation could be one in which the action takes place too fast for words to be spoken, such as keeping a small child safe in today's traffic conditions. There can be a feeling that words are not part of the mental processing of the situation. The kinaesthetic thinking preference means someone has a preference for using thinking based on the kinaesthetic sense.

When one person instinctively uses the kinaesthetic thinking preference and another the verbal one, communication between them can be difficult. If your student regularly finds conversations disrupted by misunderstandings, it might be worth discussing what is happening with anyone who shares situations with him; he probably needs to establish an effective way of dealing with lack of words.

Experience is in some ways more fundamental than reading or hearing about something. The experience is what actually happens; reading and hearing are reports about something; they are descriptions, never the actual experience. You can read about a foreign city, you can walk round it or you can live with people in the city for a period of time. It depends on the individual person, but many find what they read and hear only comes alive in the experience. We empathise with others through our own experience. The body of experience that accumulates through life can often contribute to learning-through-doing and taking-action.

The kinaesthetic sense is fundamental to a lot of experience, but that does not make it someone's thinking preference; for some people it is the least preferred sense. The distinctions between 1) kinaesthetic learning as a thinking preference, 2) learning-by-doing and 3) taking-action are drawn out in the *INSIGHT BOX: PRACTICAL SCIENCE EXPERIMENT*.

INSIGHT BOX: PRACTICAL SCIENCE EXPERIMENT: p 392

Key point: Different reasons for practical work

- Kinaesthetic learning is the best way of learning anything when kinaesthesia is a person's strongest sense (Stacey, 2019).

- Learning-by-doing can be done and may be necessary whatever someone's *THINKING PREFERENCES* are.

- *TAKING-ACTION* is about practically using knowledge and skills irrespective of *THINKING PREFERENCES*.

SENSES: p 74
Stacey (2019)

TAKING-ACTION: p 388

THINKING PREFERENCES: p 72

Learning-through-doing may be:

1 part of learning a practical skill

2 to help your student understand some elements of knowledge.

A skill is a pattern of repeated processes; skills are often used automatically, i.e. without conscious thought.

Driving and cooking are two examples of practical skills that one can learn; making music is also accomplished through doing.

Knowledge in science is built on experiments[1] that scientists have done, and students of science can understand their subjects by carrying out experiments, which they then relate to the theories they are learning; engineering is an example of a subject that is essentially practical, even though there may be a lot of theory to learn.

Both skills and knowledge can be repeated until they are securely learnt; such repetition uses the feedback loop in *A MODEL OF LEARNING*.

A MODEL OF LEARNING: p 145

Skills and knowledge can be used exactly as they were learnt or they can be developed to suit other situations.

§3, DOING AND THINKING PREFERENCES discusses how thinking preferences can be used to help learning-through-doing.

§3: p 285

Learning-by-doing is discussed in:

   §4, LEARNING A SKILL

§4: p 288

   §5, KNOWLEDGE LEARNT-BY-DOING.

§5: p 290

Practical suggestions for learning-by-doing are set out in:

   §6, PREPARATION FOR DOING,

§6: p 291

   §7, STRATEGIES FOR DOING

§7: p 293

   §8, PROBLEMS RELATING TO DOING.

§8: p 297

3 Doing and thinking preferences

Learning-through-doing should suit kinaesthetic learners very well. Other types of learners also have to acquire knowledge or skills through doing and some may find it hard.

The practical work of learning-through-doing can be easier if your student's other thinking preferences are used. *EXAMPLE: USING A PREFERENCE-FOR-IDEAS TO DEAL WITH PRACTICAL WORK* describes using a preference-for-ideas to help with practical work.

EXAMPLE: USING A PREFERENCE-FOR-IDEAS TO DEAL WITH PRACTICAL WORK: p 290

---

[1] Even the scientific knowledge that springs from abstract thinking, such as Einstein's theory of relativity, would not be taken seriously if experiments and experience did not eventually fit with the theory.

Similar approaches can be developed with all the other styles of thinking preferences; the *INDEX* lists examples of use of the different thinking preferences. The *TEMPLATE: E1 - LIST OF OPTIONS FOR THINKING PREFERENCES* has key words for many different ways that thinking preferences can be used.

thinking preference examples in *INDEX:* p 589

TEMPLATES

If learning-by-doing does not come naturally to your student, he needs to think how to use his thinking preferences so that his way of thinking is the primary process and the doing is assisting it.

The following suggestions are ways different people could use thinking preferences to assist practical work:

- Visual thinkers can use any of the visual techniques to hold the steps of the physical movements together, or to hold the final outcome in mind; then they can focus on using the pictures while completing the movements.

- Verbal thinkers can do likewise with words; quotes from appropriate sources could add a different enjoyment.

- People who need a framework should take the time to create one that appeals to them.

- Consider what motivates your student to do the practical work:

    o Is it something he wants to share with others? He should find a way to keep them in mind during the practical work.

    o Does he do it for sheer love of the action?

    o Does he want to give a good performance of something? Suggest he feels the good performance growing as he practises the movements. (Similar questions can be asked about creating objects.)

    o Does he want to impress others? What is likely to impress them? What impresses him about other people's way of doing anything? Suggest he builds his reactions into the practical work.

    o Is he in competition with others?

If the practical work is being done in order to enhance theoretical ideas, it might be more effective for your student to apply his thinking preferences to them rather than the practical movements.

Your student can use any of the insights about *Thinking Preferences* to alter how he regards practical work. He should make sure he is working positively and maintaining his self-confidence, see *Building Confidence and Self-esteem*.

Thinking Preferences: p 72

Building Confidence and Self-esteem: p 78

Record your student's progress and notice what approach helps him diminish his reluctance for practical work. What makes the practical work grow into an effective skill or helps him to understand the knowledge he is trying to gain?

When your student is learning a skill, the initial stages can be very important and they can be part of the way he uses the skill once it is fully developed.

Insight: Importance of initial stages of learning

For some dyslexic/ SpLD people, if the initial stages don't use their thinking preference, the skill will always be vulnerable to degeneration. Even when the skill is learnt correctly later, it is often the *Oldest Memory Trace* that is used.

Oldest Memory Trace: p 568

For example, an experience of many dyslexic adults is that they can learn to spell but, when they are thinking about ideas rather than words, the oldest, incorrect spellings get used, not the later, correct ones.

When your student is learning-through-doing in order to understand ideas and gain knowledge, the initial stages are probably not so critical, but using his thinking preferences will considerably improve the way he can be active in the learning process.

The feedback loop is a stage of *A Model of Learning:* p 145

Using his thinking preferences will also be important in the feedback loop when repeated work is used to make sure that his learning is establishing the best neural networks for the processes involved.

Ⓖ p 575: neural networks

If he is someone who is never going to master practical work easily, focus on the tasks he has to do, and let others do the rest. There will be other contributions he can make instead. The work you do together in this area may be part of negotiating ACCOMMODATIONS.

ACCOMMODATIONS: p 128

4 Learning a skill

There are different stages in learning a skill:

- there is a time when you don't have the skill; and possibly don't know it exists
- in the initial stage you start learning
- in the middle stage you practise
- at the final stage you perform or use the skill; effectively you are applying the skill.

The final stage may involve the same techniques as the middle stage or even the initial stage, so the ideas in this chapter also apply to APPLYING A SKILL. Once learnt many skills are used in different situations, see ADAPTING A SKILL TO A NEW SITUATION.

APPLYING A SKILL: p 404

ADAPTING A SKILL TO A NEW SITUATION: p 404

Examples of skills include:

driving   riding a bike   handwriting

touch typing   using a computer

cooking   sewing   playing sport

carpentry   operating machinery

DIY (Do It Yourself)   crafts and art work

playing a musical instrument   medical operation procedures

working on an archaeological dig

Some of the skills your student learns-through-doing should become automatic, in that he needs to use them without consciously thinking about them. The way he builds his skills will make a considerable difference to how automatic they can become; see AUTOMATICITY.

AUTOMATICITY: p 153

Example: Touch typing automatically

When you touch type automatically, you think of the words you want to write and you concentrate on the sense you are making or you look at the page of text you are typing into the computer.

You do not think about the movement of your fingers to find the correct letters; you do not look at the keyboard. Finding the letters is done automatically by your brain using efficient neural networks.

A dyslexic/ SpLD learner needs to avoid any inefficient initial stages in the learning process: they are likely to persist in the same way early incorrect spelling does.

The right kinds of programme have been discussed in *Learning to Touch Type*. Touch typing can be learnt with a barrier that prevents the learner from seeing his hands in order to prevent *Sight Interference with Learning Movement*.

Learning to Touch Type: p 147

Sight Interference with Learning Movement: p 148

Mimicry can be an important part of learning-through-doing.

Some people are very good at it.

Sometimes the mind builds on the mimicry and the skill develops in a relatively smooth way.

Sometimes the mimicry brings good initial results, and could be seen as beginner's luck, but subsequent performance doesn't seem to build on that success; it is as if the learner has to go back to the beginning and build other understanding around the practice until it becomes well known.

Story: Mimicry not producing long-term learning

A player new to bowls had good results when she could copy advanced players' actions. However, she wasn't internalising the actions and after the first few sessions, her performance deteriorated. She had to re-think how she was moving and learn in a different way to get back to her previous level of performance.

5 Knowledge learnt-by-doing

The purpose of some practical work is to assist the understanding of theories. Such practical work rarely happens without visual or verbal information being given, which caters for visual or verbal learners. The style of presentation will be important, see *GENERAL CONSIDERATIONS* for indirect communication and *INSTRUCTIONS*. Discuss with your student how well he can understand the information he is given and how well his needs are being met.

GENERAL CONSIDERATIONS: p 122

INSTRUCTIONS: p 125

Deliberately using *THINKING PREFERENCES* may be part of your student's learning strategies for dealing with learning knowledge and skills through-doing.

THINKING PREFERENCES: p 72

Example: Using a preference-for-ideas to deal with practical work

A historian may like thinking about theories and concepts (Myers-Briggs, Intuiting) in wide-reaching ways, and he may have no instinct for visual representation of concepts nor for kinaesthetic learning. As part of his coursework, he has been told to construct a time line[2].

---

[2] A time line is a line covering a specified length of time and you put different events on it at the time they happened; you can also show how long they occurred for. One benefit of time lines is that gaps between events, or lack of gaps, show clearly.

If he is thinking about the influences on and between the events as he makes the time line, he will be engaging his thinking preference; the task of creating the time line will have an immediate purpose for him and his lack of enthusiasm for doing and for visual aids will not be detrimental.

If he further draws out the historical details that can be seen from the time line, his abstract thinking will be enhanced, which could further diminish his reluctance to create time lines.

Similar approaches can be used for all the *THINKING PREFERENCES*.

Some students hate practical work, but even they can find ways to alter their thinking so that they can find some way of making progress and lessening the stress. Use the *TEMPLATE: B4 - ACTION, RESULTS, NEXT STEP* to record different tasks that your student does; include some that go well and some that have problems. Then reflect on the tasks that go well to see how to assist the tasks that don't work; see *USING CHALLENGES*.

TEMPLATES

USING CHALLENGES: p 80

6 Preparation for doing

The ideas in *PREPARATION FOR READING* and *PREPARATION FOR LISTENING* will apply to learning-by-doing as well.

PREPARATION FOR:
READING: p 243
LISTENING: p 271

Exercise for student: Find the preparation for-doing best suited to you

Don't use the cross references before you brainstorm.
Brainstorm:
> your *THINKING PREFERENCES*
> the *TECHNIQUES FOR USING THE MIND* that suit you
>> best
> the methods you use to keep you *THINKING*
>> *CLEARLY*
> your choices of *MATERIALS AND METHODS* for
>> organising

THINKING PREFERENCES: p 72

TECHNIQUES FOR USING THE MIND: p 156

THINKING CLEARLY: p 79

MATERIALS AND METHODS: p 565

Check the paragraphs on *PREPARATION FOR READING* and *PREPARATION FOR LISTENING* Which ideas suit you and will be useful for the task in hand?	*PREPARATION FOR:* *READING:* p 243 *LISTENING:* p 271
Consider *MENTAL REHEARSAL* and how it would suit you to use it. What is the task in hand? How can you relate what works well for you to the task in hand? What are the steps in your preparation?	*MENTAL REHEARSAL OF MOVEMENTS* below

6.1 Mental rehearsal of movements

Mentally rehearsing movements is a way of using the kinaesthetic memory. It can be done in a range of ways:

- from just short of a full performance, or full action
- to minimal action
- to purely mental rehearsal in which no physical movement takes place.

It can be used in preparation for learning-by-doing, taking-action or any practical work, where 'practical work', and similar phrases, means any work or actions that are carried out in a physical way.

This style of preparation is well known by top sports people[3]. It is a kinaesthetic method for *MIND SET*.
Rehearse the movements you have learnt:

MIND SET: p 158

- You can do it by repeating the actual movements.
- You can repeat a minimal version of the movement: for example, to learn a dance sequence with a right-hand star*, you don't have to have other people to do a complete right-hand star, you can just put your right hand up, as if clasping another's hand, and you can move your body an inch or two in the direction of a right-hand star.

*right-hand star: in English Folk Dancing, this is a movement in which 4 dancers hold their right hands together and dance round in a circle.

---

[3] Examples of other careers and hobbies which include doing are: Playing music; Dancing; Medical procedures; Teaching; Building trade; Animal husbandry

- You can imagine yourself doing the movements: you can either visualise yourself doing them, or you can feel the movements in your body (**visual** or **kinaesthetic**).

- You can shut your eyes, to increase the attention you are able to pay to movement as you rehearse.

- You can rehearse the mental processes[4] that you are using, to help the movements become better established in your mind.

7 Protocol for doing

This section sets out a protocol for dealing with doing, whether that involves learning or accomplishing a task.

It may be very important for your student to organise his materials and space so that they work for him. He may have to reach agreement with others, as his way of using materials and space may interfere with others working with him or nearby.

Key point: Protocol for doing

It can be rather like having a recipe, but for practical work:

- Find your instructions.

- Know what you are doing.

- Know which ideas help you from *DOING AND THINKING PREFERENCES*.

- Know your *REGIME FOR MANAGING YOUR DYSLEXIA/ SPLD*.

- Set up the space for the practical work; see *ENVIRONMENT*.

- Draw up a timetable and set out an order for the practical work.

- Find your materials and tools.

DOING AND THINKING PREFERENCES: p 285

REGIME FOR MANAGING YOUR DYSLEXIA/ SPLD: p 540

ENVIRONMENT: p 70

---

[4] Mental processes: you might be using a story to link the movements (**verbal**);
you might have a **verbal** list of single words for groups of movement;
you might have cartoon pictures for the movements (**visual**).
These are examples of mental processes that could be rehearsed.

⬆

- Carry out the practical work.
- Record anything that needs recording, so that you benefit next time you do the action.

The protocol can be adapted for preparation or mental rehearsal of doing.

EXAMPLE: BUILDING A FLAT PACK: p 294

EXAMPLE: RESEARCH FOR A REPORT OR DISSERTATION: p 296

A couple of examples follow: *BUILDING A FLAT PACK* and *RESEARCH FOR A REPORT OR DISSERTATION*.

The first describes a practical task of everyday living. The principles behind the example could apply to the directly practical stage of any task, including learning-by-doing.

The second deals with research, which could relate to everyday living, education or employment. Research could range from 1) a simple browse on the internet looking for information to 2) an in-depth investigation for a complex project that takes many years to complete.

Example: Building a flat pack[5]

- Find a space where you can unpack the flat pack and build the item. Take into account that you need to be able to get the item from the building space to its final place.
- You will probably need to be organised in the way you unpack; you will need to make sure you don't lose anything; and you need to identify everything correctly.

- Find the instructions. Some people can build flat pack items without referring to the instructions; others have to follow the instructions meticulously.

⬇

---

[5] A flat pack is a product, often furniture, which you have bought as a kit that needs assembling. The kit is packed so that the pieces lie flat in a box.

- Know where your capabilities lie and either glance at the diagrams to spot any tricky operations or follow the instructions closely. If you will be following the instructions carefully, does it help to read all the way through, or should you work one step at a time?

- Assemble all the tools you need.

- Mentally prepare yourself, if you don't like building flat packs, or if you are short of time: relax, breathe correctly, remember what you want to gain from the item.

- Build the item and move to its resting place.

- Record any lessons you learnt and file them for the next time you build a flat pack: it's not worth struggling at the same point again.

The first time anyone undertakes a task like building a flat pack, he is learning the processes involved. Once he is familiar with them, building a flat pack item will feel much more like an everyday task. He may habitually forget some detail, e.g. to check everything is there and he has all the tools, so making a note as a reminder could be worth the effort, but otherwise there would be no need to write anything.

Scientific experiments can be carried out with the same mental approach; but since the experimenter is learning (either as a student or a researcher) through the experiment there is likely to be more to record during the whole experiment.

RESEARCH FOR A REPORT OR DISSERTATION focuses on the first 2 bullet points of the protocol: understanding any instructions and knowing what to do. The instructions might be in the form of constraints on the work. Knowing what to do includes assessing any skills involved.

e.g.

Example: Research for a report or dissertation[6]

See *MAJOR PROJECTS*, p 400, for building a full action plan for other projects (including a dissertation or report).

There are several different end points for a piece of research:

- You may be finding out what happened during a period of time or during a set of actions taken by others.

- You may be doing scientific research, experiments, to further knowledge.

- You may be doing research as part of an undergraduate degree.

In the first two, you may have time and financial constraints (*an instruction*), but the object of the exercise is to find the truth (*an instruction and goal*) and if you research unproductive avenues, you should have the resources to re-start the research. In the third situation, you are demonstrating that you can carry out research (*an instruction*); in this case, you are unlikely to have the resources to re-start the research; how you do the research is as important as producing an end result. For all three, a null result (see *MARGIN NOTE*) might be just as useful as a definite positive or negative result.

MARGIN NOTE:
a null result clarifies that there is no need to pursue the line of research.

The methods that you have used will be a significant part of the report. You will need to take notes as you proceed, so that you can include the methods in the report. Others need to know how reliable your work is (*an instruction*); your methods should be capable of being reproduced by other people (*an instruction*).

The end point is to make information available to others in a report of some kind (*an instruction*).

---

[6] Other names used for dissertation are: thesis, project, survey. These are major pieces of work for a qualification.

The stages of the research will include:

- determining the subject for research (*goal*)
- planning the research
- doing the research
- drawing conclusions and making recommendations (*goal*)
- writing up the whole process, from selection to conclusion (*an instruction and goal*).

Break down the stages into manageable sections; make sure each section has a genuine interest for you, see *DOING AND THINKING PREFERENCES*.

Look at *SUMMARY: CHECK-LIST OF SKILLS, PROCESSES, MIND TECHNIQUES, ETC.* Discuss with your support tutor which ones will be useful, which you are familiar with. Identify any areas that need work in order to be helpful to you.

Apply the rest of the protocol and adapt *BUILDING A FLAT PACK* to carry out the rest of the research.

DOING AND THINKING PREFERENCES: p 285

SUMMARY: CHECK-LIST OF SKILLS, PROCESSES, MIND TECHNIQUES, ETC.: p 220

BUILDING A FLAT PACK: p 294

The above example has applied the beginning of the protocol to research for a complex project; the more objectively and deliberately the different stages are conducted, the more likely the research will proceed well.

Finding information from the internet is also research and it can be more satisfactory if a systematic approach is adopted, though it may need a bit less planning and writing.

8 Problems relating to doing

Not everyone finds doing and taking-action easy. Some of the experiences of difficulties, and the solutions, have been discussed more fully under *Kinaesthetic Learning* in *Finding Your Voice with Dyslexia and other SpLDs* (Stacey, 2019). *Space, Place and Direction* in *Organisation and Everyday Life with Dyslexia and other SpLDs* (Stacey, 2020) also discusses problems and solutions that have a bearing on doing and taking-action. Very brief résumés can be found in *SPACE, PLACE AND DIRECTION* and *ENVIRONMENT*.

Stacey (2019)
Stacey (2020)

SPACE, PLACE AND DIRECTION: p 69

ENVIRONMENT: p 70

Your student needs to know the source of any problem before he can find the right solution. He can brainstorm to focus on the practical task and explore the problem he is experiencing. He can use the ideas in METHODS OF EXPLORING BEHIND THE OBVIOUS and the CHECK-LISTS FOR EXPLORING BEHIND THE OBVIOUS to find out what is at the heart of his difficulties.

Ⓖ p 575: brainstorming

METHODS OF EXPLORING BEHIND THE OBVIOUS: p 65

CHECK-LISTS FOR EXPLORING BEHIND THE OBVIOUS: p 67

Summary: Problems relating to doing

Among the possibilities are your student:

- disliking practical work
- not understanding the instructions
- not thinking the right way for him
- not having the right ENVIRONMENT
- not having the right layout to work in
- not having enough time for the work
- not having good control of his movements or no sense of space
- not being organised
- having other problems relating to using the kinaesthetic sense.

'Other' is a very useful category for brainstorming with your student.

ENVIRONMENT: p 70

See kinaesthesia in SENSES: p 74

'Other' has been used several times in the book. If someone's behaviour pattern, or something else, doesn't quite fit with what's been categorised before, it is worth using TEMPLATE: E7 - THE BOX 'OTHER' in which to record the observations. It is better to leave something inconclusive in this way than to try to fit the behaviour in somewhere. It is better to have somewhere to record the observations than to leave them out.

Ⓖ p 575: other

TEMPLATES

When you and your student have identified the source of the problem, search for a solution. *Methods of Exploring behind the Obvious* may help you both put all the information together to work towards a solution.

Methods of Exploring behind the Obvious: p 65

9 Summary: learning-by-doing

Summary: Learning-by-doing

- Learning-by-doing is suitable for learning knowledge as well as skills.
- Kinaesthetic learners (and workers) need to use their kinaesthetic sense as a priority, whether for knowledge or skills.
- Those who don't take easily to practical work should be enabled to use their other thinking strengths to assist with learning-by-doing.
- Mental rehearsal of movements helps to establish the movements in long-term memory.
- Communication can be disrupted when gestures are used by one party instead of words.
- It is worth going to the root of any problem to find out exactly what is causing it; any solutions developed will be more effective.

References

Stacey, Ginny, 2019, *Finding Your Voice with Dyslexia and other SpLDs*, Routledge, London

Stacey, Ginny, 2020, *Organisation and Everyday Life with Dyslexia and other SpLDs*, Routledge, London

Website information

Series website: www.routledge.com/cw/stacey

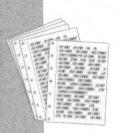

7 Taking and Making Notes

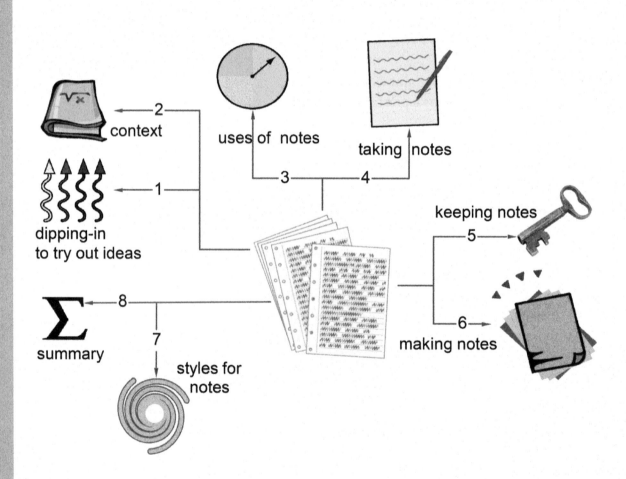

context —2—

uses of notes

taking notes

—1—

—3— —4—

dipping-in
to try out ideas

keeping notes

—5—

—8—

—6—

summary

making notes

—7—

styles for
notes

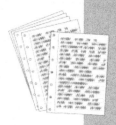

Contents

THINKING PREFERENCES, p 72, are highlighted in orange in this chapter.
Examples of their use are listed in the *INDEX*: p 589

List of key points and summaries

K = key points
S = summaries

Templates on the website

TEMPLATES

Information for non-linear readers

Before the context of the *Useful Preface* and *Chapters 1* and *2*, there is information that I hope will help non-linear readers as they approach the chapters. For chapters 4 – 14, this information would be identical except for which parts to scan and read. I have put all the information together into *Guidance for Non-Linear Readers, Chapter 3*. It is worth reading *Chapter 3* at some stage of working with this book.

Guidance for Non-Linear Readers:
p 222

1 Dipping-in to try out ideas: reading and scanning lists

Start with *Dipping-in to Try Out Ideas: General Pattern*.
Read:
>   *Context*, p 303
>   *Key Points* and *Summary* boxes, page numbers listed above
>   *Styles for Notes*, p 316

Scan:
>   the sections marked with the green line as important to discuss
>>   with your student.

Dipping-in to Try Out Ideas: General Pattern:
p 228

1.1 Key points: for policy-makers and general readers

Key points: For policy-makers and general readers

- The style of notes can make the difference as to whether any notes can be used by a dyslexic/ SpLD person.

- Dyslexic/ SpLD people should be shown a wide range of styles for making notes and allowed to experiment with them.

- They should be allowed to use the styles that work for them.

- For some, taking notes is a strategy that supports other skills, such as reading and listening.

- For others, taking notes is a very difficult task.

- Accommodation may be needed if:
  o students' notes are part of an assessment process
  o their notes are to be used by others
  o they find taking notes difficult.

2 Context

Taking notes and making notes can be two different tasks. You tend to take notes while something is happening, a lecture or a meeting. The main situation carries on and you don't have time to stop and think very much about the content of the notes. You may be able to use a style of notes that works for you and you may have to switch styles as the event progresses, but keeping up with the event limits your opportunities to make changes.

Making notes is often a more deliberate process: you are putting information down in a shortened form and you have time to edit the notes so that they are as you want them to be. You may be reading a book, researching a topic on the internet or preparing for a forthcoming event. Dyslexic/ SpLD students usually find that the way they make notes is very particular to themselves.

Notes have a variety of uses. Sometimes notes will be just for the note taker and sometimes they will be shared with others.

Key point: Notes that are for your student

Notes are often a private affair, reminding your student of some ideas. She can mis-spell to her heart's delight; she can use symbols rather than words; she can show relationships between ideas by the way she uses the space around the words; she has to worry about neatness only in so far as it matters to her.

When notes are shared with others, they need more attention. The way notes are to be used should determine the styles that can be used for them. How they are to be kept probably depends on when they are to be used.

This chapter discusses notes in terms of their uses, taking them, keeping them and making them. It ends by presenting a range of different styles for notes.

3 Uses of notes

Some notes are taken just to assist processing information, to keep attention on listening or reading: their use is in the taking. Other notes are taken for a future use which will determine whether the initial notes taken are a draft version that has to be made into a more permanent set and whether the set needs to be kept.

Notes are used for many different reasons.

They can be kept as a record of discussions and decisions for a particular group of people.

They may be used to pass information from one person to another.

They might be used to remember the key points of a subject, where the source is a lecture or a book or the internet.

They might be part of learning a skill.

They could be used as prompts when giving a lecture.

They could be a to-do list.

The list roughly falls into:

- those that are for short term use, don't need to be very full and will be thrown away fairly quickly

- those that other people need to understand and which will probably be kept for a considerable time

- those that are for your student's use only; that she will use at a later date and that she needs to be able to understand when she uses them again.

USING NOTES WHILE TALKING lists several situations when notes are useful in the short term, such as consulting a doctor. The notes need to be instantly understandable and bring to mind exactly what your student wants to remember.

USING NOTES WHILE TALKING: p 372

There are some situations in which your student has to make notes for others to read. If she is working with other professionals, for instance in the healthcare professions, she may be making brief notes to pass on vital information to be used by others. Many people develop a 2-stage approach to the task, when time allows. They take notes for themselves in the immediate situation and later make these into a version that can be used by others.

On some practical courses, the notes written during the practical work are assessed as part of the practical assignment. These are notes taken by your student for her own use, but someone else is assessing whether they are fulfilling the role required of them: to give your student enough information for later use. Your student will need to discuss with the assessors how she deals with any obstacles or hazards that she faces. You can help her to describe the problems using *METHODS OF EXPLORING BEHIND THE OBVIOUS*.

Ⓖ p 575, obstacle, hazard

METHODS OF EXPLORING BEHIND THE OBVIOUS: p 65

In making notes only for herself, your student can experiment with different styles of making notes and use the ones which allow her to recall most easily; she can test her recall using *RECALL AND MEMORY EXERCISES*.

RECALL AND MEMORY EXERCISES: p 159

4 Taking notes

Key points: Skills for taking notes

The skills needed for taking notes are:

- listening well or observing what is happening
- knowing the purpose of the notes
- understanding the main issues
- being able to let details go when that's appropriate
- capturing the main issues fast enough to keep up, whether by writing or typing
- being confident of the style used for the notes, that it works for your student.

COMPREHENSION: p 162
KNOW THE GOAL OF ANY TASK: p 181

LISTENING: p 262

You need to work with your student on all the skills in *COMPREHENSION*, *KNOW THE GOAL OF ANY TASK* and *LISTENING*.

Being able to keep up while taking notes is often quite difficult. Knowing why the notes are being taken helps with deciding what is important to take down.

4.1 Preparation

Preparation makes a significant difference to the ease with which your student can take notes.

- She needs to make sure she has the materials that suit her: the paper and pens or pencils; the electronic device she uses.

- She can arrange to get notes or handouts early, so that she has time to use them in her preparation.

- Doing *MIND SET* will switch her brain on so that it is ready to chunk information together and use her *WORKING MEMORY* to its full *CAPACITY*.

MIND SET: p 458

CAPACITY OF WORKING MEMORY: p 157

Finding the right time to do the preparation can make a difference. Some people benefit from mind setting for a short time the day before a lecture or meeting. In the time after the preparation, their minds put the information together so that they understand the topics better during the lecture or meeting. Then *CHUNKING* happens more easily and the notes taken are much better.

CHUNKING: p 158

4.1.1 Adding to lecture notes

Some lecture notes will be suited to the way your student thinks and have everything she needs to record; she just needs to remember where they are and use them when needed.

Some are a good basis for her to add clarifying details.

Your student should thoroughly check that the lecture notes have everything she needs and not rely on first impressions.

The point made in the *KEY POINT: YOUR STUDENT UNDERSTANDING HER OWN NOTES* could be relevant: notes enable recall of all the information for only a certain length of time and beyond that they trigger recall of very little.

KEY POINT: YOUR STUDENT UNDERSTANDING HER OWN NOTES: p 308

4.2 Practice

It is good to practise taking notes by listening to a half-hour radio programme with a 'listen again' facility. That way your student can take notes and then assess how well she has represented the speaker's ideas. She may also be able to see what strategies she is using when she doesn't quite get the right words.

4.3 Problems

Key points: Problems while taking notes

There are a variety of problems with taking notes.

- Some dyslexic/ SpLDs try to take down every word and they don't understand what they are writing.
- They take down information that is irrelevant, so they take too many notes.
- They focus on the mechanics of writing; they can't listen at the same time and they lose the context.
- They can't keep up with the lecture or meeting and have gaps in their notes.
- They forget what they are writing because they can't hold information in working memory.
- They can't remember how to spell words and they lose the thread of the topic while trying to work it out.
- They can't read their writing later.
- They stop concentrating.
- They get distracted.
- Their minds get switched off.
- They get bored or tired.

ACCOMMODATIONS:
p 128

You need to work with your student to find out exactly what her problems are; see *METHODS OF EXPLORING BEHIND THE OBVIOUS*.

METHODS OF EXPLORING BEHIND THE OBVIOUS:
p 65

Story: Being involved mattered

One student was working on organising her subject with me. She showed me the hand-written notes the lecturer had made available on the university website and the photos she had taken of his writing on the board. We were discussing her understanding of the subject as well as her organisation.

The remarkable thing was that she could fluently tell me about the lecture from her photos and she could tell me nothing from the lecturer's handouts. There was very little to choose between the two: the text was the same and both were handwritten.

The indication was that her presence in taking the photos was part of her recall mechanism. Having seen this kinaesthetic possibility, we then went on to see whether we could build on the insight.

Your student may become good at taking and making notes, but never quite fast enough to keep up with certain situations, such as lectures in a college course. Appropriate provisions might be for her to have notes taken by a recognised note taker or to be allowed to record the lectures, see *ACCOMMODATIONS*.

ACCOMMODATIONS: p 128

Key point: Your student understanding her own notes

There is often a time issue about remembering what the notes mean.

- Many dyslexic/ SpLD people recognise that there is a limited period of time during which they can remember what the notes meant and what else was being discussed at the same time.

- If the notes were made to be used later, it is important that they are re-drafted while they can still be understood.

- Students either need to add to the original set or they need to re-make the notes in a way that will make sense after some considerable time.

At this point it is probably worth your student getting the spelling right, so that she produces the correct words in her work. She can still use symbols and space to convey meaning, and she need only worry about neatness if the notes are to be shared with others.

4.3.1 Seeing, listening and writing

The interplay of the senses while taking notes is worth mentioning separately as a problem.

Many dyslexic/ SpLD people (and others) cannot listen, see and write at the same time. They need to use recording devices to capture the spoken word so that they can process the information later or they need someone to take notes for them, see *ACCOMMODATIONS*.

ACCOMMODATIONS:
p 128

Others need to see as they listen and write. Sometimes students arrange to go with a friend to a lecture so that they can look at the friend's notes while writing their own. They don't necessarily copy the notes of the friend; it can be that the eyes are engaged on the same task as their fingers.

5 Keeping notes

Once your student has decided that she is going to keep her notes rather than throw them away, she should think carefully about how she will keep them and how she will access the information in the future. You need to discuss different filing systems with her to help her decide what will suit her best; there is a list of questions in *PAPERWORK, INCLUDING FILING* which you can use to help her make decisions.

PAPERWORK, INCLUDING FILING: p 71

Sometimes it works better to write directly into a book, such as an A4 book or a small notebook that fits easily into a pocket or bag. Your student might use a book for general notes of ideas that she wants to capture during the day. She will probably use these notes in a relatively short length of time. She might have a log book that is capturing ideas that all relate to a definite project. These notes might be referred to after some length of time.

As discussed in *Strategies for Listening*, notes may be taken simply to assist listening and they are never going to be used again; your student can throw them away as soon as they have served their purpose.

Strategies for Listening: p 275

It is a good idea to have some way of finding information relevant to a particular topic again. At some stage your student can decide which are the main themes in a set of notes. The earlier she does this, the less work she will have putting the themes in all the useful places. *Generating Useful Questions* will help your student to decide what the important themes are.

Generating Useful Questions: p 530

Your student could:

- use the left-hand margin to write the keyword of each theme

- box or highlight key words within her notes

- write the theme of each note at the beginning, possibly on a line above the note; if necessary leave a line to add the theme later

- use right-hand margins for key themes; an example of this method is given in *Example from a Log Book*

Example from a Log Book: p 544

- put the date on her notes; combining her notes with other work done at the same time and with information in her diary may help her to decide on the main themes of her notes.

Whichever method your student uses, she can use colour coding as well, if that helps her.

5.1 Source, page numbers and date

Your student should always put the source, page number and date of working on every page of her notes, then she can organise them quickly to put them away, or to move them so that she has space to work. If she doesn't have such a system (e.g. source, page number and date) and the notes get out of order, she either keeps them in a random order and then doesn't use them or she wastes valuable time just working out how the pages fit together.

Key point: Collect full references as you work

Make sure you have the full details of sources, so that you don't have to go hunting for them just before a deadline. They are much easier to collect as you work.

Use some software to help you. You may only need a word document, or electronic notebook, etc., in which to collect the information. You may need a full professional reference package.

Make sure you distinguish between any of the author's words that you copy and words that you contribute from your own thinking. If you want to use the ideas again, e.g. for an essay, you must be clear about which words came from an author's work.

6 Making notes for later use

Notes already taken can be converted, made, into a set that can be used by your student at a later date or that can be used by others. As previously mentioned, the conversion needs to happen while your student can still remember what the original notes were about, see *KEY POINT: YOUR STUDENT UNDERSTANDING HER OWN NOTES*.

KEY POINT: YOUR STUDENT UNDERSTANDING HER OWN NOTES: p 308

If other people are going to use the notes, your student probably has to write them rather than use a non-verbal style of notes. She may be able to use bullet points or other layout devices to suit her style of making notes, but she probably won't be able to use various other *STYLES FOR NOTES*. If people are going to check her notes, she may have to demonstrate that the style she has chosen works for her. Otherwise, if the notes are purely for her later use, she is free to use whichever style suits her best.

STYLES FOR NOTES: p 316

6.1 Making notes and *THINKING PREFERENCES*

Making notes is one of the stages of the *MODEL FOR LEARNING* in which *THINKING PREFERENCES* can play an important part. If your student has a preference for visual processing, her notes are likely to use visual symbols and ideas. If her preference is more strongly verbal, her notes will be based on words and language.

MODEL FOR LEARNING: p 145

THINKING PREFERENCES: p 72

The kinaesthetic component comes from the action in making the notes and any way that the kinaesthetic sense has been added, see *EXAMPLES: ADDING KINAESTHETIC SENSE*, below.

The need for a framework, or the logic of the topic, will come from the organisation of the notes.

The other *THINKING PREFERENCES* influence the perspective and content of the notes. Your student can use knowledge of her *THINKING PREFERENCES* to add details that will make the information more meaningful to her, see *STORY: THINKING PREFERENCES ADDED TO NOTES*, next page.

THINKING PREFERENCES: p 72

Notes taken by different people from a single presentation of information are likely to vary depending on people's interests and experiences, both of which could be coloured by their *THINKING PREFERENCES*. Whatever her *THINKING PREFERENCES*, your student needs to make sure she is getting all the necessary information and not just what is interesting to her.

KEY WORDS: p 176

Using the *KEY WORDS* exercise should help her to distinguish the most important points and avoid her feeling the need to write down every word because she doesn't know which are the most important.

Working to her strengths will make the tasks of taking and making notes much more enjoyable for your student and therefore easier to recall.

Examples: Adding kinaesthetic sense

One person liked gym. She would actually do cartwheels while working on one part of a subject, headstands on another, somersaults on a third, etc. Then in exams she just remembered the movement used while making notes and revising and all the information came to her mind.

Others take their notes for a walk, usually on a route they know well. They then mentally attach information from the notes to different objects along the walk: trees, gate posts, bus stops, etc. To recall the information they mentally go along the route to find it. The initial walk can be real or imaginary.

Rooms or places can be used in the same way[1] to create a holding system for information. Changing the season or the decoration can be a way of expanding the possibilities.

MAKE UP A STORY shows how one student linked marketing information to an imaginary walk. It is another example of adding the kinaesthetic sense to notes.

MAKE UP A STORY: p 319

Story: Thinking preferences added to notes

An engineering student was making notes eight months before her final exams and wanted to use the best methods for her. Her thinking preferences already discovered were:

- holistic thinking, especially overviews without details
- her own experience (kinaesthetic) was a key to memory especially when used with analogies that caught her attention
- she liked looking for similarities and patterns that could aid classification (Multiple Intelligence, Naturalist)
- verbal skills suggest rhymes would work, see below
- visual memory was good to use.

---

[1] Romans used to mentally hang information about the room where they were speaking. Then they would say, "In the first place, ...; in the second place, ...".

Way forward:

- to work from the overview of each topic on one page

- to make sure everything, overview and further details, was noted in a way that caught her attention

- to use:
  - analogies and her classifying strengths
  - word play and visual strategies
  - all with personal experience attached wherever possible.

Story: Architecture in mind maps

One student put a whole year's architecture modules in mind maps that he put on his walls. He found he had to remember only one key idea on each map and then he could remember all the rest of the map.

Example: A rhyme, almost a rap, for the kings and queens of England from 1066

Willie   Willie   Harry   Steve
Harry   Dick   John   Harry 3
1 2 3 Neds   Richard 2
Harry 4 5 6   then who?
Edward 4 5   then Dick the bad
Harrys twain   then Ned the lad
Mary   Bessie   James the vain
Charlie   Charlie   then James again
William & Mary   and Anna Gloria
4 Georges   William   and Victoria
Ned   George   Ned   and George again
Now Bessie 2   and that's the end.

There are many different adaptations of these ideas, including using objects. Any system used should be one that resonates with the way your student thinks. She is not adding extra detail to remember, she is adding something that enables her to remember all of it much more readily.

6.2 Language and *Thinking Preferences*

The language your student uses could reflect her preference for using visual, verbal or kinaesthetic processes. It could reflect any other thinking preferences that she has. Because notes are taken when she is thinking about something other than the notes, namely the subject of the notes, the notes can show more of her thinking preferences, see the *Key Point Box* below.

Key point: Different language used to describe notes

One student **saw** how he could use colour to make his notes dynamic.   visual

Another could **tell** she didn't like colour, but singing them **sounded** attractive. verbal

A third **felt** encouraged that his own experience would be so helpful.   kinaesthetic

A fourth **understood** how to structure her notes.   rationale

---

6.3 Humour

Humour is well worth using in notes, if possible. It can make the ideas much more memorable; the dog is more memorable sitting on the bike in *Figure 7.1*.

Any form of humour can be used, so long as it comes easily to your student and supports what she is trying to remember. It is not working if the humour is remembered and the information it is attached to is forgotten.

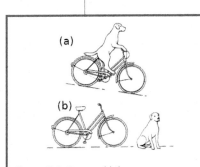

Figure 7.1 Dog and bike
a) connected; b) disconnected
(Russell, 1979)[2]

---

[2] Figure used with permission from Peter Russell and Routledge.

7 Styles for notes

Styles of notes need to be demonstrated rather than discussed, and the impact will vary from person to person, for example:

- many people have no response to using colour; others are very enthusiastic about the difference it makes

- some people would find images of rooms in different conditions a delight to play with, as in *EXAMPLES: ADDING KINAESTHETIC SENSE;* for others, it would be a huge extra effort.

EXAMPLES: ADDING KINAESTHETIC SENSE: p 312

Key point: Permission to think well

When I take a person through a range of styles there will often be the reaction: "I used to do that, but it didn't seem right, as an adult." Or "I always wanted to do that, but didn't feel I had permission."

The choice of style will be particular to each individual student. Encourage your student to try some of the styles she doesn't immediately feel drawn to; she may find she can adapt them to make them work well for her and then she has a different way of creating notes in her repertoire.

Key point: Use interesting but unimportant topics for new techniques

I usually suggest that students try new ideas on something that isn't essential to them, but is interesting. If they are trying a new technique and worrying about getting everything, they will not give the new way a fair trial.

Key points: The styles of notes covered

Verbal:
Lists with clear headings
Annotating notes
Make up a story
Mnemonics (ⓖ p 575)
Singing or talking to a recording
          device
Use music
Tabular notes

Visual:
Mind map
Symbols, including those from
          diagrams
Sections or words highlighted
Colour to separate ideas
Flow chart
Diagrams
Pictures
Index cards
Drawings
Creating blocks by adding borders

Myers-Briggs Personality Type and making notes

Examples: Verbal, visual and
Myers-Briggs Personality Type and making notes

The different styles are discussed below, with examples and suggestions for using them, and with comments about their use.

The blue line outlining the examples is used in the rest of the chapter, but the example logo is not.

7.1 Verbal

Lists with clear headings	Some people write fairly full notes. The use of clear headings helps to make it obvious what the main theme is and when the theme has changed. People develop their own shorthand symbols to reduce the number of words they write; e.g. → for 'leads to'. People can often use indentation from the margin to indicate a change in the level of hierarchy of ideas.

Annotating notes If your student likes writing notes on sheets of paper or in a notebook, it can be useful to have a margin in which she specifies the topic of each note.	Identifying the issues as she works should keep your student actively engaged with the subject. The annotation means she can more easily scan her notes to find information as she needs it later. If she is systematic about the words she uses for the issues and she takes notes on to a computer, she can use the sort facilities to gather the issues together. She should have a column for the page number as well, in case she needs to consult the source again.
Thick and thin nibs Some people have pens which have two writing orientations, one giving a thick line and one a thin line. The thick is used for the major ideas and the thin for the less important ones.	The process of deciding which to use means the person is actively engaged with the subject, which is an added bonus, not an extra task; it will keep her alert.

Make up a story

A module about marketing was put into stories.

This story shows the contrasts between local shops and supermarkets:

A person went to visit a friend in a town flat[1] and they went out for a walk. They passed Mr G's local shop[2] and decided to buy something for tea. As they went in, they saw Mr G talking[3] to a customer. As they walked round, they saw sales promotions[4] and the way the shelves[5] were stacked. As they came back to the counter, they saw the ham on special offer[6] and they noticed that Mr G was packing up a box[7].

See the comparison of the same information in *TABULAR NOTES*, p 321.

The issues in the story are:

1) local shops are in residential areas

2) whether shopping is planned or spur of the moment

3) how well shop keepers know their customers

4) price differentials

5) stock variety and turn over

6) specialities

7) the development of home deliveries from a time when local shops delivered to house-bound customers to the current time when working families use the internet to organise home deliveries from supermarkets.

Story: Marketing module in stories

The student who came with the problems about his marketing module had passed all the other modules using textbooks and lectures. The marketing module should have been the easiest because he had been employed for several years in marketing and knew the issues from experience. Trying to learn it in a theoretical way just didn't work. He was working for the last possible re-sit and would fail the whole degree if a solution couldn't be found. His tutor was very concerned about his situation. Once the story above had evolved, he put the whole module into stories and passed his degree.

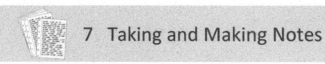

Mnemonics Mnemonics are sounds, words or phrases used to recall something.	Some people make up their own mnemonics; some people find they can remember them but not make them up.

Examples:

To remember the order of the planets:
See My Very Easy Method Just Set Up Nine Planets
Sun, Mercury, Venus, Earth, Mars, Jupiter, Saturn, Uranus, Neptune, Pluto.

To remember palaeontology eras[3]:
Peter Piper Met the Canadian Team in Quebec
Precambrian Paleozoic Mesozoic Cenozoic Tertiary Quaternary

Singing or talking to a recording device	People who struggle with writing are often recommended to use recording devices to dictate their notes as a first step. In doing so, some have found that the act of recording their notes has been all that is necessary to get the information into long-term memory. One student got so bored with talking to the recorder that she sang, and again that was all that was needed to fix the information in long-term memory.
Use music	Some people like to have music playing as they work and have discovered that they easily remember what music was playing during work on a particular topic; then recalling the music brings back all the work done on the subject.

---

[3] Palaeontology is the study of fossils to find out about life on earth and the structure of rocks. The eras are time spans that are defined by specified events.

Tabular notes

Tabular notes are particularly useful when comparisons are to be made. A different student would have used a table for the marketing example in *MAKE UP A STORY* above.

MAKE UP A STORY: p 319

Tables (see *MAKE UP A STORY* above for a comparison with a different style)

Issues	Local shops	Supermarkets
Position	Residential areas	Out of town
Timing	Spur of the moment as well as planned	Planned
Relationships	Shop keepers can know customers quite well	Staff unlikely to know customers
Price	Tend to be higher	Can reduce costs by bulk buying and through loss leaders
Stock	Range of goods might be limited and might run out of items	Wider range of goods, larger premises for storage
Specialities	Known specialities, often home made	Homemade quality not often available
Home deliveries	Customer can ring and get personal service when ordering for a home delivery	Online shopping is impersonal

Tables can be used to gather information from different sources. If your student has several books or articles to read about a particular subject, identifying the issues and then making notes in a table form works well. *B5-8 - RECORDING TEMPLATES – 1-4* can all be used for recording and collating information in this way.

TEMPLATES

COMPANION @ WEBSITE

7.2 Visual

Mind maps

There are several examples of mind maps in this book, including *Figure* 7.2.

There are several software packages for making mind maps.

Advantages: your student can use space, colour, shapes, images to show meaning and relationships; information doesn't get camouflaged by words; there's usually room to go back and add new ideas as her understanding increases.

Not all dyslexic/ SpLD people can work with mind maps.

Some can only work with ones that look neat and they find many of the software packages produce suitable maps.

For some people the spatial layout is of prime importance, and they can only use those software packages that allow the user to determine positions.

For some, creating the mind map by hand is a crucial part of the process.

Symbols, including those from diagrams

All sorts of symbols can be used to replace words.

Arrows are very common, but your student can use anything that has a definite meaning for her; her symbols don't need to be understood by anyone else.

Sections or words highlighted

In this book, words referring to *Thinking Preferences* have been highlighted to catch the attention of readers.

Highlighting is used in the examples in *Skilled Thinking*, p 167, to pick out the different thinking processes involved.

Many people highlight sections as they read. One common provision for dyslexic/ SpLD students is a book allowance so that they can annotate the material as they read; used well this is a good strategy.

The danger is that they end up with everything highlighted and their understanding is not assisted in any way. Highlighting needs to be used effectively, with discrimination. Being able to sort out *Main Themes vs. Detail*, p 178, helps in using highlighting well.

Example: Sections highlighted

The *EXPANDED MAP OF THIS CHAPTER, FIGURE 7.2*, has different symbols to add a visual element to the words. It is using colour coding to highlight the different sections.

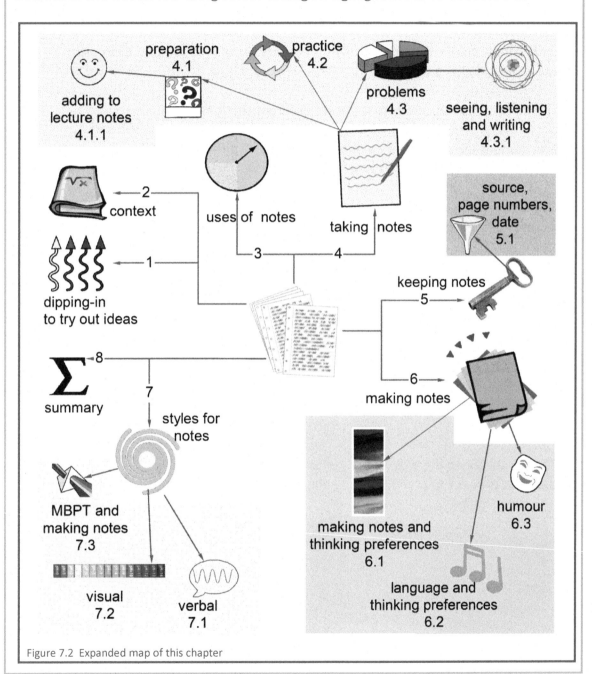

Figure 7.2 Expanded map of this chapter

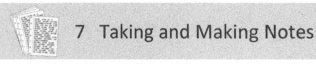

Colour to separate ideas

Sometimes it is purely a question of separating one idea from another
    sometimes the colours used have significance
    sometimes the order of the colours is important.

In this book, colour is used to show different types of information: examples, exercises, insights and tips.

The mind maps use colour to separate different sections.

One student used different coloured paper for his different subjects; many use different coloured ring binders to contain their notes.

Some people use pens with 4 colours so that they can separate ideas even during lectures or meetings.

The *INDEX CARD* example uses colour to separate ideas, see *FIGURE 7.7*, p 329.

Colour used to separate maths concepts

One maths student made his notes and then put coloured boxes round different aspects of maths.

There is a logic to the way he used the order of the rainbow in his colour coding.

Red = definitions
Orange = proofs
Yellow = examples
Green = lemmas (statements used in proofs)
Blue = propositions
Purple = theorems
Pink = remarks and corollaries (something that
    follows on from the work just done)

Example: colour used to sort out spelling

as in

school

foreign origin
Greek letter
(has parallels
with Mozart)

origin:
single Greek
letter —
often
'ph' for 'f' sound

schizophrenia

to split   mind

used in other
combinations

schizophrenia — the disorder

schizophrenic — adjective
(describing word)

schizophrene — a person with the
disorder

different 'en' sounds

same spelling shows common root

Figure 7. 3 Schizophrenia: coloured spelling

FIGURE 7.3 shows colour used to annotate notes for learning to spell 'schizophrenia'.

It was important to include the family of words: to see the constant spelling and know the different sounds.

Flow charts

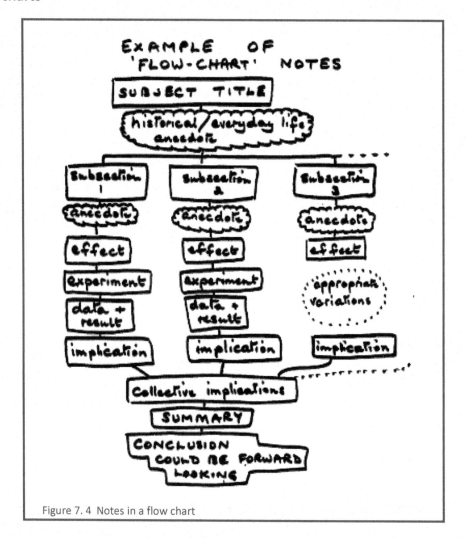

Figure 7. 4 Notes in a flow chart

Flow charts are useful to show how different stages of something relate to each other, for example:

- how your student progresses through a project
- how different attitudes influence a sports club's decisions
- how a new drug becomes licensed for use.

FIGURE 7.4 shows the patterns of information in a textbook.

Diagrams

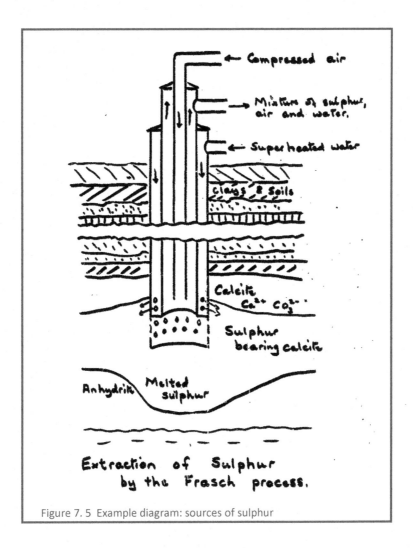

Figure 7. 5 Example diagram: sources of sulphur

Diagrams contain a lot of information; they may have no words, or they can have labels for significant parts, or they can be accompanied by an explanation. They can be much easier to remember than equivalent text.

Several diagrams have been used in the book.

For example, *FIGURE 4.4 GOOD PARAGRAPH SHAPE*, p 250. Once your student understands the explanation of the diagram, all she needs to remember is the diagram. She will then have all the ideas about looking for main themes in paragraphs as a strategy for reading; she won't need to remember the words.

Pictures

Story: Abstract concepts in concrete images

A group of students challenged me; they said I was talking of concrete ideas and their subjects were much more abstract. I looked along the shelves to find the most abstract subjects I could and came across *The Tao of Physics* by Fritjof Capra (1999). *Dualism in Eastern Mysticism and Quantum Physics* seemed a good representative of abstract ideas. FIGURE 7.6 shows how the abstract ideas can be represented by concrete objects and symbolism.

Capra (1999)

Abstract concepts in concrete images

Dualism in Eastern mysticism:
looking into a garden you can see:

- a healthy tree and a diseased one: good and evil

- daffodils tied to provide bulbs for next year: life and death

- runner beans growing up cane supports: male and female.

Dualism in quantum physics:

- in dreams you shift from one scene to another, the wavy line shifts the observer from garden to kitchen: wave and particle nature dualism

- the clock represents the 4th dimension, time, being added to the 3 dimensions of space

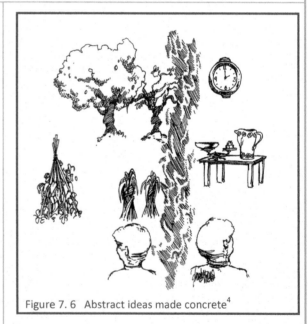

Figure 7. 6 Abstract ideas made concrete[4]

A different person would have other experiences to draw on; what matters is that the connections work for the person using them.

[4] Used with permission of the illustrator, Rory Walker.

- the scales represent the mass weight dualism
- the jug represents destructibility and non-destructibility, from a delightful scene in the film *Mon Oncle* in which Jacques Tati accidentally knocks over a jug that bounces and then experiments with a cut-glass jug, which doesn't bounce.

Index cards

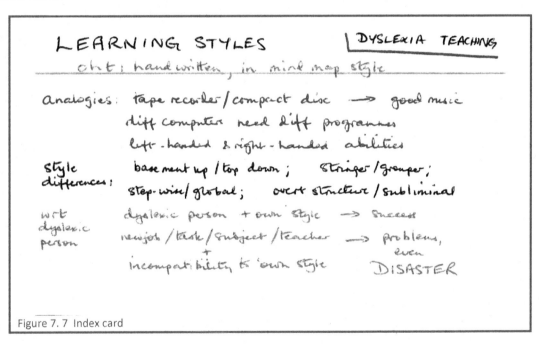

Figure 7. 7 Index card

Index cards are often used as part of memorising routines or for revision. The size means the information is reduced to the essentials. The cards can be carried around and used in spare moments. They can have a prompt on one side and the information to be remembered on the other.

This example also has the topics separated by colour.

Drawings

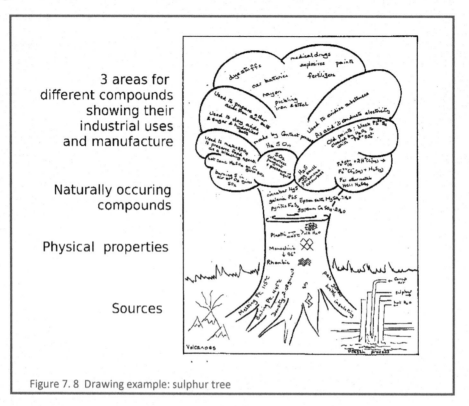

3 areas for
different compounds
showing their
industrial uses
and manufacture

Naturally occuring
compounds

Physical properties

Sources

Figure 7. 8 Drawing example: sulphur tree

A drawing need not be related to the topic it is used for. It just needs to work for the person using it.

This tree has the information needed about sulphur for a 5th-form exam. The analogy behind the drawing is the parallel between a tree getting nutrients from the ground and the supply of sulphur being crucial for the use of sulphur.

The trunk of the tree supports the crown of the tree; the physical properties of sulphur determine how it can be used; and the naturally occurring forms are closely linked to the physical properties.

The crown of the tree has three separate areas containing three sulphur chemicals and related information. These chemicals are like the leaves of the tree, they disperse as they are used in industry.

Holding the information in a visual way can keep it all together and make it easy to remember.

Creating blocks by adding borders

The effect of having borders has to be seen; trying to describe it often does not convey the impact it makes on those it helps. I have a sample page without borders and then put a transparency with the borders on top. The act of covering the original page increases the impact.

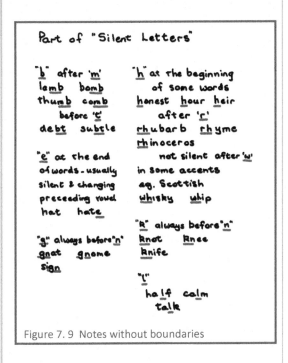

Figure 7. 9 Notes without boundaries

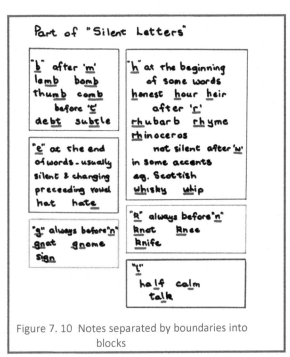

Figure 7. 10 Notes separated by boundaries into blocks

When borders work, the page on the right is a relief. The information has been simplified into 6 blocks and is just visually much more acceptable.

Blocking can also be used around certain words within a section of text. It is used in *EXAMPLE: AN EXAM QUESTION ABOUT ATMOSPHERIC MANAGEMENT*.

EXAMPLE: AN EXAM QUESTION ABOUT ATMOSPHERIC MANAGEMENT: p 192

The same separation of ideas can be achieved by colouring in the blocks, as has been done for the *EXPANDED MAP OF THIS CHAPTER*.

EXPANDED MAP OF THIS CHAPTER: p 323.

7.3   Myers-Briggs Personality Type and making notes

Myers-Briggs Personality Type (MBPT) theory includes contrasting pairs of mental functions which can lead to knowledge being presented in very different ways.

Many practical (S) people have to gain qualifications and their courses require work written about theories (N). Often their courses include work experiences which have to be written up according to theory or *National Guidelines*. The students with S in their type have difficulty relating the practical work to the theories.

One way to deal with the problem is to list their work experience chronologically on one side of a piece of paper, and to list the theories, models and concepts of the course on the other side. They then draw lines across the page to show which of the experiences is relevant to each concept of the course. I work with pencil so that we can rub out lines and re-draw them until the links are easy to follow. Colour, symbols or letters can be used to code the themes and then mark the events. Letters and columns have been used in the example below because the line-drawing method doesn't work on this size page.

If the concepts are listed in a useful order for a report, these two lists then become a report plan.

In the example below, the student can decide the order she wants to write the report, then follow down the columns in turn and make sure that she has included everything in the accepted structure.

Myers-Briggs Personality Type (MBPT): p 76

Example: Practical vs. theoretical, MBPT S vs. N

Chronological order of events to interview a client	These columns show the links						Course theoretical issues
	A	B	C	D	E	F	A-F indicate groups in essay
talking to supervisor beforehand						✓	current National Guidelines of professional practice likely to include:
collecting client's notes	✓			✓	✓		A latest model for the care of clients
reading through notes	✓		✓	✓	✓		A data protection
travel to appointment					✓		B constructing questionnaires
greeting client					✓		B interview techniques
consent forms filled in	✓						client's condition:
questionnaire for interview		✓					C clinical description
discussion during interview		✓					C full range of possible symptoms
other issues around interview					✓		C impacts on life style
summary for client	✓						D medical solutions
updating records	✓						D equipment solutions
follow-up work	✓		✓				D career solutions
contacting other professionals	✓		✓	✓			E client's details: name, address, age, etc.
setting out programme for client			✓	✓			F personal reflection:
feedback to client		✓		✓	✓		F organisation
summary of what happens next	✓		✓	✓			F engaging with supervisor
reflection with supervisor					✓		F disability issues

8   Summary: taking and making notes

Summary: Taking and making notes

- *TAKING NOTES* is the initial stage of capturing ideas.

- Making notes is a second stage of creating notes that either others can use or your student can use at a later date.

- Several skills can be learnt that help with *TAKING NOTES*.

- It is worth developing strategies for keeping notes and finding information again.

- Good preparation facilitates taking and making notes.

- Practising taking notes while listening to a recording allows your student to review her strategies and progress.

- Picking out the main theme of each note helps clarify the notes.

- The purpose of the notes will influence the style that can be used and how the notes are kept.

- Knowing a wide range of styles that can be used allows greater choice.

- It is worth your student experimenting with several styles, and adapting them, to find which ones resonate with her.

- New techniques and styles of notes are best trialled on topics that are not important while still being interesting. If the topics are important, students may become anxious that the new style won't work and they will stop really trying it out.

TAKING NOTES: p 305

- Using the style that suits your student is not adding extra details for her to remember; it is giving her easier ways to use notes and remember them.

- Accommodation in respect of notes may be needed in some education and employment situations.

References

Capra, Fritjof, 1999, *The Tao of Physics,* Shambhala Publications, MA
Russell, Peter, 1979, *The Brain Book: Know Your Own Mind and How to Use It*, Routledge, London

Website information

Series website: www.routledge.com/cw/stacey

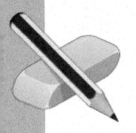

8 Writing

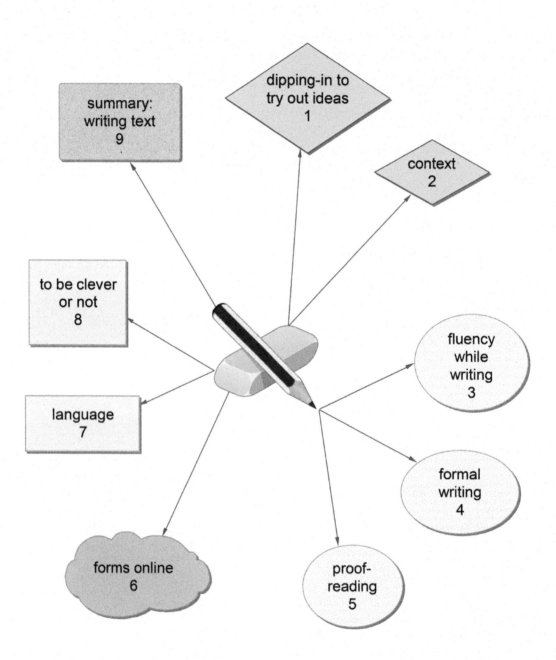

summary:
writing text
9

dipping-in to
try out ideas
1

context
2

to be clever
or not
8

fluency
while
writing
3

language
7

formal
writing
4

forms online
6

proof-
reading
5

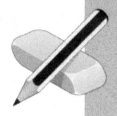

Contents

List of key points and summaries

K = key points
S = summaries

Templates on the website

TEMPLATES

Information for non-linear readers

Before the context of the *Useful Preface* and *Chapters 1* and *2*, there is information that I hope will help non-linear readers as they approach the chapters. For chapters 4 – 14, this information would be identical except for which parts to scan and read. I have put all the information together into *Guidance for Non-Linear Readers, Chapter 3*. It is worth reading *Chapter 3* at some stage of working with this book.

Guidance for Non-Linear Readers: p 222

1 Dipping-in to try out ideas: reading and scanning lists

Start with *Dipping-in to Try Out Ideas: General Pattern*.
Read:

> *Context*, p 339

> *Fluency while Writing*, p 340

Dipping-in to Try Out Ideas: General Pattern: p 228

Scan:

> *Formal Writing*, p 345

> all the *Summary* and *Key Point Boxes*, as listed above

> *Language*, p 355

1.1 Key points: for policy-makers and general readers

Key points: For policy-makers and general readers

- There are a variety of influences that will help a dyslexic/ SpLD person to write as well as possible.

- Having a good pattern to follow helps dyslexic/ SpLD people produce good work.

- The difficulties can be different for the separate SpLDs.

- It is important to listen for any problems not related to writing that may be hampering progress.

- Help should be given with kindness and with respect for the difficulties being experienced.

2 Context

This chapter is about the techniques of writing, which include:

- many issues that influence the ease with which your student can write and express his ideas
- the components of the final document
- proof-reading.

The chapter also includes:

- dealing with forms online
- teaching language through your student's writing tasks
- some thoughts about your student trying to be too clever.

The chapter assumes that:

- your student has decided on his goal, see *Goals for Written Work*
- he has planned what he wants to write about, see *Planning Related to Knowledge*
- his notes are in a style he finds easy to use, see *Styles for Notes*.

See *Goals for Written Work:* p 187

Planning Related to Knowledge: p 202

Styles for Notes: p 316

Key points: To help with techniques of writing

Your student will benefit from knowing:

- how he writes well
  - what motivates him
  - what his *Thinking Preferences* are
  - how the environment affects his ability to write
  - what he uses to write
  - the style of writing that he likes
- what components are needed in the document he is writing
- how to proof-read effectively.

Thinking Preferences: p 72

Key point: Difficulty with writing

Getting their ideas into coherent text can be one of the most difficult tasks for some dyslexic/ SpLD people. The suggestions in this chapter will go some way to providing a framework for writing, but when there is a deep-seated barrier to the process of writing it may need to be addressed first, see *DON'T WORRY, WE KNOW YOU CAN'T DO THIS* and *BEHIND THE OBVIOUS*.

DON'T WORRY, WE KNOW YOU CAN'T DO THIS: p 59

BEHIND THE OBVIOUS: p 64

3 Fluency while writing

One of the common characteristics of dyslexia/ SpLD is that writing is not consistently fluent. Sometimes, your student can find the words he wants; his writing captures exactly what he wants to say, and is as beautiful as he wants it to be. Other times, he struggles. The words don't come, let alone flow; his ideas seem to disintegrate.

There are many issues that make the difference between writing with ease and struggling to produce anything. The ones I've found to be most important are how clearly your student has sorted out his ideas and the details of his environment, including the implements he is using. Other individual requirements also occur and you need to work with your student to find out anything else that is interrupting his ease of writing.

Once your student has found his most fluent way of writing he can record everything that is contributing to the situation. He could use *B6 - RECORDING TEMPLATE - 2* with the headings given in the margin. The code in column D would briefly indicate what he has written in B, e.g. 'ideas' could be the code for anything that related to the way he is handling his ideas or 'strat' could be used for strategies such as colour coding. Being systematic in this way will allow him to group together details for each influence on his writing-fluency.

Some practical details should be relatively easy to put in place whenever he is writing.

TEMPLATES

B6 - RECORDING TEMPLATE - 2:
Title= document
A = section
B = what is helping fluency
C = why it's helping
D = code (see text)

Other details may be more difficult to manage especially when he is struggling with writing. The ideas from *USING CHALLENGES* can be used to transfer approaches from times when he is writing fluently to those times when he is struggling.

USING CHALLENGES: p 80

3.1 Clarity of ideas

Even when your student has identified his goal and has a clear plan of what he wants to write, the writing process can still show areas which he finds hard to engage with.

THINKING PREFERENCES, and the motivation that accompanies some of them, can be missing from goal-setting and planning. It is almost as if the missing element then blocks the writing process. The problems and solutions are particular to the student concerned and need to be uncovered by exploring *BEHIND THE OBVIOUS.* The *EXAMPLES: STUDENTS USING THEIR THINKING PREFERENCES TO ASSIST THEIR WRITING*, below, shows some of the strategies that have been used.

THINKING PREFERENCES: p 72

BEHIND THE OBVIOUS: p 64

Examples: Students using their *THINKING PREFERENCES* to assist their writing

Thinking Preference	strategy
visual sense	created visual images for all his ideas
MBPT – feeling	had a frieze of people from magazines to assist his report writing
practical kinaesthetic	worked out the usefulness of different section
MBPT – feeling	maintained an advocacy role for a powerless group

The following *Tip Box* also has some useful questions and suggestions to help your student to assess the way he is writing..

Tips: Writing fluently

- Use your *Thinking Preferences* to maintain fluency.

- Is your main interest, or motivation, engaged with the piece you are writing? If necessary, change something so that it is.

- When you started, did you have a purpose? See *Goals for Written Work*. If not, has one developed while you have been working? You may not be aware of a shift in purpose and you may be writing in a way that doesn't fit the new one. If you brainstorm around your progress, you could find something is preventing you from writing as well as you know you can.

- Keep referring back to your plan and title; doing so can help you to keep focused. Some people put the title on the desk in front of them, or in the header of their document.

- On the other hand, for some the preparation is useful work but if they keep checking too frequently, they feel trapped. Find out the level of checking that helps you.

- If a piece of writing feels really easy, it may mean you have gone off on a tangent and you are writing everything you know about a topic. You could then find that most of it has to be deleted, since it isn't relevant (even though it is absolutely fascinating).

Thinking Preferences: p 72

Goals for Written Work: p 187

3.2 Writing style

When helping students with the way they write, I have found I need to be very sensitive. Many have a long history of painful experiences and it is not easy for them to make changes. You need to consider the way they set about writing and the way they express their ideas.

For the initial writing, your student needs to be comfortable with his approach and confident that he will make progress.

Different approaches may be:

- long-hand or straight on to an electronic device

- being neat or having a rough style

- fast to get ideas down or slower to be accurate

- sort out details as he writes or leave a lot of sorting to later

- other, work with your student to identify anything else that is important.

Your student may need to give himself permission to work the way that suits him and not try to follow other people's ways.

Your student might have definite ideas about the final style that he wants for his documents. One way he can decide on his own style of writing is to notice those books and articles that he finds easy to read, and then analyse what it is that helps him to read them. He can then include these elements in his writing. He should find out, by trial and error, when is the best time to pay attention to the style. If he works on it too early he may spend time perfecting text he later discards.

Even when he is writing informally to a friend, he wants the friend to understand what he writes, so thinking about his style of writing can help his informal communication.

3.3   Practical elements of writing

At a practical level, the tools and materials that your student uses can make a significant difference to the ease with which he can write, as can the environment around him.

Among the practical, physical elements to consider are:

- a favourite pen or pencil
- a particular colour for the paper; lined or unlined; texture of the paper
- what e-device to use
- the colours of text or background on any e-device
- whether to stand or sit
- whether looking out of a door or window is important
- the colour of the furniture around him.

It is worth paying attention to the details of the writing implements and paper that your student uses. A thicker pen with a non-slippery grip takes some of the tension out of handwriting. It is possible to buy grips to slide onto pens or pencils to make them easier to hold. He may find he prefers to write on some types of paper and not others. Encourage him to respect any details like this that make writing easier and more fluent for him.

Using assistive software[1] and other devices can make a considerable difference to the ease with which a dyslexic/ SpLD person can write. Some talk more fluently than they write and recording what they want to say is often the first stage of getting their ideas written. Your student should try different technologies to find the ones that will help him.

Being comfortable while he uses a computer will also help: the organisation of the desk he works at, the computer screen colours, the font style and size, see *READING FROM A COMPUTER, E-READING* for other suggestions about customising the computer environment.

READING FROM A COMPUTER, E-READING: p 240

Your student may find standing to work helps him to remain alert, see *BEING ALERT*.

BEING ALERT: p 91

---

[1] Assistive technology: spell checkers, homophone checking, text-to-speech, thesaurus, meanings of punctuation marks

The *ENVIRONMENT* around his workspace can have a significant impact on his abilities to write. It is not worth struggling with physical constraints when altering them can help him write more effectively.

ENVIRONMENT: p 70

Examples: Impact of the environment

One student felt trapped as he tried to write. He moved his desk so that he could look out of the open door to feel the freedom of the world beyond the room, then he was able to write.

Other students have been affected by the colour around them.
One put yellow objects and paper around her room.
Another painted her study room purple.
Both then felt more comfortable and able to write.

4   Formal writing

This section lists many forms of writing then discusses components of formal writing. The *SUMMARY: FORMS OF WRITING*, below, lists the different forms and indicates which components of formal writing apply to each of them.

Short and informal communication is not covered beyond a reminder for your student to think of the long-term implications of what he writes and who is allowed to read it.

Formal letters, emails, essays and essay-type exam answers are relatively short pieces of writing with a length of a few pages.

Reports, dissertations and theses are much longer. They can be regarded as a series of essays that belong together. Often, they are easier to write when they are divided into sections with a defined topic.

Summary: Forms of writing

Letters, emails – informal

- worth your student being clear about what he wants to say and who is reading the letter or email

Letters, emails – formal

- a first line in bold acts as a title for a letter; the subject line acts as one for an email
- separate paragraphs for different points
- summary or clear request for action

Essays

- all of this chapter applies, except the abstract and executive summary;
- the bibliography and references may merge into one set

Exam answers in the style of essays

- usually, these should be as near to an essay as possible bearing in mind that under most conditions, your student can't look something up

Articles

- all of this chapter applies, except the executive summary

Reports

- all of this chapter applies, though possibly not the abstract
- often there needs to be an executive summary which picks out the main points with recommended actions

Dissertations, theses

- all of this chapter applies, except the executive summary
- check the instructions for the work to see whether an abstract is required or not

In the discussion of the component parts of a piece of writing, 'essay' is used to cover all the different forms.

Summary: Components of formal writing

- title
- structure
- introduction (often re-written when the rest is finished)
- introduction to the subject
- body of the essay
- conclusion
- summary
- executive summary
- abstract
- references
- bibliography
- layout.

Title

A well-chosen title can give a good focus for the essay. Sometimes the title is given; sometimes it is in the form of a question. If a title isn't given it can be useful to create one.

Structure

1. The basic structure of an essay is: introduction; several paragraphs (the body of the essay) picking up topics as ordered in the introduction; summary; and conclusion. "Say what you are going to do. Do it. Say what you have done. Finish off."

2. For clarity, headings can be used and different points can be numbered and indented. Even if no headings are allowed in the final work, your student may find their use keeps his writing on track during the early stages.

Introduction

N.B. This may not be an introduction to the subject; it might be an introduction to this particular essay.

1. The introduction is used to tell the reader what is coming in the complete essay. It should clearly contain all the major topics of the essay (your student should check with his tutors as the introduction is different for some subjects, for example, history, philosophy and medicine).

2. The introduction usually has some order, such as: the problem is set out (very briefly), or the question restated; topics ("topics" means whatever is appropriate to the problem and the subject your student is studying) are listed in the order of importance; the conclusion which the essay leads to is briefly stated.

3. The introduction is often written properly when the essay is otherwise finished. A good draft introduction is sometimes needed at the outset because your student needs the order of the topics to write the essay.

Introduction to the subject

Your student will need to introduce the subject, say why it is interesting and how he is going to write about it. Where this will be done and how much depth is needed should be decided during the planning stage of the work. The introduction to the subject varies from being a couple of sentences right at the beginning of an essay to being a complete chapter in a thesis or project report.

Body of the essay

1. Topics are discussed in the order they are set out in the introduction, with one paragraph, at least, per topic. Use all the topics in the introduction.

2   Each paragraph: First sentence says what the paragraph is about. The rest of the paragraph expands that sentence as is appropriate to the essay. The final sentence draws the paragraph together and/or links it to the next paragraph. This is the diamond shape in *FIGURE 4.4: GOOD PARAGRAPH SHAPE*.

FIGURE 4.4: GOOD PARAGRAPH SHAPE: p 250

An alternative is to use the mnemonic PEAR, which stands for:

P	make your <u>P</u>oint
E	<u>E</u>vidence
A	<u>A</u>rgument or <u>A</u>nalysis (depending on type of essay)
R	<u>R</u>eflect or lead on to next pa<u>R</u>agraph

3   If your student is one of those dyslexic/ SpLD people whose focus of attention wanders, it will be especially important for him to keep asking himself "Can the reader follow?" "Have I missed out steps in the logical sequence?"

Summary

Fairly briefly, your student should pick out the main threads and say what he has done.
Notes 2 and 3 of *BODY OF THE ESSAY* also apply.

In a formal letter, it is often a good idea to have a summary which states, diplomatically, exactly what he wants the other person to do. *DIPLOMACY CAN BE HARD* for dyslexic/ SpLD students and may require active learning.

DIPLOMACY CAN BE HARD: next box below

Insight: Diplomacy can be hard

Some dyslexic/ SpLD find it quite hard to be diplomatic. The thought of writing extra words is not a good one; several of us wish others wouldn't be so WORDY! Our succinct way of expressing ourselves can be misinterpreted as unsociable, unfriendly or undiplomatic.

Conclusion

The conclusion shows where the essay has led to, or where the subject of the essay might lead to in the future.

Notes 2 and 3 of *BODY OF THE ESSAY* also apply.

Not every essay needs both a summary and a conclusion; your student can combine both aspects together in one section.

Executive summary

Large reports often start with an executive summary which summarises the major points of the report together with actions that need to be taken. The idea being that busy executives can read this summary and know the broad outline of the issues and the recommendations.

Rewriting the introduction

Once the essay is finished, check whether the order of the topics in the essay is the same as that indicated in the introduction. If these two orders are not the same, change one of them. Check that the introduction, summary and conclusion are consistent. Alter whatever is necessary; normally it is the introduction.

Some people only start with a very sketchy introduction, because they know they will re-write it once the first draft has been completed.

Abstract

Usually publications, long essays and projects have an abstract after the title. The abstract contains the main topics with no details, though it may contain succinct results. The purpose of the abstract is to tell the reader what points follow in the essay.

Tip: Introduction vs. abstract

In the introduction your student tells the reader why the subject is interesting and how he is going to present the discussion.

In the abstract, he gives a factual list of the main points.

References

Any idea or text or picture, etc. that comes from someone else's work needs to be referenced properly. There are conventions for the way references are given; once your student understands the conventions, references can be easier to use and to write. Your student should find out what convention his field uses and use that one. It is worth asking the library if they have a handout for the system he needs to use.

Tip: Collecting references

Collect your references as you go, with all the necessary details. Finding them at the end of a piece of work can be much more laborious.

Bibliography

A bibliography is a list of books which deal with the subject of the essay or which would give a reader more knowledge of the subject. In a course-essay or dissertation, the bibliography also shows the tutor the range of your student's reading.

Layout

Good layout, or presentation, improves the ease with which your student's essay can be read. Layout includes headings, paragraph spacing, use of numbering and indentations, and many other details of word-processing. To select a layout style, your student could look at those books or articles that he finds most easy to read and choose one as a model. One important principle is that the layout is consistent throughout the essay. When he finds a layout he likes, your student can create a template which he uses for all subsequent work. He can have templates for letters as well.

5 Proof-reading

Your student may do some proof-reading before he has produced a final draft.

He may find reading over what he wrote in a previous session acts as a *MIND SET* at the beginning of a new session and helps him to continue fluently.

MIND SET: p 158

He should probably guard against spending time perfecting his work; he may want to revise his work because his ideas develop as he writes.

The pattern of proof-reading set out in *FIGURE 8.1* is applicable at whatever stage the proof-reading is done.

Summary: Proof-reading

- Dyslexic/ SpLD people read their minds and not the words on the page.

- 24 hours or more time might be needed between writing and proof-reading.

- The time delay helps proof-reading because the ideas have had time to fade in the mind.

- Proof-reading needs to be prioritised: ideas, grammar and punctuation, then spelling.

- Assistive technology can read back.

- Recording while reading aloud, then listening works for some.

---

1 Allow at least 24 hours between finishing your essay and the final proof-reading. It seems to take time for dyslexic/ SpLD people to forget what they want to write, i.e. the ideas in their heads, and to see what they have actually written. You need to be able to see and read what you have actually written in order to proof-read it and to make the alterations that are necessary to convey your ideas effectively.

2 Allow time to elapse between sessions spent working on a draft; this will probably help the essay writing because you are allowing the ideas in your head to die down and not dominate your proof-reading.

3 Prioritise your proof-reading, see *FIGURE 8.1*. First, work on getting your ideas correct; then the structure of the piece of writing; then grammar and punctuation; and lastly spelling. There is no point in correcting spelling of sections that you are going to delete or re-write.

4 You can use a computer to read the text to you, or you can read it out loud. Reading it out loud might be helped by recording yourself and then listening as a separate task.

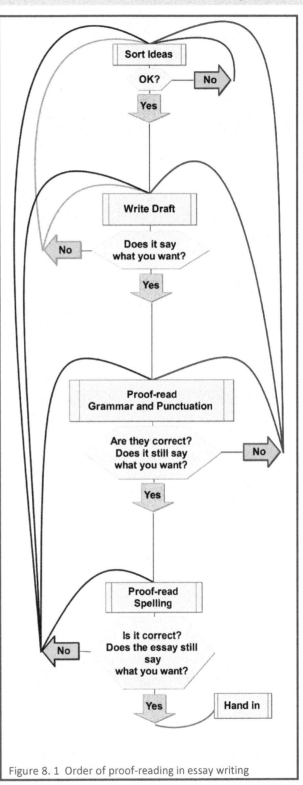

Figure 8. 1 Order of proof-reading in essay writing

6 Forms online

Filling in forms online is another task for which your student needs to observe very accurately what the problems are. For me one problem is that I'll click on a button before the meaning of the words has fully penetrated my mind. Other people find they don't know what to write; or that they spend time answering one part, say A, and then a later part alters what they should have put at A. Another irritating situation is to get to the end and find that several parts of the form didn't need to be filled in.

Use *Behind the Obvious* to help your student sort out the issues and how to solve them.

Behind the Obvious:
p 64

Tips: Tactics for dealing with forms online might include:

- Printing the form before your student fills it in.

- Reading all of it before he starts; this is often not possible, as he can't move on to another page without completing sections. He could try putting in fake answers or "temporary text as I need to read the form"! Doing so should enable him to move through the form, **just don't send or submit it**.

- Dividing his screen into two parts, one with the form and one with word processor for his answers. Copy and paste, or type, the questions into the word processor window; note any space or word limits. Then, when he has the whole form, he will be in a position to write the answers. Once he has finished them, he can copy and paste them into the online form.

- Asking a sympathetic person to help, one who is able to use most of the *General Approaches* to disentangling difficulties.

General Approaches:
p 81

---

7 Language

The way your student uses language alters the impact of his ideas. The following are some of the ways language can be problematic for dyslexic/ SpLD people. They have come to light while working on particular issues with individual students.

With most students, I do not mention these issues unless they become relevant to the student: it is confusing to have the solution to a problem that affects other people.

Key point: Listen for the real request for help

Your student may be aware that something is not working the way it should in his writing, but he may not be able to say exactly what is wrong.

As you give advice, listen to his reactions and monitor his ability to use your suggestions. Examples of ways writing can be undermined can be found in:

- second bullet point of *SOME UNOBVIOUS PROBLEMS* (starting: 'A student wanting writing strategies...')

- *DON'T WORRY, WE KNOW YOU CAN'T DO THIS*

- *INSIGHT: DIPLOMACY CAN BE HARD*.

If the standard writing techniques are not helping, use *METHODS OF EXPLORING BEHIND THE OBVIOUS* to help uncover underlying issues.

SOME UNOBVIOUS PROBLEMS: p 64

DON'T WORRY, WE KNOW YOU CAN'T DO THIS: p 59

INSIGHT: DIPLOMACY CAN BE HARD: p 349

METHODS OF EXPLORING BEHIND THE OBVIOUS: p 65

The order of words

The order of words can subtly alter the meaning of a sentence. For example, compare the following two sentences:

1. It helps to read all of a form before you start filling it in; online, this is <u>often not</u> possible, as you can't move on to another page without completing sections.

2. It helps to read all of a form before you start filling it in; online, this is <u>not often</u> possible, as you can't move on to another page without completing sections.

The only difference between 1) and 2) is that the order of 'not' and 'often' are reversed.
1) means: frequently you can't read all the form.
2) means: occasionally it is possible to read all the form.

The impact of the sentence is changed.
From the first, you don't expect to help yourself this way;
from the second, you look out for the opportunity to do so.

The tone of sentences

The following four sentences express a basic fact in different ways and each has a different impact. The context is that reading exam scripts helps a support tutor to uncover a student's real dyslexic/ SpLD problems in exams; and that reading the scripts is not possible.

Sentence stating fact	Impact
Exam Boards are often not willing to give permission for scripts to be seen.	The Exam Board is seen as obstructing progress.
You may not always persuade Exam Boards to let you read scripts.	You are seen as working for progress while the Exam Board is unwilling to help.
You may not always be able to read exam scripts.	A more neutral statement, but the focus is on the inability of the tutor to read the scripts.
Exam scripts may not be available for reading.	A neutral statement of the basic fact, with no reason given and no people mentioned.

Your student may need to consider how the tone he uses is received by his readers.

The main idea of a sentence

When the main idea of a sentence is put at the beginning of the sentence, it is easier to understand the meaning. *EXAMPLE: POSITION OF THE MAIN IDEA IN A SENTENCE* demonstrates moving the main idea of a sentence. The first sentence is the same in both A and B; the second sentence is different. The meanings of the second sentences are underlined; it is at the end in A and at the beginning in B.

Example: Position of the main idea in a sentence

A

It is worth distinguishing between kinaesthetic learning as a thinking preference, and learning-by-doing and taking-action. The chapter on *TAKING-ACTION* has an *INSIGHT BOX: PRACTICAL SCIENCE EXPERIMENT* to <u>draw out the distinctions</u>.

B

It is worth distinguishing between kinaesthetic learning as a thinking preference, and learning-by-doing and taking-action. The <u>distinctions are drawn out</u> in the *INSIGHT BOX: PRACTICAL SCIENCE EXPERIMENT*, in the chapter on *TAKING-ACTION*.

In the first version, you don't know why you are reading the sentence until you get to the end of it. In the second, the main idea is stated at the outset.

Sentences

Sentences have structure. Each sentence has a subject and each part of the sentence relates to the subject. A new idea needs a new sentence. Sometimes two sentences can be joined to emphasise a comparison or contrast. Words such as: 'however', 'therefore', 'but', 'and', 'since' and many more, are used to join simple sentences together to make complex sentences. This class of words is called connectives or conjunctions. Realising sentences have a structure can help your student to write.

Spelling and grammar

Your student may be one of those dyslexic/ SpLD people who find that they write most easily by concentrating on ideas and ignoring grammar, punctuation or spelling for the first draft; grammar, punctuation and spelling are then worked on during subsequent drafts.

Or your student may be one who finds it useful to mark words or sentences that he is not sure about while writing an essay.

> When writing by hand, "sp" for spelling and "gr" for grammar can be written in the margin.

> When using a word processor with a search facility, "**" for spelling and "^^" for grammar can be inserted in the text.

> Then, when the essay is finished, he can easily find the words or sentences that he wants to check.

He can use any system that suits him.

The aim is to reduce mental stress, related to spelling and grammar, while producing an effective essay.

TEACHING LANGUAGE in a practical way is often effective while helping your student to express his ideas clearly.

TEACHING LANGUAGE: p 94

Key point: Accommodations

ACCOMMODATIONS: p 128

Depending on the core difficulty that gives rise to the different SpLDs, the problems encountered can be different:

- dyslexics can struggle with using words and language effectively

- dyspraxics can struggle with the mechanics of writing, the fine motor control

- AD(H)D can struggle with keeping their attention on the task in hand

- dyscalculics may only struggle with the words associated with arithmetic and maths.

Careful identification of the problems should enable the right accommodations to be arranged.

It helps if the abilities of the individual are part of any discussion: he feels valued and the people arranging accommodations realise the reason for them.

8   To be clever or not

Some people really want to demonstrate the strength of their intellect through their writing and they concentrate on showing how clever they are.

I think this is not a good strategy for dyslexic/ SpLD people, especially when their readers know more than they do. The work produced is often not well constructed and when I probe to find out what is intended, I often uncover some very muddled thinking.

Normally, I'm not an expert in the subject and I can't understand text unless it is fundamentally sound. A more expert person will unconsciously use his knowledge to interpret the surface cleverness of the essay and not realise that the writer is lacking understanding. In this way the student doesn't learn, because the need for more clarity in the student's thinking is missed by the expert.

Key point: Intelligence vs. cleverness

At the end of the day, your student ends up more knowledgeable because he has written to demonstrate his depth of knowledge rather than the quality of intelligence. When the depth of his knowledge is good, his intelligence will show anyway.

9 Summary: writing text

Summary: Writing text

Check that your student:

- has identified his goal and planned his structure
- can be comfortable while writing
- can maintain his fluency while writing
- uses suitable assistive technology
- has selected the right components from *Formal Writing* for the piece that he has to write
- has broken the task into manageable-sized sections or chapters.

Does he know how to deal with forms online?

Are any *Accommodations* appropriate?

Formal Writing: p 345

Accommodations: p 128

Website information

Series website: www.routledge.com/cw/stacey

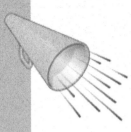

9 Talking

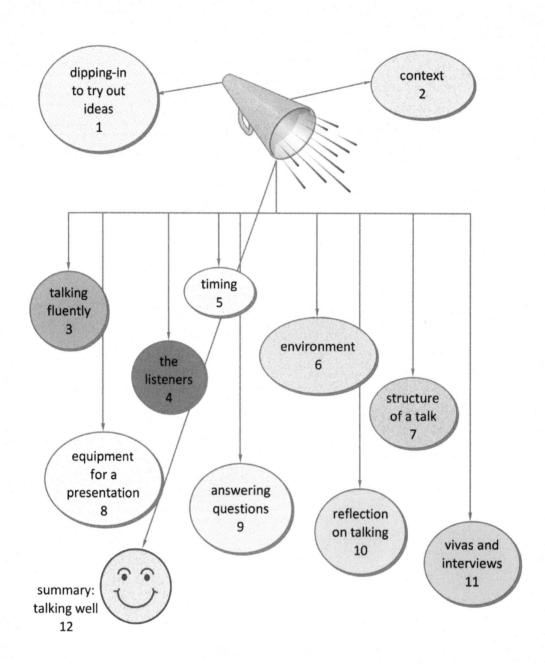

Contents

THINKING PREFERENCES are highlighted in orange in this chapter.

Examples of their use are listed in the *INDEX:* p 589

List of key points and summaries

K = key points
S = summaries

Information for non-linear readers

Before the context of the *Useful Preface* and *Chapters 1* and *2*, there is information that I hope will help non-linear readers as they approach the chapters. For chapters 4 – 14, this information would be identical except for which parts to scan and read. I have put all the information together into *Guidance for Non-Linear Readers, Chapter 3*. It is worth reading *Chapter 3* at some stage of working with this book.

Guidance for Non-Linear Readers: p 222

1 Dipping-in to try out ideas: reading and scanning lists

Start with *Dipping-in to Try Out Ideas: General Pattern*.
Read:
    Context, p 364
    Talking Fluently, p 368
    The Listeners, p 374

Scan:
    the rest of the chapter.

Dipping-in to Try Out Ideas: General Pattern: p 228

1.1 Key points: for policy-makers and general readers

Key points: For policy-makers and general readers

- Talking is vulnerable to the effects of dyslexia/ SpLD.

- Some dyslexic/ SpLD people find talking the best way to communicate.

- There are many strategies that can be used in order to speak fluently.

- Friendly, sympathetic listeners can help dyslexic/ SpLD people develop their best ways of talking.

2 Context

This chapter is about talking as a means of communication.
As always, there is a range of competence in talking:

- Some dyslexic/ SpLDs are natural talkers. Their ideas flow well in speech; they are confident; they can get on well and easily with many people. Their gift for language may be less well established when it comes to writing.

- Other dyslexic/ SpLDs find the spoken form of language just as problematic as the written one.

- Competence in talking is not static, which is probably true for anyone. As they become less competent, the added factor for dyslexic/ SpLDs is that they become more vulnerable to the effects of their dyslexia/ SpLD.

The chapter has suggestions for talking well in many circumstances.

Talking can take place in both informal and formal settings.

Key points: Some different situations involving talking

- One-to-one conversations
  face to face, on the phone

- Informal chat

- Formal discussion

- Giving out notices

- Presentations or lectures or talks

- Meetings

- Seminars

- Vivas[1]

- Job interviews

In all situations, the ideas discussed in the first four sections can be relevant:

Talking Fluently, p 368

The Listeners, p 374

Timing, p 374

Environment, p 377.

---

[1] A viva is an oral exam.

The following four sections apply to more formal settings:

Situations which involve several different people talking in discussion are covered in GROUP WORK: MEETINGS, SEMINARS AND DEBATES.

GROUP WORK: MEETINGS, SEMINARS AND DEBATES: p 446

Key point: You can't unsay your words

There's a significant difference between writing and talking. For most pieces of writing your student can do as many drafts as she needs; doing many may be tedious, but usually she can alter what she has written, even for emails and text messages.

When it comes to talking, she can rehearse lectures and presentations beforehand. She can go over her ideas for conversations.

However, she can't undo what she says in the same way that she can alter what she writes before she lets others see it.

For formal situations, it is assumed that your student knows her goal, see KNOW THE GOAL FOR ANY TASK, and she has done her PLANNING. She can be MONITORING PROGRESS in the way she talks to see how defining her goal and planning help her to talk well. She may notice ways she wants to change them.

KNOW THE GOAL OF ANY TASK: p 181

PLANNING: p 200

MONITORING PROGRESS: p 535

Even in informal situations, your student may find it helpful to keep her main point in mind and to find out whether the listener has the same mental image as herself, see the STORY: MEET YOU AT THE TOP OF THE ROAD, below. Different conclusions, e.g. about what she has agreed to do, happen even after quite informal conversations, especially when people are using different internal interpretations.

Story: "Meet you at the top of the road"

Two people A and B have agreed to meet "at the top of the road". A is walking along a path to the road. B is coming to the road from a roundabout. They have to agree a time for meeting because parking is difficult. B was quite frustrated when he had to wait a long time for A. Since this happened several times during a week, they decided to compare what they meant by "the top of the road".

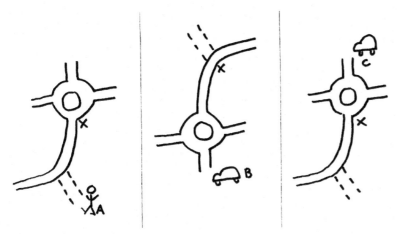

Figure 9. 1 Where is the top of the road?
X marks the top of the road for the 3 people A, B and C

A and B have internal, mental maps with themselves at the bottom, at the point where they enter the road; which is why they wait for each other for ages.

B told the story to C and discovered that in C's internal map she is at the top of her map, again where she enters the road. She would have met with A as soon as they have both arrived.

In this story, the visual maps were different, but there can be other differences, see *DIFFERENCES IN THOUGHT PROCESSING*.

DIFFERENCES IN THOUGHT PROCESSING: p 114

The language your student uses makes a difference to the success of her conversations and formal talking. As her success increases, so should her confidence increase.

Amongst many ideas are:

- Using positive, direct sentences keeps her ideas clear.
- If she includes too many secondary ideas (technically, subordinate clauses), people are likely to lose the thread of what she says.
- There is a skill in knowing when to stop.
- Using negative expressions instead of positive ones can lead to the wrong outcome. "Get some fruit; we don't need apples" could mean the shopper-without-a-list brings back apples and nothing else – that's all she's heard.

MONITORING PROGRESS as soon as possible after talking will help your student to develop a sense of how well she is talking; it may help her to develop the skill of METACOGNITION.

MONITORING PROGRESS: p 535
METACOGNITION: p 63

It will be hard for your student to ignore the emotional element of her memory of herself as a speaker. She could try recording more important conversations, meetings or talks to allow her to be more objective about the way she talks. She can use the responses of other people as feedback to help her develop her talking skills.

3 Talking fluently

By talking, your student is expressing ideas through language, including words. Many people automatically think about ideas in verbal ways; they gain confidence and self-esteem from the way in which their language flows with ease.

Story: Self-respect from using words

In one of the first workshops I ran, a tutor said "Do you mean I've got to respect other ways of thinking? My self-respect is in the way I use words."

Key point: Translation from non-verbal thinking

Many dyslexic/ SpLD people don't think in words[2]. They think in any of the non-verbal ways described in *THINKING PREFERENCES*. In order to use words, the ideas have to be translated from one format to another. It is like using a second language.

THINKING PREFERENCES: p 72

Story: From non-verbal thinking to words

No-one else can see, but when I give a talk I know a lot of my mental processing is dealing with the words to use. It is always difficult the first time I do a translation from my non-verbal understanding into words.

There is a bonus. I can't rattle off what I want to say; the time taken for me to find words allows time for other people to understand what I'm saying.

As with everything else, what works for one person won't work for another. Your student has to find what works for her in a friendly setting before talking in a testing situation.

You need to:	Further discussion:
be able to focus your mind on your ideas	*METACOGNTION:* p 63 *FOCUS OF ATTENTION, CONCENTRATION:* p 159
use your *THINKING PREFERENCES*	*THINKING PREFERENCES:* p 72
know what you are interested in and what point(s) you want to make	*MIND SET:* p 158

---

[2] There are many dyslexic/ SpLDs who are gifted speakers; it would be interesting to know whether they think in words or not.

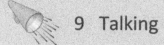

You need to:	Further discussion:
practise using good breathing and relaxation	*THINKING CLEARLY:* p 79
use your notes (applies mostly to formal settings)	*USING NOTES WHILE TALKING:* p 372

With the ability to focus her mind, your student can select those thoughts and actions that are going to help her; she can keep to the point of what she wants to say; she can maintain the clarity of her ideas.

Insight: Ideas lead, words follow

I find that when I focus on the ideas I want to talk about, I can leave the words to follow. I don't get distracted because I can't think of the best word or a word that is hovering on the edge of my conscious mind.

My way of focusing on ideas involves my *THINKING PREFERENCES*. I will frequently use the situation or student who first showed me the importance of the topic I'm talking about.   My notes will contain a reference to the person or situation, rather than a wordy description of the idea I want to put across.

Ways to use your THINKING PREFERENCES:	
Using your hands	adds a kinaesthetic element; you can draw in the air as you talk; you can point to things
Role play or add a dramatic element to your delivery	as you talk, you can add characterisation to your words in a dramatic fashion: you could be using episodic memory of an actual event; you could be using people intelligence from the characters and the story; you could be using the kinaesthetic sense through the role play

Real experience	keep your mind focused on the real experience behind the concepts you are talking about, or the person whom you most connect with the concepts; you could be using visual or kinaesthetic senses when you do so
Visualisation	you could be seeing pictures
Logic	you could be using the logical connections of the ideas to hold them in mind while you talk

The above ideas will work for both formal and informal situations.
The ones below are more appropriate to formal situations.

Visual aids	either for you in your notes, or for the audience in a slide show: you can draw pictures or symbols; you can use colour; you can use a mind map; you can use the spaces in between ideas to show relationships. These methods are likely to be a combination of visual, kinaesthetic, holistic and logic
Lists	either for you in your notes, or for the audience in a slide show: list of key ideas. You could be using: verbal, kinaesthetic, linear and logic THINKING PREFERENCES

This list is not exhaustive. Your student can experiment with her THINKING PREFERENCES to find the best way to keep her mind focused while she talks.

Using MIND SET before your student starts talking will help in many situations:

MIND SET: p 158

      What is she phoning someone to find out about?

      What are her questions?

      How can she capture their response?

      Is the other person raising new ideas?

Just taking time to switch on to a conversation before she starts makes it more successful. Obviously the more formal the setting the more a technique like MIND SET will help. The aim is to recall to mind what your student is interested in and what points she needs to make. When she rings someone, it is good to be aware that the other person also needs time to bring information to mind.

Maintaining good *BREATHING* is especially helpful when talking as it allows your student to increase the *CAPACITY OF WORKING MEMORY*. A good state of *RELAXATION* also helps while talking. Both techniques need to be well practised to be fully effective when she needs them.

BREATHING: p 557

CAPACITY OF WORKING MEMORY: p 157

RELAXATION: p 558

In formal settings, there may be other influences that impact on your student's fluency:

- Some people are helped by being smartly dressed. Others find being smart has school uniform connotations and memories of failure, therefore being smart is not helpful.

- Some find wanting to impress gives a buzz to the way they talk; others find it gets in the way and they talk more fluently when they concentrate on enjoying their subject.

- The way the environment is set up can affect fluency, see *ENVIRONMENT* below.

ENVIRONMENT: p 377

Confidence can grow when your student notices what makes a difference to her; she can choose what suits her best and then she can enjoy her increasing fluency.

3.1 Using notes while talking

There are many situations when it is a good idea to make notes in advance, for example when:

- seeing a doctor or another professional person
- taking purchases back to a shop
- wanting information from someone, even a friend
- giving a talk or presentation.

If your student is clear about the ideas she is putting across, her listeners will be able to understand her better. Good notes will help her maintain fluent speech.

Your student can experiment to find the *STYLES FOR NOTES* that suit her best and how she will use them reliably and comfortably. She can use the size of paper that suits her, or use an electronic device.

STYLES FOR NOTES: p 316

Many dyslexic/ SpLD people cannot reliably read text they have written when other people are present. Your student should find out how well she can read text in front of an audience.

How your student handles any notes or other materials while she is speaking is also important, especially if she knows that she will not read reliably in this situation. The placing of my materials has to be right; the use of symbols rather than words helps, as does colour coding.

It is worth doing a live trial; trying out notes on her own may not show all the difficulties she faces. She can ask a few people she trusts to let her experiment.

3.2 Practising

For presentations, lectures, giving out notices and any situation when your student has to deliver information by talking, it is worth practising beforehand. It is important to actually speak during practising; simply rehearsing mentally is often not enough.

She could record herself; she could ask someone to listen to her; she could use a mirror; she could use some photos out of a magazine to represent listeners. All these methods have been used by people I've supported. The result is that your student then speaks with more confidence and greater fluency.

3.3 Key points: talking fluently

Key points: Talking fluently

Main issues to consider:

- Does your student think without words?
- Can she focus on her ideas?
- Can she use any non-verbal strengths to keep her ideas in mind?
- What external factors affect her fluency?
- Are her notes right for her?
- Has she practised?

4 The listeners

Your student needs to think about the people who are listening to her and how they will impact on the ease with which she speaks. In *PLANNING RELATED TO KNOWLEDGE* there are several prompts to help her think about people before she talks to them.

PLANNING RELATED TO KNOWLEDGE: p 202

Your student should notice how people's attention affects her fluency. Some people are helped when they see enjoyment or understanding on the audiences' faces; others have to avoid looking at faces. If she feels it is rude not to look at people she can try looking towards them but not at them; in a formal situation, she can look just above their heads.

Story: Eyes closed while talking

When I'm saying something that is taking all my attention, I find I have to shut my eyes until I get to the end of the idea. It feels as if I have to switch off my vision in order to concentrate. When I open them again, I often ask whether the last bit made sense.

In formal situations, your student may need to be aware of people's comfort or discomfort. People often find it difficult to concentrate if the lighting is wrong, if the temperature or the air conditions are not suitable. It isn't going to help your student if people can't listen well because the physical conditions are not good. Your student will probably realise all is not well with the audience but she is more likely to think she is not talking well, than to consider the impact of the environment on her audience.

5 Timing

Timing is important when it comes to looking after the listeners, whether in an informal setting or a formal one.

Insight: Monitoring time while talking informally

Relations are coming to see you after they've been to a hospital appointment. You have arranged for someone to ring you at a time well after your relations will have left.

In the event, the relations are much later than expected; you don't know that they will have left by the time of the call.

The quality of chatting with your relations will be lessened if you are sitting there with half your mind working out what to do about the time, especially if one of the peculiarities of your dyslexia/ SpLD is that you have no internal sense of time.

For situations like this informal example, your student can experiment with different ideas to find the approach that helps her most, which will probably vary from one situation to another.

Suggestions:

1. Your student can explain the situation about the phone call at the start of the relations' visit; see how it fits with the time they expect to go; decide in advance what she will do when the call comes; relax and enjoy the relations' visit.
2. If the call comes while your relations are with her, your student can apologise to the caller, say her day hasn't gone according to plan and ask for a time when she can phone back.
3. Your student can mention the call a bit before it is due to happen; discuss whether her relations will stay on or go.
4. Do nothing and hope the caller gets delayed.

The criterion for your student's choice would be: what she finds a comfortable approach that doesn't leave her making decisions that she later has to undo or that she feels bad about. If I don't think through situations like this as soon as I see a problem looming, my dyslexia hampers my conversation both with the relatives and with the caller.

Insight: Monitoring time while talking formally

You are giving a talk and you are running out of time. People have to leave without hearing the conclusion and the summary of the main idea of your talk. What they take from your talk is likely to be less complete than if you had ended with your conclusion.

Timing a presentation of any kind, like the formal example above: your student is the one who should be controlling the timing. She may be given warnings that time is running out by a chairman, but it is up to her to manage finishing on time.

When there is no one else keeping time, your student can think about how she will know when time is running out. She can use a count-down watch, a kitchen timer, a visible clock-face, or the time on a computer depending on what suits her. She needs to make sure she can see or hear whatever she uses.

She can time a trial run to know approximately how long the talk takes. Does she speak at the same rate during the live presentation as she does during a rehearsal? If she finds she goes faster, then there will be time for questions. Or your student could have supplementary material to use. If your student goes slower, or she has a tendency spontaneously to include extra material, or the audience ask a lot of interesting questions, she could decide in advance what she will miss out if time runs out.

Four suggestions for ending at the right time:

1   She could give herself 5 minutes notice: to finish what she is saying and then give a brief conclusion.

2   She could arrange her talk with a poster of the ideas she wants people to go away with; it could be a flip chart with the key words written on it. Then she can decide how she will finish the talk fairly quickly when time runs out, using the poster and the key words.

3   She can know her concluding slide(s) on the electronic presentation, how to get to them immediately and how much time she wants for them. Then when the time comes to finish, she moves confidently into the conclusion.

4   Similar to 2) and 3), but she could have an ending section that has some ideas she wants to include as well as the technical conclusion. She times how long this ending section and the conclusion take and knows where it is in her notes and slides; then at the right time she simply moves to the ending section.

6 Environment

The environment plays an important part for many dyslexic/ SpLD people: whether your student can see out of the room; whether there are distracting details in the room; the layout of the room may be unsuitable for her, see ENVIRONMENT. It is useful for your student to recognise anything that is not helping her. She may be able to change it. If she can't, then she needs to do what she can to minimise its effect on her dyslexia/ SpLD. Use ideas in BEHIND THE OBVIOUS and SUPPLEMENTARY ISSUES to help your student decide how the environment is helping or hindering her.

ENVIRONMENT: p 70

BEHIND THE OBVIOUS: p 64
SUPPLEMENTARY ISSUES: p 68

Many dyslexic/ SpLDs find being in the middle is very difficult:

- if they have people speaking either side of them
- if they have to refer to visual material on either side of them while they are speaking
- if they are listening to someone and there is visual material on either side of the speaker.

These kinds of situations can result in the dyslexic/ SpLD person feeling very split and confused; it can be difficult to minimise the effects of dyslexia/ SpLD in these conditions.

Solutions

In all situations, your student can try to be comfortable (without making others uncomfortable) and in a place that is going to help her rather than hinder. Finding the right place can be especially important for meetings.

For more formal situations, she can get to places of importance early so that she will have some choices about the environment.

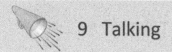

Insight: Furniture moving before a talk

With presentations, I move the furniture around as much as possible so that I am working from one end, with all the materials and equipment on one side of me. If I can't do that, I have enough confidence now to acknowledge the problem in advance. Doing so usually keeps everything under control.

When I look at a place I'm unsure about and hope that I will have no problems, I often become gradually anxious. The anxiety pushes me into a problem and by the time I know I've been too optimistic, my confidence has gone and I don't cope with the situation at all well.

Summary: Listeners, timing, environment

Has your student thought about her listeners:

- Who are they?
- What do they know?
- What do they want to know?
- What does she want them to learn?

Is your student in control of timing?
How will she end a formal talk?

Does the environment feel comfortable

- to her
- to her listeners?

Is there anything that can make it more comfortable?

7 Structure of a talk

In most situations it is useful for your student to have a structure to her talk. In speeches she probably won't need to spell out her structure.

In talks and presentations, when she wants people to understand and remember what she says, it is often good to say what her structure is. *PLANNING RELATED TO KNOWLEDGE* sets out the thoughts your student can use for planning her structure. A table at the end of the section suggests possible allocations of time between the subtopics of her talk. It might help her to number the points she is making. In the introduction, she can outline the plan for the talk; she then follows the outline as she gives the talk and she can summarise ideas in the same order as she concludes.

PLANNING RELATED TO KNOWLEDGE: p 202

Your student can listen to the way other people deliver lectures or talks and decide what she finds easy to listen to and follow; then reflect how she could make that style work for her.

8 Equipment for a presentation

Organising equipment is very similar to organising *OBJECTS NEEDED*. The comments here are specifically to do with aspects relevant to giving a talk.

OBJECTS NEEDED: p 71

It is a good idea for your student to arrive in time to try out the equipment before starting and to check that it is working well. If she is using slides, she can help people to sit in the best place for them by putting "Please sit where you can read" on the slide that is visible while people are gathering.

The quality of your student's slides in a presentation (or any other material that has to be read from a distance) will make a considerable difference to the way her talk is received, which in turn will impact on her confidence. She can make slides as bullet points, keywords, diagrams or pictures. Continuous text is not usually a good idea.

Your student shouldn't deliver her talk by reading the slides out loud.

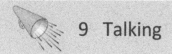
If she can, your student should try out any presentation slide show beforehand in the place she will be talking or a similar one. Really look at the details and size of text on slides and see if she can see and read them from the back of the room. Some programmes alter the font size for lists or bullet points; your student needs to make sure the size isn't made too small. It is better to have several readable slides than one unreadable one.

The colour of different projection systems can vary and make details invisible, so your student should keep looking at the screen from time to time as she works through a presentation. People are more likely to support her if she recognises when something is not as good as she intended.

Story: Check the microphone

The sound equipment needs checking too. I have to make sure any microphone is not going to cause me problems. I need both hands free to express my ideas otherwise I don't talk fluently.

Writing on a white/ black board:

1. Can she? She can try it first with some friends watching. She can observe what happens and how she feels. She can then decide whether there are any dyslexia/ SpLD issues that she needs to deal with.

2. Possible solution: have written sections prepared so that they can be Blu-tacked into position.

Using a flip-chart:

When your student is using several pages and moving between them, she can label them at the bottom so that it is easy for her to find the one she wants.

9 Answering questions in a talk or presentation

Questions can present several different challenges, whether they are raised at the end of a talk or during it.

- If your student finds questions difficult to process, it is possible to say that people are welcome to talk to her afterwards, rather than asking questions at the end.

- She could ask someone to write questions down for her so that she can see and hear at the same time; the person could then read out the question for those who didn't hear when it was asked.

- If someone asks a question during the talk and your student knows she answers it later in the presentation, she could write it down, or get her scribe to do so, and say she will check at the end whether the person felt their question had been answered. I often do that on a surface that is visible during the talk.

- If asked a question to which your student doesn't know the answer, it's best to be open; it is less embarrassing than being caught out. If she knows the answer, but can't recall it, again say so; she may find the answer then comes.

10 Reflection on talking

It is worth reflecting with your student on how well she talks, especially in formal situations, though the 'particular situation' in *FIGURE 9.2* can range from talking to friends to giving presentations.

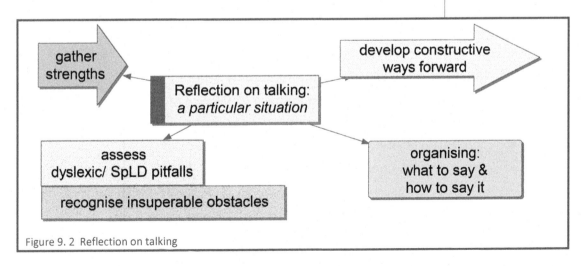

Figure 9. 2 Reflection on talking

A linear equivalent to *FIGURE 9.2* would include:

What are her strengths?

What is her motivation for talking?

How does dyslexia/ SpLD affect her?

Are there any dyslexia/ SpLD obstacles that need *ACCOMMODATIONS*?

Ⓖ p 575 obstacle

ACCOMMODATIONS:
p 128

What is the organisation of her ideas?

What else needs organising?

Is practice needed?

How will she maintain confidence?

What are the next steps towards talking well in the given situation?

Ideas in *BEHIND THE OBVIOUS* may shed light on strengths, pitfalls and obstacles. You need to be aware that the presented problem may not be the real cause, so keep an open mind.

BEHIND THE OBVIOUS:
p 64

Summary: Giving a talk

- Keep a clear goal in mind.
- Use a structure for the talk.
- Organise the slides; make sure they can be read.
- Think how the talk will be interpreted by others.
- Include *THINKING PREFERENCES* in the organisation of the talk.
- Use notes that work well.
- Manage time competently.

- Practice.
- Know how to maintain confidence.
- Plan getting to the right place, and plan to get there early.

- Make sure equipment is working.

- Arrange the room and furniture to be comfortable.

- Fully understand any questions; or invite people to raise them afterwards.

11 Vivas[3] and interviews

Vivas and interviews have much in common and there are some notable differences.

Colour coding has been used to help distinguish between the two: viva interview, when appropriate.

Key points: Vivas and interviews

During vivas and interviews your student is not in control of the situation in the same way she might expect to be in control when she is giving a talk. She is in a position of demonstrating to her listeners that she knows what she's talking about.

Your student will have to:

- listen carefully to their questions and understand them

- recall knowledge that she has

- organise that knowledge so that it is answering the question

- give her answer clearly, succinctly and fluently.

For some purposes your student may have to give a presentation as well; most teachers have to deliver a lesson during the interview process.

---

[3] A viva is an oral exam.

There is one important factor in which interviews differ from vivas: in the interview your student wants the interviewers to feel she would work well in their employment setting, whereas in an exam viva, how much the examiners like her should not be an issue.

Some people, even dyslexic/ SpLD people, find the process easy, and some find it very hard.

Preparation

Your student can prepare for the viva or interview:

1   by revising the subject matter

2   by making sure all her techniques are well rehearsed.

It might also be necessary to arrange appropriate exam provisions for a viva. PREPARATION is discussed more fully in relation to exams.

PREPARATION: p 413

Subject matter for vivas

In a viva your student will be asked about the subject she has been working on.

If the viva is part of, for example, the final exam for her undergraduate degree then she can revise the material for her degree.

It's a good idea to think especially about the areas that she knows she answered incompletely.

If possible, she can ask her subject tutor to organise a practice viva for her; one of her peers might be able to give her one.

When she goes into an examination viva, your student wants to be confident of the processes of listening to questions, recalling information and speaking her answers.

She probably needs to have two mock vivas before she experiences the real exam viva.

If your student has written a postgraduate thesis, then she will be asked questions about the content of her thesis.

She should remember that she is probably the most knowledgeable person on the subject.

In her preparation, it might be worth thinking about the specialities of her examiners.

Her thesis supervisor will probably organise a practice viva for her.

It is worth getting the best advice she can about the subjects that she should prepare for the viva.

Subject matter for job interviews

The notes that your student made while searching for a job, see *JOB APPLICATION*, should give her information about the job that she wants to do and about the business that she wants to join.

JOB APPLICATION: p 504

The essential and desirable criteria for the job and the information in "Your duties are ..." will tell her what the employer is looking for in the new employee.

By way of preparation, your student could use *MIND SET* and *RECALL AND MEMORISING EXERCISES* and apply them to the information about the job and her letter of application.

MIND SET: p 158

RECALL AND MEMORISING EXERCISES: p 159

She also needs to think slightly wider so that any further questions from the interviewer will be ones that she can answer relatively easily.

Your student can use any impression she gained about the cultural setting of the prospective employment to think how she would fit into the organisation, what experience she has had that demonstrates her ability to get on with people, to be self-motivated, etc.

The way in which she answers these questions can influence whether she gets the job or not.

Again it is a very good idea to practise being interviewed.

Your student needs to find someone who is capable of asking searching questions.

In giving her answers, she needs to bear in mind that she is demonstrating to the questioner that she has the qualities and skills he is looking for; and that she has the personality that will make a good employee.

The environment

If your student is someone who is affected by the environment, she needs to think how she is going to deal with the sort of environment she doesn't like.

* Is there some visualisation that could help her?
* Can she dress in a particular way that gives her confidence?
* Can she practise talking in places that don't help her just so that she can be familiar with the kind of difficulties that she experiences?

Use BEHIND THE OBVIOUS and ENVIRONMENT to explore any issues.

BEHIND THE OBVIOUS: p 64

ENVIRONMENT: p 70

Arriving

It usually helps to arrive in good time. It is unlikely to help your student if she arrives in a rush right at the last minute.

Viva and interview techniques

The most important aspect of techniques is for your student to keep THINKING CLEARLY.

THINKING CLEARLY: p 79

BREATHING: p 557

RELAXATION: p 558

* She needs to practise the various techniques of BREATHING and RELAXATION well in advance. She can decide which one she feels most confident with; practise it as early as possible so that her use of it is very fluent.
* Knowing what her best ways of thinking are will help; again practising their use will increase her confidence.
* She needs to be able to keep her thoughts on target, clear in her head and relevant to the questions she has been asked.

It is possible that the interviewer will use long sentences which your student finds difficult to reduce to the most important point. She may need to ask for clarification. She may get halfway through an answer and realise that she's not answering the main point. It is probably better to stop and check with the interviewer whether her first or second interpretation was the correct one.

Your student may be asked to give a presentation as part of the viva or interview; as mentioned at the beginning of this section, teachers in particular are usually asked to give a lesson. All of this chapter is relevant to the preparation of her presentation.

At the end of many interviews, people are asked if they have any questions. It is a good idea to think about any questions in advance of the interview. Your student will need a way of using her *THINKING PREFERENCES* so that she can recall these questions.

THINKING PREFERENCES:
p 72

Your student wants to improve her chances of giving a good interview. If she doesn't get a job, she can try to phone and find out why, asking objectively for any guidance for her next interview.

12 Summary: talking well

Summary: Talking well

- Spoken words can't be unspoken, edited or re-checked in the same way that written words can.

- There are many factors that can assist or hinder speaking fluently.

- Focusing on ideas and letting the words follow improves communication.

- People have different mental interpretations of words.

- Strategies for talking well can be developed and practised in friendly company.

- Talking happens in informal and formal situations; for both it is worthwhile to know how to talk well.

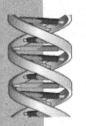

10 Taking-Action

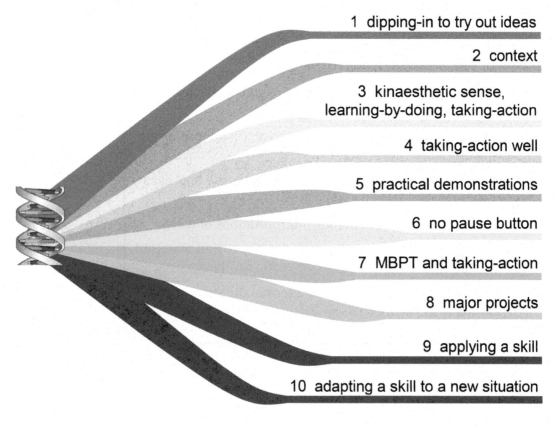

1 dipping-in to try out ideas

2 context

3 kinaesthetic sense,
learning-by-doing, taking-action

4 taking-action well

5 practical demonstrations

6 no pause button

7 MBPT and taking-action

8 major projects

9 applying a skill

10 adapting a skill to a new situation

Ⓖ p 575 MBPT

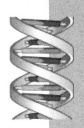

Contents

THINKING PREFERENCES are highlighted in orange in this chapter.

Examples of their use are listed in the INDEX: p 589

List of key points and summaries

Page		Box title:
390	K	FOR POLICY-MAKERS AND GENERAL READERS
394	K	A FRAMEWORK FOR TAKING-ACTION
397	S	SUMMARY: TAKING-ACTION WELL
399	K	DIFFICULTIES IN TAKING-ACTION
404	K	MAJOR PROJECTS
405	S	SUMMARY: SKILLS AND TAKING-ACTION

K = key points
S = summaries

Templates on the website

B7   RECORDING TEMPLATE - 3

TEMPLATES

Information for non-linear readers

Before the context of the *USEFUL PREFACE* and *CHAPTERS 1* and *2*, there is information that I hope will help non-linear readers as they approach the chapters. For chapters 4 – 14, this information would be identical except for which parts to scan and read. I have put all the information together into *GUIDANCE FOR NON-LINEAR READERS, CHAPTER 3*. It is worth reading *CHAPTER 3* at some stage of working with this book.

GUIDANCE FOR NON-LINEAR READERS: p 222

1 Dipping-in to try out ideas: reading and scanning lists

Start with *DIPPING-IN TO TRY OUT IDEAS: GENERAL PATTERN*.
Read:

DIPPING-IN TO TRY OUT IDEAS: GENERAL PATTERN: p 228

> *CONTEXT*, p 391
>
> *KINAESTHETIC SENSE, LEARNING-BY-DOING AND TAKING-ACTION*, p 392
>
> *TAKING-ACTION WELL*, p 393
>
> *NO PAUSE BUTTON*, p 397

Scan:

> the rest of the chapter

1.1 Key points: for policy-makers and general readers

Key points: For policy-makers and general readers

- Taking-action engages the kinaesthetic sense.
- Some dyslexic/ SpLD people function best when the kinaesthetic sense is engaged.
- Some find taking-action in practical ways extremely difficult.
- Education and workplace policies and practices should cater for those who naturally take-action in practical ways.
- *MYERS-BRIGGS PERSONALITY TYPES (MBPT)* with strong Judging attitude often enjoy taking-action speedily.
- *MYERS-BRIGGS PERSONALITY TYPES (MBPT)* with strong Perceiving attitude often delay taking-action as they prefer to continue finding out more about relevant issues.

MYERS-BRIGGS PERSONALITY TYPE (MBPT): p 76

2 Context

Taking-action is about practically using knowledge and skills, as mentioned in *Key Point: Different Reasons for Practical Work*.

Key Point: Different Reasons for Practical Work: p 284

Reading and writing, and listening and talking are pairs in systems of communication, including acquiring and applying knowledge and skills. Attention is given to the way visual and verbal processing are involved and what can be done to improve the quality of the communication. Little attention is paid to the contribution of kinaesthetic processing.

Sense-based Thinking Preferences: p 75

In order to focus on kinaesthesia and kinaesthetic processing, I have used 'doing' and 'taking-action' as a pair in parallel with reading and writing, and listening and talking.

From my work with other dyslexic/ SpLD people, I know kinaesthetic processing needs to be taken into account as a *Thinking Preference*. For many dyslexic/ SpLD people, it can be their strongest preference.

Thinking Preferences: p 72

Your student will be using kinaesthetic processing in some way when he is taking-action to apply knowledge and skills whether it is a thinking preference for him or not.

After distinguishing between 1) kinaesthetic learning as a *Thinking Preference*; 2) learning-by-doing; and 3) taking-action, the chapter discusses taking-action in sections:

It discusses issues relating to skills in sections:

3 Kinaesthetic sense, learning-by-doing and taking-action

The INSIGHT: PRACTICAL SCIENCE EXPERIMENT is an example demonstrating the distinctions between 1) the kinaesthetic thinking preference, 2) learning-by-doing and 3) taking-action, with organisational skills mentioned since they can be a key part of practical work.

The elements listed in the box are annotated to emphasise the distinctions:

SENSE-BASED THINKING PREFERENCES: p 75

- the italic style picks out 'experiment' since it can be replaced to suit another situation
- highlighting picks out THINKING PREFERENCES and an SpLD
- underlining picks out aspects that relate to knowledge and skills, or acquiring and applying them.

Insight: Practical science experiment

Elements	Comments
Kinaesthetic learners root their learning in the *experiment*.	kinaesthetic sense
Strongly verbal/ visual learners with weak kinaesthetic sense won't like the *experiment*. Dyspraxic people may find the necessary skills impossible.	no help from kinaesthetic sense
A tutor with <u>knowledge</u> can decide how an *experiment* is to be set up.	taking-action: using knowledge for a practical end
The *experiment* might be a <u>demonstration</u> or a <u>practical</u> for students to undertake.	learning aid suited to kinaesthetic thinking preference
Someone, tutor or technician, may need the <u>technical skills</u> to set up the *experiment*.	taking-action: knowledge and skill
Students will learn <u>technical skills</u> and <u>knowledge</u>	learning-by-doing

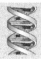

| The person setting up the *experiment* and the ones doing it can all be using <u>organisational skills</u>. | organisation |
| If the skills involved in the *experiment* are repeated many times, they can be learnt to the point that they are <u>automatic</u>. | one result of learning-by-doing is automaticity |

This scenario could be changed to apply to other situations just by replacing the title *Practical science experiment* and the task *experiment*.

For example, there could be a practical session to show people how an aspect of gardening works: the title for the box would be *Practical Gardening Workshop* with the word *session* replacing *experiment*.

3.1 Making decisions

As a phrase in everyday life, 'taking action' (without a hyphen) can also mean 'to act on a decision'. The decision could be something like, "I need to send an email to XX about YY." Taking action would involve all the processes related to emails, which may include identifying goals and planning the email content. The primary attention goes to the thoughts relating to the context, as in WRITING and TALKING. The physical, kinaesthetic, sense is of secondary importance.

WRITING: p 336

TALKING: p 362

In this chapter, the practical, physical element is of primary importance.

4 Taking-action well

Taking-action covers anything:
- from reaching out to pick up a piece of fruit
- to:
  - going shopping
  - building a house
  - managing a company.

Most actions have a reason behind them, though not all. Some actions happen spontaneously and need no deliberate thought. Some actions require a great deal of thought and planning.

Key point: A framework for taking-action

Taking-action can involve:

- physical action
- deliberate thinking, though not always
- motivation or goal
- planning.

This section is concerned with taking-action that involves deliberate thinking, has goals and needs planning.

Many of the processes involved in taking-action have been discussed elsewhere. The table below re-caps what is important and includes references to other sections in the book.

Components of taking-action well		
Framework element	*section*	*page*
Deliberate thinking		
Engaging with ideas in this table will involve deliberate thinking.		
Deliberate thinking will enable your student to be in control of his taking-action.		
You need to work with your student to find out: • exactly how he deals with taking-action • what his strengths are • what areas of skills need to be worked on.	BEHIND THE OBVIOUS	64

Framework element	section	page
Physical action		
There are several elements to the kinaesthetic sense; be aware of them and discuss whether they are strengths for your student.	Senses Context of Doing (up to Key Point Different Reasons for Practical Work)	74 282
The examples and comments about the kinaesthetic sense and its use will help your student to recognise its impact in his life. They may help him develop his use of the kinaesthetic sense. They are gathered together in the Index.	Index	589
He may decide that other Thinking Preferences are more important to him.	Thinking Preferences Doing and Thinking Preferences	72 285
He may have difficulties with the physical realm of life.	Core Issues Problems Relating to Doing Space, Place and Direction Environment	62 297 69 70
Preparing for taking-action can make a significant different to the way practical actions are carried out.	Preparation for Reading Preparation for Listening Preparation for Doing Mental Rehearsal of Movements	243 271 291 292
Sometimes taking-action has a series of steps that need to be carried out. It may have some that are repeated. Being conscious of the steps and organising them can bring a smooth flow to taking-action.	Protocol for doing	293

Framework element	section	page
Motivation or goals		
Knowing his goal will help him take-action effectively.	KNOW THE GOAL OF ANY TASK GOALS FOR ACTION	181 184
Any instructions from others need to be understood and, if necessary, clarified.	INDIRECT COMMUNICATION DIALOGUE	119 107
Planning		
Planning also makes taking-action more effective.	PLANNING PLANNING RELATING TO SKILLS	200 208
He will have to decide his priorities for taking-action.	PRIORITISING	197
A detailed timetable is often essential.	MAJOR PROJECTS	400

Work through the COMPONENTS OF TAKING-ACTION WELL with your student and help him in any areas that are not working for him.

Work with him to establish his best way of approaching taking-action. It might help him to devise a scheme, such as that in FIGURE 10.1, which he can use as the basis for his plans for taking-action.

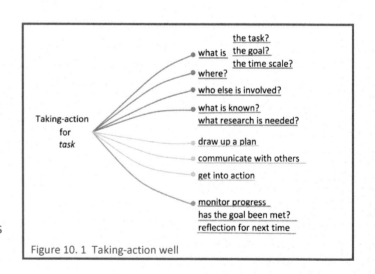

Figure 10. 1 Taking-action well

> ### Summary: Taking-action well
>
> - Know the reason for the action.
>
> - Know the practical skills required and check they can be provided.
>
> - Think about the place where the action will happen and make it as suitable as possible.
>
> - Plan with an appropriate level of detail.
>
> - Draw up a timetable, if that's helpful. Include any activities that might interfere with the progress of the planned action.

5 Practical demonstrations

The usual purpose of practical demonstrations is to communicate knowledge or a skill.   Therefore, the ideas about communication in *GOALS FOR WRITTEN WORK* and *GOALS FOR SITUATIONS INVOLVING TALKING* will also be relevant to how your student prepares for giving practical demonstrations. In the practical situation he needs to bear in mind that not everyone will like using the kinaesthetic sense and he needs to include a flexibility that will cater for those with different *THINKING PREFERENCES*. In *FIGURE 10.1*, part of the answer to What is the goal? should be to communicate with people who may not like practical demonstrations.

GOALS FOR WRITTEN WORK: p 187

GOALS FOR SITUATIONS INVOLVING TALKING: p 196

THINKING PREFERENCES: p 72

6 No pause button

There are many situations when, once you have started, you can't pause at all or you may have to wait for a suitable moment to pause:

- when you are driving, the traffic conditions may prevent you from stopping

- when you start a piece of music in a performance or exam, you cannot stop

- in sport, once play has started, you often can't stop.

Some situations have danger attached, for example taking the wrong action while driving could result in an accident; others are not life-threatening but have significant emotional impact, so it is worth assessing the risk.

In preparation for such situations, it is useful for your student to think in advance how he will deal with realising that he would like to pause.

- How will he keep his mind focused on his task?
- How will he deal with any emotions he is feeling?
- How will he retain a sense of his goal?

He should think about questions like these and work out his solutions well in advance.

Your student also needs to observe how taking, or avoiding, precautionary measures impacts on him.
Some people hope that wanting to pause will never happen to them and then find the unconscious worry undermines their performance and makes the moment of wanting to pause more likely. Such people should work out their strategies in advance to disperse the worry.
At the other end of the spectrum are those who have fewer need-to-pause moments if they don't work out any strategies for dealing with the need to pause.

USEFUL ABILITIES OF THE MIND: p 63

Your student needs to observe objectively how different situations and reactions impact on him. To help him, he could combine ideas from USEFUL ABILITIES OF THE MIND with those from BEHIND THE OBVIOUS.

BEHIND THE OBVIOUS: p 64

7 Myers-Briggs Personality Type and taking-action

MYERS-BRIGGS PERSONALITY TYPE: p 76

The Myers-Briggs system of personality includes two pairs of attitudes. One pair describes the way people like to interact with the world around them. People are either:

perceiving types (P) who like to gather information from the world around, the environment or other people. They like to observe what's happening and will continuing observing and gathering information for a long time. They find it hard to stop and go into action: the next moment might bring something that changes everything that went before.

judging[1] types (J) who like to go into action immediately. They either have an impact on the physical environment or they organise the people around them. They find gathering information an unnecessary delay. For them, an immediate decision based on no information feels better than a delayed decision.

I have portrayed the extremes of these two types. People can naturally be somewhere in between the extremes. With a little time for consideration, people who have extreme tendencies can modify their decision-making processes. However, under pressure people tend to operate from the extremes.

I have found it useful to help a student to recognise when he is operating at one end of the dimension and when his decision-making tendency is being unhelpful in taking-action.

Key points: Difficulties in taking-action

- Your student may not like practical action.
- He may be disorganised and not take-action effectively.
- If his Myers-Briggs Personality Type has a strong element of Judging, he may take-action before finding out all the necessary factors.
- If his Myers-Briggs Personality Type has a strong element of Perception, he may delay taking-action too long because he wants to find out more.
- Some actions have no pause button and have to be carried on beyond the moment when your student would like to stop.

---

[1] Judging is not about assessing value, good or bad, but about deciding.

8 Major projects

Major projects are part of everyone's life at some time; very few of us get away without being involved somewhere. Many of them involve action of some kind.

Examples are:

re-decorating a room; moving house
organising: a child's birthday party, a wedding
putting on a play; leading a school trip
organising: a holiday, a complex work project
doing the research for and writing up: a report, a dissertation, a thesis, a book.

Most major projects are easier to organise and carry out when they are broken down into manageable components, without losing sight of the overall task.

Often, major projects grow out of actions your student already does and the skills he needs to use are well established. Sometimes, he will need new skills or he will have to considerably adapt the skills he has. Dealing with major projects will involve many different parts of the book. The initial stages are likely to include some of the following, if not all.

Adapting DIPPING-IN TO TRY OUT IDEAS: GENERAL PATTERN (p 228) to major projects	
Step of the GENERAL PATTERN and additional sections with page numbers	Reason
MATERIALS AND METHODS: p 565	To choose the most suitable.
Step 1 and KNOW THE GOAL OF ANY TASK: p 181	To define the purpose of the project. To identify your goal. To register any guidelines you have to follow.
DIALOGUE: p 107 GROUP WORK: MEETINGS, SEMINARS AND DEBATES: p 446	To keep in contact with other people involved in the project. To manage discussions well.

Step 2 and *B7 - RECORDING TEMPLATE - 3*	To assess the overview; break into subsections. To capture your present knowledge of the project. Template headings: A = date B = project C = what has to be achieved, break this into sub-projects D = what action is necessary E = priority rating.
Step 3 and *GENERATING USEFUL QUESTIONS:* p 530 For examples of useful questions, see *INDEX,* p 589.	To identify: • what you already know and can do • where research will provide the answers • what you will need help for from another person • who will help you.
Steps 4 and 5, and *PRIORITISING:* p 528	To sort out: • the priorities • where you want to start • the timetable, with deadlines. To keep sight of how the different subsections fit together.
Step 6 and *PAPERWORK, INCLUDING FILING:* p 71	For each subsection: • carry out research and actions • keep records of progress, further work or questions • file your records.

The subsections need to be small enough that they feel achievable.

When helping students to draw up a timetable, I always ask about other activities that will need time: social events, household chores, plans for holidays, etc.

We also try to be realistic about the time available in the day or evening. It may be better to err on the pessimistic side and have time in hand than to be too optimistic and run short of time.

As always, you need to be aware of people's differences. Some people need to feel they are running out of time in order to get started.

When everything has been put in, it is often very surprising to find how little time there is for a project, especially when the deadline seems a long way away.

This realisation can get people moving when previously they were feeling reluctant to do so.

Major projects are often quite stressful. There are many factors contributing to the stress: some relate to other people or the environment; some may be centred on your student.

Story: Work from the right perspective

One student started working with me half way into the research for her master's degree. She was a mature student who had managed several projects successfully during her working life. She was finding her research work very difficult.

She was researching the rights of native peoples throughout the world.

She kept expressing dissatisfaction with the attitudes of some organisations and telling me how she didn't like her project, which she had chosen to do.

I made various study skills suggestions but they clearly weren't sufficient.

We worked with the principles of *BEHIND THE OBVIOUS* and found that the phrasing of her goal and her research questions did not reflect her own attitudes; they were written using the terminology of her discipline and rather impersonal.

BEHIND THE OBVIOUS: p 64

We rephrased the goal and research questions to reflect her experiences of working with native people and her desire to bring more harmony to their relationships with the rest of the world. After that, she was able to engage with her research and see a positive outcome for her Master's thesis.

The conflict we resolved was between the logical, Thinking approach of her discipline and her innate Feeling approach – two of the contrasting mental functions from MPBT.

MYERS-BRIGGS PERSONALITY TYPE: p 564

Gradually build up an effective way of dealing with major projects so that your student can move through them at the best pace for him, while meeting the various deadlines and constraints from the situation around him.

It may be a continual learning process, but if your student engages with it without making it heavy labour, he will probably find it much more rewarding.

The philosophy of *The E-Myth Revisited* (Gerber, 2001) has much to offer. The author looks at business systems in order to construct them so that they aim to satisfy the needs of customer, employee and employer all together. One idea is to 'work on the business, not in the business'. Translating the idea to working on major projects, one might say, 'be aware of the progress and purpose of the project rather than be overloaded by the day-to-day detail'.

Gerber (2001)

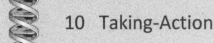

Key points: Major projects

- Break the major project into manageable subsections.
- Make sure the motivation for the task suits your student.
- Timetable the whole project, include non-project tasks.
- Prioritise.
- Monitor progress.
- Keep engaged with other people involved with the project.

9 Applying a skill

Most people have to *LEARN A SKILL* over a length of time. As they learn it, they gradually become more proficient in using it. It may be a skill that is always used the way it was learnt, or it may be a skill that is intended to be used in many different situations, some of which will involve the skill being modified as it is used.

LEARN A SKILL: p 288

The final stage of learning a skill results in the usable skill. Many of the ideas and processes leading up to the final stage may still be useful in using the skill. Gradually, as it becomes more automatic, your student should find that he has to pay less attention to using the skill, and that the thought processes he used during learning become reduced and fast.

If he uses the skill regularly, your student will probably find that it is one he can rely on and that it doesn't deteriorate. There are some skills that remain good however little one uses them: once you've learnt to ride a bicycle you don't forget how to.

Other skills will fade if they are not used. They can be re-established by *MENTAL REHEARSAL OF MOVEMENTS*.

MENTAL REHEARSAL OF MOVEMENTS: p 292

10 Adapting a skill to new situations

A skill may need to be altered to fit a situation different from the one in which it was learnt; see *DEVELOPED USE OF KNOWLEDGE AND SKILLS*.

DEVELOPED USE OF KNOWLEDGE AND SKILLS: p 154

Your student may have to assess the situation and the skill to work
out how to achieve the desired adaptation.
He should be cautious about any new aspects and make sure they
don't interfere with the skill he has carefully learnt.
For example some people can't switch easily between two
racquet sports, such as tennis and badminton; they find
they become worse players in both games.
Other people can switch easily without any affect on their
performance.

A strong episodic memory may be problematic in adapting a skill to a
new situation: it may be difficult to break the skill into component
parts, which can then be used in different arrangements.

Ⓖ p 575: episodic
memory

Over-practice of the components in a random order may help to
establish the components in their own right rather than as part of the
whole original skill.

Summary: Skills and taking-action

- Skills are often involved in taking-action.

- A skill becomes proficient and automatic with practice.

- A skill can be used just as learnt.

- A skill may need to be adapted to new situations.

- Episodic memory may hamper using components of a
  skill.

- Care may be needed to preserve a learnt skill when
  adapting it to a new situation.

References

Gerber, Michael E., 2001, *The E-myth Revisited: Why Small Business
Don't Work and What To Do About It*, HarperCollins Publishers,
NY, 2nd ed.

Website information

Series website: www.routledge.com/cw/Stacey

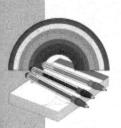

11   Exams

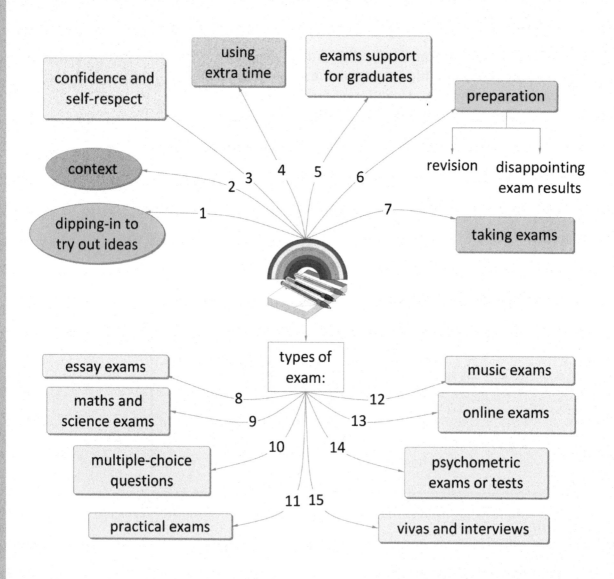

confidence and self-respect

using extra time

exams support for graduates

preparation

revision   disappointing exam results

context

dipping-in to try out ideas

2   3   4   5   6

1   7

taking exams

types of exam:

essay exams

maths and science exams

multiple-choice questions

practical exams

8

9

10

11

15

12

13

14

music exams

online exams

psychometric exams or tests

vivas and interviews

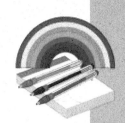

Contents

THINKING PREFERENCES, p 72, are highlighted in orange in this chapter.

Examples of their use are listed in the *INDEX:* p 589

List of key points and summaries

Page		Box title:
408	*K*	*FOR POLICY-MAKERS AND GENERAL READERS*
411	*S*	*EXAMS*
413	*S*	*PREPARATION*
414	*K*	*STEPS IN PREPARATION FOR EXAMS*
416	*S*	*REVISION OVERVIEW*
428	*K*	*BEFORE AN EXAM*
430	*K*	*EXAM-TAKING PROTOCOL*
442	*K*	*EMPLOYERS MISSING GOOD EMPLOYEES*

K = key points
S = summaries

Templates on the website

TEMPLATES

B9   A CALENDAR MONTH FOR PRIORITISING – 5 WEEKS

Information for non-linear readers

Before the context of the *USEFUL PREFACE* and *CHAPTERS 1* and *2*, there is information that I hope will help non-linear readers as they approach the chapters. For chapters 4 – 14, this information would be identical except for which parts to scan and read. I have put all the information together into *GUIDANCE FOR NON-LINEAR READERS, CHAPTER 3*. It is worth reading *CHAPTER 3* at some stage of working with this book.

GUIDANCE FOR
NON-LINEAR READERS:
p 222

1 Dipping-in to try out ideas: reading and scanning lists

Start with *DIPPING-IN TO TRY OUT IDEAS: GENERAL PATTERN*.
Read:
    CONFIDENCE AND SELF-RESPECT, p 411
    KEY POINTS: STEPS IN PREPARATION, p 414
    REVISION , p 415
    TAKING EXAMS, p 428
Scan:
    the sections on the different types of exam, starting on p 432
    USING EXTRA TIME, p 412
    DISAPPOINTING EXAM RESULTS, p 424

DIPPING-IN TO TRY OUT
IDEAS: GENERAL PATTERN:
p 228

1.1 Key points: for policy-makers and general readers

Key points: For policy-makers and general readers

- Understand the difficulties dyslexic/ SpLD students face when trying to demonstrate their knowledge and skills under exam conditions.

- Facilitate the strategies they use for preparation and taking exams.

- Provide reasonable adjustments so that they can show what they can do.

- Focus on the knowledge and skills that are being tested and not on the formalities of testing.

2 Context

Exams are intended to test your student's knowledge or skills.

- Some exam results are pass or fail; and there is a variety of values for the pass mark.

- Some exams have grades.

- Some exams are competitive – only a number of the highest achievers will go forward with a pass.

- Some are online.

- Some are paper-based.

- Some are practical.

- Some exams need to be re-taken every, say, 5 years, for example gas-fitter exams.

This is not a comprehensive list of the characteristics of exams.

Essentially: your student needs to demonstrate his knowledge or skills in a specified way.

Many of the details of the specified ways put dyslexic/ SpLDs at a disadvantage because the impact of the dyslexia/ SpLD hinders their ability to show their knowledge and skills. There should be a clear distinction between the exam[1] as a communication channel and the knowledge and skills to be demonstrated. Exam provisions should be organised to remove the disadvantages, or at least diminish them.

The acceptability of exam provisions, including extra time, varies from one situation to another. Justifying them, designing a workable system that seems fair, and monitoring the system are all complicated tasks. Some students feel that extra time is not right and they undervalue their achievements if they use it.

Dyslexia/ SpLD are not syndromes that go away once some skills and strategies have been learnt. People can be more reliable in the ways they manage the ASPECTS OF DYSLEXIA/ SPLD, but they always need to reserve some MENTAL ENERGY TO MANAGE DYSLEXIA/ SPLD.

ASPECTS OF DYSLEXIA/ SPLD: p 568

MENTAL ENERGY TO MANAGE DYSLEXIA/ SPLD: p 541

---

[1] Or any other assessment process.

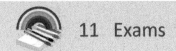

The conditions of the exam need to be suitable:

> Any negotiation of appropriate provisions should take place as soon as possible, see NEGOTIATING ACCOMMODATION.

NEGOTIATING ACCOMMODATION: p 550

Your student needs to know the format of the exam.

> Length of time, number and style of questions, how many he has to answer; what paper he will be writing on; how any practical exam is arranged; where the exam will take place and what sort of room, or situation, he will be in.

Your student needs to learn in the best way for his mind:

> see INDIVIDUALS WITH DYSLEXIA/ SPLD and FOUNDATIONS FOR KNOWLEDGE AND SKILLS.

INDIVIDUALS WITH DYSLEXIA/ SPLD: p 57

FOUNDATIONS FOR KNOWLEDGE AND SKILLS: p 134

Your student needs to keep his thinking at its best:

> see BUILDING CONFIDENCE AND SELF-ESTEEM.

BUILDING CONFIDENCE AND SELF-ESTEEM: p 78

Your student needs to practise so that he is confident as he enters the exam and he knows what he is going to do to take the exam.

This chapter starts with some comments about

> CONFIDENCE AND SELF-RESPECT, p 411
>
> USING EXTRA TIME, p 412
>
> EXAM SUPPORT FOR GRADUATES, p 413

PREPARATION: p 413

REVISION: p 415

TAKING EXAMS: p 428

A third of the chapter is about the PREPARATION in the run up to exams, including REVISION, and TAKING EXAMS. TAKING EXAMS covers the final preparation for the day of the exam, reading exam papers and good techniques for managing how your student answers the questions. TAKING EXAMS also includes ten KEY POINTS: EXAM-TAKING PROTOCOL, most of which are generally applicable.

KEY POINTS: EXAM-TAKING PROTOCOL: p 430

The sections §8 - §14 have extra comments, relating to key points 6 and 7 in EXAM-TAKING PROTOCOL, about taking exams in various formats:

§8: ESSAY, p 432   §9: MATHS AND SCIENCE, p 432
§10: MULTIPLE-CHOICE QUESTIONS, p 434   §11: PRACTICAL, p 436
§12: MUSIC, p 437   §13 ONLINE, p 439
§14: PSYCHOMETRIC, p 440
VIVAS AND INTERVIEWS are also a format for exams.

VIVAS AND INTERVIEWS: p 383

The sections about the less common formats also include discussion of likely problems and possible strategies your student could use to manage them. The problems and strategies are important when negotiating any appropriate exam provisions. Your student may need to accumulate evidence, similar to keeping good records in *ACCOMMODATIONS,* to back his arguments in the negotiations.

ACCOMMODATIONS:
p 128

Summary: Exams

- Accommodations (exam provisions) put in place as soon as possible.

- Revision materials accumulated throughout the relevant study.

- Self-confidence established and maintained.

- Realistic revision timetable drawn up, and modified if need be.

- Revision planning should be encouraging.

- Exam-taking skills and strategies need to be taught.

- Early practice in near exam conditions will show problems to be solved.

- Frequent practice will help to reduce exams to a less daunting task.

It might seem odd to advocate more exams rather than less. My experience comes from working in a university where there were exams every term, i.e. students had one or two exams three times a year. Students then had the opportunity to test out their strategies on a regular basis. The frequent exposure opens the possibility of moving from the frame of mind in *STORY: DON'T WORRY, WE KNOW YOU CAN'T DO THIS* to that in *STORY: I KNOW HOW I LEARN.*

*STORY: DON'T WORRY,
WE KNOW YOU CAN'T DO
THIS:* p 59

*STORY: I KNOW HOW I
LEARN:* p 58

3 Confidence and self-respect

Exams are stressful times, but they aren't the only stressful events that may occur in a person's life. One useful approach to exam stress is to regard it as an opportunity to learn de-stressing mechanisms and to test their robustness. *BUILDING CONFIDENCE AND SELF-ESTEEM* has some brief ideas about dealing with stress.

*BUILDING CONFIDENCE
AND SELF-ESTEEM:* p 78

A possible source of stress is comparison with other people. It would be best if your student is cautious about how he compares his performance with that of others, remembering that other people's minds work differently. Non-SpLD people may be able to recall knowledge and skills outside the exam situation in a way that his mind just doesn't. Before exams, during a series of them, and after exams, encourage him to engage only with those discussions that he knows help him. It's up to him to do all he can to preserve his confidence and self-respect.

You and your student need to be aware that dyslexic/ SpLD people can be very vulnerable to exam results that are lower than expected, even if they are above average. For example, there may be one subject that a student likes and is good at. His self-esteem may draw a lot from his skills in this subject. If his exam results for this subject are lower than he expects, his self-esteem and confidence can take considerable work to be re-established.

4 Using extra time

There are various ways that people use extra time. If your student is allowed extra time, the most important thing is to experiment to find what helps him best. Possibilities include:

- taking his time to read the paper carefully, to choose the right questions and plan

- taking his time to answer questions carefully

- dividing all the time equally between the number of questions to be done

- answering all the questions to be done; it is not good practice to leave a question out

- re-reading at the end, adding further ideas, checking the work, checking the spelling.

Encourage him to use every exam situation to his benefit to learn how to use his mind under difficult circumstances. Use the ideas in BEHIND THE OBVIOUS to reflect on his problems with exams and help him develop strategies and skills for dealing with them.

BEHIND THE OBVIOUS:
p 64

Extra time is sometimes just a buffer against the difficulties of dyslexia/ SpLD. If your student knows he has the extra time, he can worry less, focus on the work and not on avoiding dyslexia/ SpLD and he may well find he can complete the exam without using all the extra time. If he had less extra time, or none, he could find himself concentrating on avoiding the effects of his dyslexia/ SpLD, which is likely to increase his anxiety, make the effects of the dyslexia/ SpLD worse and he would find himself needing all the extra time, and possibly wishing for even more.

5 Exam support for graduates

If your student has been at university recently and is doing exams towards getting a job, he may need support to negotiate suitable provisions. The careers department[2] of his old university may be able to help him; or his nearest university may be able to help him as an ex-student of another university. He should be allowed exam provisions similar to those he has had in the past.

6 Preparation

Anxiety is probably the main problem with taking exams. The best way to tackle it is with thorough preparation and good exam techniques.

Summary: Preparation

The preparation includes:

- knowing the format of the exam, including any exam paper

- knowing what is expected of the candidate

- good revision

- your student looking after himself

- developing the right skills

- as much practice as possible.

---

[2] At the time of writing, careers departments can help students for a couple of years after they have left university and there are agreements to help students of other universities. Find out what help is available to your student.

Good exam techniques cover the last stages before an exam and what your student will do in the exam; they are discussed in *TAKING EXAMS*.

TAKING EXAMS: p 428

Make sure you know what your student is anxious about and that you are both addressing the root of his anxiety, see *BEHIND THE OBVIOUS*.

BEHIND THE OBVIOUS: p 64

Insight: Anxiety about not knowing everything on the exam paper

For school exams, everybody is taught all the topics and students are usually expected to be able to answer questions on any of the topics. Often at university, students choose which topics they are going to study and the exams are set to cover all possible choices; therefore it is expected that they will be unable to answer questions on every topic.

One student was becoming very anxious because there were too many questions that she couldn't answer; she wasn't looking at them and thinking: "I chose other topics and that's a topic that I shouldn't expect to be able to answer". Her level of anxiety was increasing quite unnecessarily.

BEHIND THE OBVIOUS: p 64
BUILDING CONFIDENCE AND SELF-ESTEEM: p 78

The ideas in *BEHIND THE OBVIOUS* and *BUILDING CONFIDENCE AND SELF-ESTEEM* can be used to search out underlying causes of anxiety.

Key points: Steps in preparation for exams:

1   Draw up your revision time-table as early as possible, and stick to it; include everything else you have to do so that it is obvious how much time you have, or how little.
2   Get plenty of sleep, good food and fresh air.
3   Learn to direct your mind. (See *METACOGNITION*)
4   Learn to relax. (See *RELAXATION*)

METACOGNITION: p 63
RELAXATION: p 558

5   Learn to breathe well. (See BREATHING)

6   *Practise the skills you need, even for exams which test knowledge.

7   *Practise in conditions that are as near as possible to those of the exam.

*There are other suggestions about 6) and 7) with the comments on different types of exam, in §8 - §14. The comments also include ideas and suggestions that are specific to the different types of exam.

BREATHING: p 557

Respect your own style of preparation:

- what suits one person does not suit another
- ignore any advice, given here or by others, that you know does not work for you
- test any suggestions that are new to you, if possible, well before an exam.

Be very cautious about trying new suggestions just before an exam or during one.

Taking exams is a time when pressure is usually considerable. At exam time, it is very helpful to be able to relax and breathe well; but your student also needs to know what to do. Practising the skills needed and in conditions as close to the real exam, points 6 and 7 above, are essential if he is going to benefit from relaxation and good breathing.

6.1 Revision

During revision, your student is reinforcing his memories of the material and skills that he has learnt; he is improving his access to those memories of that knowledge or those skills; he is improving the skills with which he uses that knowledge or those skills.

Your student may be preparing for practical exams in which skills are being examined as well as knowledge. Some practical revision will be to practise over and over again until your student is no longer thinking of the details of the movements:

- for music and dance he might then focus on the interpretation
- in driving he would concentrate on the situation
- in gas-fitter exams he would focus on the job to be done.

The forklift truck indicates those sections that could be most helpful and any relevant margin notes.

—The forklift truck shows ideas relevant to practical revision.

Summary: Revision overview

 People do revision in many different ways depending on their THINKING PREFERENCES.

You want to:

- find the processes that help you recall knowledge and skills from your mind
- find methods of working that suit you and encourage you
- find ways of prioritising the material, or skills, you are revising so that you are covering everything in a way that increases your confidence
- practise the skills you need to take the exam: reading exam questions and understanding them, planning, time-keeping, writing (or talking) the answers, doing the practical, keeping your mind on the topic
- organise a revision timetable that you can stick to and which you find builds your confidence.

 Several times as your student goes through the revision process, get him to reflect on his progress and how he feels about it. The reflection will give him some information that helps him make changes for the next time. The more he objectively assesses how he is doing, the more he will find the right way for him to approach revision, and other difficult situations.

6.1.1. Techniques for revision

RESOURCES FOR WORKING TOWARDS EXAMS lists the important sections, with page numbers, that are relevant to studying and revising. As your student works with recall and a good set of notes he can reflect on the topics he finds easy to recall and use; from the reflection, he will be able to establish which processes are the ones that work best for him for the course that he is revising.

Resources for working towards exams

METACOGNITION: p 63	*REGIME FOR MANAGING DYSLEXIA/ SPLD:* p 540
RECALL AND MEMORY EXERCISES: p 159	*ORGANISATION:* p 70
MIND SET: p 158	*COMPREHENSION:* p 162
CHUNKING: p 158	*TAKING NOTES:* p 305
BREATHING: p 557	*PLANNING:* p 200
RELAXATION: p 558	*INPUT, OUTPUT AND MOTIVATION:* p 72
THINKING PREFERENCES: p 72	

The following examples of *THINKING PREFERENCES* making a difference to the way people think may help your student to explore his choices:

- *SUPPORTING MATHS LEARNING*: the paragraph starting 'There can be solutions that come from your student's *THINKING PREFERENCES*' where different learning needs are spelt out

  paragraph in *SUPPORTING MATHS LEARNING:* p 104

- *DIFFERENCES IN THOUGHT PROCESSING*: where different internal interpretations are suggested for a single sentence

  DIFFERENCES IN THOUGHT PROCESSING: p 114

- *STORY: USING A VARIETY OF THINKING PROCESSES*: where different *THINKING PREFERENCES* are used for the various stages of working with a topic

  STORY: USING A VARIETY OF THINKING PROCESSES: p 150

- *EXAMPLE CONTINUED (AN EXAM QUESTION ABOUT ATMOSPHERIC MANAGEMENT)*: the analysis of the exam question helps people with different *THINKING PREFERENCES* in a variety of ways.

  EXAMPLE: AN EXAM QUESTION ABOUT ATMOSPHERIC MANAGEMENT: p 192

It is suggested in *GOALS FOR A COURSE* that your student uses the course materials to establish the knowledge and skills that he is learning from a course. If your student goes through a course knowing the goals and making effective sets of notes, he will have good revision materials at the start of his revision process.

GOALS FOR A COURSE: p 198

The methods of working that suit you might be one or several of:

- using mind set at suitable times so that your revision efficiency is improved

- working with a revision partner, or group

- working on your own

- spreading your topics, or skills, uniformly across your revision timetable

- assessing the relative importance of your topics, or skills, and how much work each one needs and then spreading them across your revision timetable according to your assessment

- having complete days on one topic, or skills

- dividing your day into two or more topics, or skills.

Insight: Mind set the evening before a day's revision

When there is a full day of revision planned, some people use the evening before to do mind set tasks in preparation for the next day. The mind set tasks might be something like organising the notes for the subject or finding the past papers or getting the textbooks together. It is often a related task but one which doesn't make heavy demands on your student's mental energies.

Ⓖ p 575 mind set

Another reason for your student to monitor his progress is that methods that he used in the past may not work for subsequent exam revision and it is better to find that out as early as possible.

6.1.2 Prioritising topics for revision

Your student should not be learning new material, though in practice the revision period may be a time when he discovers which bits of the subject he has missed. He will need to decide how important they are to his subject and whether he should learn them or leave them.

Your student should think about all the subjects he needs to revise and whether he is going to give equal time to all of them, or whether some subjects need more or less time than others.

 It is important to get the priorities right when choosing which subject to revise and when. If your student starts with the subject that he knows least well or that he most dislikes, he may find that revision is hard, it takes more time than he would hope, and he quickly disengages from the process. However if he leaves this subject to the last, he is likely to panic that it is getting no attention.

One suggestion that gets taken up by students very frequently is to start with the favourite subject, or the one your student knows best, and after that to revise his least favourite subject.

The idea being that he develops his skills and enjoys his revision on his favourite subject

he then applies the skills to the least favourite subject and enjoys working with them

the combination of the two subjects could mean that the revision of the least favourite subject feels easier for him to do.

Your student then alternates: second best, the second worst, third best, third worst; he works in from the extremes until he's covered all his subjects.

6.1.3 How much can be written in an exam?

As your student revises, he can check his exam techniques as well. For example as part of 'writing the answers', he needs to be able to balance his main points with detail; he needs to manage time; and he needs to answer the question set. The following *Tip: To Work Out How Much You Can Write, and to Keep on Target* can help him improve his techniques.

Tip: To work out how much you can write, and to keep on target

This example is based on a nominally three-hour exam in which you might be expected to answer four questions, giving a nominal average of 45 minutes per answer.

The *ILLUSTRATION* assumes that you use the 25% extra time[3] to brainstorm, to plan, and to proof-read at the end.

- Choose an exam question that you know something about; write freely on it for 15 minutes, using anything that comes to mind no matter how vague or off the point: you're writing on the topic to see how many words you write in those 15 minutes.

- Count the number of words and multiply by 3 to give the number of words you can write quickly in 45 minutes: in the *ILLUSTRATION*, 900 words.

- The number of main points you might expect to put in an essay is between 4 and 8: 6 in the *ILLUSTRATION*. The number of main points will be the number of paragraphs in your answer.

- Dividing the total number of words by the number of main points gives you a rough idea of how many words per paragraph: in the *ILLUSTRATION*, 150 words.

- Then create a document with 6 headings 'main point' spaced out, with each space stating the number of words; this is the 'Guiding layout' in *FIGURE 11.1*.

- Print this document and put it alongside you as you do practice papers.

ILLUSTRATION: You write 300 words in 15 minutes;
thus 900 words in 45 minutes; you aim for 6 paragraphs of 150 words per paragraph.

Your guiding layout:
900 words per answer
main point 1   150 words
main point 2   150 words
main point 3   150 words
main point 4   150 words
main point 5   150 words
main point 6   150 words

150 words of your 300 words shows you how much you can write for a main point. The number of lines for 150 words gives you an estimate of the space for each paragraph.

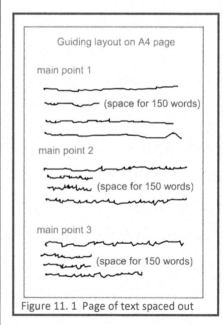

Figure 11. 1 Page of text spaced out

---

[3] I have included 25% extra time to demonstrate what it can be used for. If your student is not allowed extra time, adjust the figures in the *ILLUSTRATION*.

- In the exam situation, you can either visualise your guiding layout(**vision** etc.), or the experience of using it will come back to you (**kinaesthetic**), or you will remember it by the words (**verbal**), or you can remember how many paragraphs fit on an A4 page and you can mark off the space for them in the margin (**framework**).

The student who worked out this method finds that he is able to keep his mind to the point when writing exam answers as a result of this strategy.

6.1.4 Revising skills

Some practical skills need to be learnt to the point that they are automatic, e.g. the different sequences in driving a car. Your student needs to find his own rhythm for learning the sequences. *PREPARATION FOR DOING*, *MENTAL REHEARSAL OF MOVEMENTS* and the *EXERCISE FOR STUDENT: MEMORISING EXERCISES* all have ideas relevant to revising skills, including the recommendation that practising skills is best done little and often. The *INSIGHT: PRACTISING TO LEARN A SKILL* has some suggestions for enhancing the right thought patterns.

PREPARATION FOR DOING: p 291

MENTAL REHEARSAL OF MOVEMENTS: p 292

EXERCISE FOR STUDENT: MEMORISING EXERCISES: p 160

Practical skills often need to be over-learnt. Your student wants to be sure that no pressure from the exam situation is going to interfere with the sequence of the skill.

INSIGHT: PRACTISING TO LEARN A SKILL: p 484
APPLYING A SKILL: p 404

Your student also needs to consider how the skills will be used, whether they are to be used as a complete set pattern or adapted to different situations, see *APPLYING A SKILL* and *ADAPTING A SKILL TO NEW SITUATIONS*.

ADAPTING A SKILL TO NEW SITUATIONS: p 404

6.1.5 Revision timetable

Setting out a timetable is a fairly regular task with many dyslexic/ SpLD students I have supported. The timetables are not just for revision purposes. The processes described here can be adapted to any task that has to be undertaken.

TEMPLATES

We use a calendar sheet such as *TEMPLATE: B9 - A CALENDAR MONTH FOR PRIORITISING – 5 WEEKS*. My template is from a spreadsheet that I update every year. It can be adjusted to cover from the present until the deadline in question. I would use several pages rather than trying to squash too much onto one. I leave space round the outside edge for relevant notes; it is better to keep them on the same page.

We include everything that is taking a significant amount of time in the student's life. We discuss things that are making him uncertain about time; how long it takes him to get up, what's causing a delay in getting to work. We include the social commitments he has; his lectures; group meetings; time for domestic chores; time to travel between places; time for meals, exercise and fun. If the specific time for something is not known, we block out a period of time to represent the task.

The aim is to be as realistic as possible about the time for revision.

I let students know that I expect there will be modifications; that we won't devise a suitable timetable the first time we do it; that what doesn't work is telling us more about the way he functions.

Story: I never start on time

One student came and said he could never start at the time he wanted to and that he wasn't getting enough revision time. He was getting depressed about his late starts and therefore not working well.

When we did a very detailed look at his timetable for the day, he realised he wasn't putting in time to eat breakfast and that eating breakfast made him start revision later than he planned.

Once he put in time for breakfast and was no longer starting later than he expected, his revision went well.

Having put all the other time-related events into the calendar, we work out how much time is left for revision. At this point, students sometimes decide they will have to reduce the number of other activities they hope to do. These get removed from the timetable.

During the discussion, we will cover the range of hours the student prefers to study. Some work better in the morning and some late at night, with all variations between.

We end with revision times clearly visible.

The final stage is to plan the revision:

- Decide what pattern of working will suit you in terms of hours per day, slots per day, subjects per day, etc.
- Count up the number of revision days or slots that you have on your timetable.
- Then write down when you plan to revise which subjects.
- It is useful to have some spare time just before the exams; you can decide how to use this time when it arrives and you see what you most need to do. You may have some topics that need extra time; you may want to go through all the subjects in a fast way right at the end.

Adapt the ideas about a revision timetable so that it suits the regime necessary to learn the practical skills to the right level of performance.

Sticking to a revision timetable is often not easy. There is always more to learn and many people have the instinct to stay on one subject and hope there will be time for the others. If he gives in to this instinct, your student could well end with one subject for which he knows very little, but for which he has to answer several questions, or which will be an integral part of a practical exam.

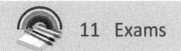

6.2 Disappointing exam results

Disappointing exam results can be usefully instructive if used in the right way: they can help your student to know more about the way he works. Comments from subject tutors that they expect your student to do better in exams quite often indicate a problem.

Story: Exam results not in line with class discussions

To let me know what his results were, one physics student forwarded the email from his tutor. The tutor expressed disappointment that the student had missed the first class grade that was predicted.

Since his marks were only just too low, the student wasn't going to do anything about it, but I offered him the chance to see if any change would make a difference.

We discussed all his methods of taking exams; his breadth of knowledge of the topics; his contributions in classes. Everything seemed to be working for him, except that he runs out of time in exams. He set about showing me how he reads questions and how he decides on the answers.

Eventually, we found that he has his own way of understanding physics and it doesn't involve the vocabulary of physics. In an exam, with questions set using the normal words, this student had to take time to realise which part of physics the question was referring to: he was having to translate between two systems: one natural to him, the other not so natural.

The student found it hard to practise using the vocabulary of physics, but he did try. Using many other exam techniques, he was able to get more done in the exams, but never to the point of having enough time. In his last exams, he didn't quite finish but he only missed the last part of one question.

With very good exams results and excellent project work, he achieved the first class that his tutor felt he was capable of getting.

You need to know exactly why your exam results are disappointing in order to find the solutions. Some possible causes are:

- you may not have done enough work or covered all the material
- the exam conditions may not allow you to demonstrate the knowledge you have learnt or the skills you have acquired
- you may have had such bad experience of exams that you are scared of them
- the exams may be so different from any you have taken before that you are not approaching them in the best way
- you may not have any strategies for taking exams that you can follow
- you may be learning the wrong way for your mind
- you may be misreading the questions
- you may be answering in the wrong way
- the exam may be competitive, with only a specified number of the top people being said to pass; in which case, the other candidates are said to have failed
- the material of the exam may be beyond your capabilities.

This list is not complete, but hopefully it covers the major causes of candidates failing exams.

There is nothing that can be done about the last reason, except to recognise when your student can't master the material and should not enter for the exam.

In the competitive exam situation, whether your student passes or fails is a little bit out of his control because it depends on the quality of the competition. How he deals with failing is more a question of self-confidence and esteem than exam preparation or technique, see *BUILDING CONFIDENCE AND SELF-ESTEEM*.

BUILDING CONFIDENCE AND SELF-ESTEEM: p 78

There should be possible solutions for all the other causes of failing exams, but you and your student need to find out the real cause, see *BEHIND THE OBVIOUS*.

BEHIND THE OBVIOUS: p 64

There have been several occasions when it has been possible for me to look at a student's script in order to see what is going wrong. The student's memory hasn't been sufficient. The exam marker and the subject tutor have only been able to look at the subject content and have not been able to appreciate signs of the dyslexia/ SpLD impacting on the student's performance. It has only been by listening to the student, knowing something of the way the student thinks and then seeing the exam answers, that I've been able to work with the student to solve the problems. Exam scripts are not always available to be read, so there need to be other ways of unravelling the problem.

If the student can sit a practice exam in as near exam conditions as possible, you and he can start to see what is happening. Sometimes watching your student answer a question will reveal the problem. You may not find the root cause of problems from what your student tells you.

Insight: What goes wrong in an exam

One physics student kept doing badly in exams. She was supposed to do a practice exam between support sessions, but other activities took precedence. She arrived at the session with the exam paper.

She talked me through the different parts of the exam and how she would approach them. She indicated the question she knew well, including telling me how she had explained the material to fellow students (this is not unknown for dyslexic people who fail exams: they coach others well, but can't pass the exams themselves). There wasn't time to wait for another round of exams to see what was going wrong. We needed to solve the problem before any more exams were sat.

I asked her to answer one of the questions she knew well in the way she would answer it in an exam. She produced several lines of physics equations and manipulation on landscape A4 paper, with a wide margin down one side. We started to analyse the processes involved in the answer. We wrote them down in the margin, as in *DISCUSSION OF KEY WORD EXERCISE*. Through the analysis, it became clear that she was leaving out all the reasoning around the equations. She felt the reasoning was so self-evident that it was unnecessary to put it down. Her answer looked like book work rather poorly remembered without any understanding; it looked as if the bare minimum was being reproduced in the hopes that it would answer the question.

No amount of changing exam techniques or revision programmes would have changed the exam results if the student had continued to leave out all the material that showed the examiners that she knew the subject very well.

The student's approach lacked recognition of the multiple goals of exams: the student has to answer questions AND show the examiners that she knows the subject, see *MULTIPLE GOALS*. The examiners can't guess knowledge and skills that aren't shown to them.

DISCUSSION OF KEY WORD EXERCISE: p 216

MULTIPLE GOALS: p 183

If the reason for the failure is something like fear, the practice exam may be sufficiently different from a real one that the fear doesn't surface and your student hasn't started to unravel the problem. In such cases, I have used a combination of techniques from NeuroLinguistic Programming (Stacey, 2019); *RECORDINGS* of the exercises can be found on the website. The *EXERCISE: SIT-STAND* shows the impact of negative expectations on the physical, psychological and mental states of a person. Combining the insight with *USING CHALLENGES* can bring about significant shifts in attitudes towards exams.

Stacey (2019)

RECORDINGS

USING CHALLENGES: p 80

It is worth investigating whether unrecognised dyslexic/ SpLD problems are at the heart of failing exams, for example the case briefly outlined in *INSIGHTS: SOME UNOBVIOUS PROBLEMS* in which panic attacks in exams were due to total lack of a systematic approach to taking exams.

INSIGHTS: SOME UNOBVIOUS PROBLEMS: p 64

7 Taking exams

The following is a final check-list before an exam; suggestions about the four points are covered in other parts of the book.

Key points: Before an exam

- The night before, check your pens, exam times, any candidate number, etc. Also check that you have anything you need relating to appropriate exam provisions, see OBJECTS NEEDED.

- Arrive in good time, see TIME and SPACE, PLACE, AND DIRECTIONS.

- Avoid previews with other candidates, and, at the end, avoid post mortems, see BUILDING CONFIDENCE AND SELF-ESTEEM.

- Maintain a good state of mind, see THINKING CLEARLY.

OBJECTS NEEDED: p 71

TIME: p 69

SPACE, PLACE, AND DIRECTIONS: p 69

BUILDING CONFIDENCE AND SELF-ESTEEM: p 78

THINKING CLEARLY: p 79

Exam papers

Many exams have exam papers; some exams are online and some are spoken (vivas). The comments here are about reading exam papers. The problems with online papers are outlined in ONLINE EXAMS, and vivas (oral exams) are discussed in VIVAS AND INTERVIEWS.

ONLINE EXAMS: p 439

VIVAS AND INTERVIEWS: p 383

Your student may have to choose a number of questions; there may be many questions that he doesn't answer or there may be just one or two that he doesn't answer. He may have no choice at all, except the order in which he answers them. He may have a compulsory question.

Answering the questions in the order your student finds easiest to the most difficult allows

- him to get going with high confidence
- his mind to subconsciously work on the other questions so that
    - by the time he is working on them
    - he knows more than he would have done had he started with the most difficult.

It is also a practice that helps him to maintain a high level of confidence.

If there is a compulsory question, he gets no extra marks for doing it first.

He still needs to be careful of timing and not write too much on the easiest question; see the *Tip: To Work Out How Much You Can Write, and Keep on Target*.

Tip: To Work Out How Much You Can Write, and Keep on Target: p 420

Long exam questions

With questions that have a lot of information, it will help your student to find out what he has to do with the information before he reads it. In law or social science exams there is often a passage that sets the scene; what he has to do is often given at the bottom of the passage. Teach your student to read what he has to do before reading the passage.

In science or maths exams there is often a lot of data; what your student has to do can be written amongst the data. He should find the instructions, read them and mark them before understanding the data.

Exam-taking protocol

Key Points: Exam-Taking Protocol is written assuming that the candidates can choose which questions to answer. Comments are included within brackets relating to situations when all the questions have to be answered.

Key point: Exam-taking protocol

1   Read any instructions carefully. Note how many questions you have to do.

2   Read the whole paper twice. Make little notes against the questions you can answer. This helps you to concentrate and also helps you to decide which questions to do. If it helps, grade the questions Y, yes I can answer; P probably I can answer; X I can't answer.
(No choice: Use any marking scheme to help you choose the order to answer the questions.)

3   Choose all the questions you are going to answer. Start with the question you know best. While you are writing the answer to the first question you are subconsciously thinking about the others, as mentioned above. If there is a compulsory question, you don't have to start with it, though you must do it.
(No choice: Choose the order to answer the questions.)

Exam management

Exam management is a continuation of reading the exam paper.
4   Use rough paper or a separate booklet to capture ideas. Have space on your rough paper for each question you decide to answer; then you can quickly jot down ideas when they come to you.
You need to balance:
- the need to work without disruption
- the benefit of capturing the ideas
- not worrying that you will forget the good ideas as they surface in your mind; the worry could disturb your fluency/ efficiency.

5   Be sure to identify exactly what the question is asking you.

6   Answer precisely the question set, no more and no less. Regard all knowledge as important only because it can be used in evidence relevant to the solution of a problem or the answer to a question.

7   If the questions have equal marks, divide the time equally between them, which
    could be done in various ways. Two examples being:

    a)   ~ 10 mins to read and choose questions & to decide on the order
          reserve 10 mins for final work = 20 mins (start & stop time)
          planning & writing time = total exam time - 20 mins (start & stop time)
          divide planning & writing time between the questions

    b)   ~ 30 mins to read paper, choose questions, decide order and plan all
              answers
          reserve 5 mins for gathering up papers = 35 mins (read & plan all +
              gathering up papers)
          writing time = total exam time – 35 mins
          divide writing time between questions
    (If the questions don't have equal marks, divide the time between them according
    to the number of marks.)

8   If you are writing in a booklet, rather than on sheets of paper, start each answer
    on a double opening. This way you have two pages to write on before you have
    the disadvantage of turning over the page; when you turn over there is a
    tendency for dyslexic/ SpLD people to forget what they wrote on the now unseen
    page; by using a double opening, you should be well into the themes of your
    answer before you have to turn over.

9   Read through your answers at the end providing you know that it is helpful to do
    so. You might remember extra points as you re-read your answers. You might see
    some errors and be able to correct them; be sure that they are errors.

10 Check that you have numbered the questions and completed any administration
    details, such as crossing-out rough-working. Assemble your answer sheets in the
    right order.

8   Essay exams

Extra suggestions to 'practise the skills you need' (*Step 6*, p 415):

- Practise reading and understanding exam questions, see *Goals for Writing*.

- Practise selecting questions, see point 3 above in *Exam-Taking Protocol*, p 430.

Read with:
Preparation: p 413
Taking Exams: p 428

Goals for Writing:
p 187

Extra suggestions to 'practise in real conditions' (*Step 7*, p 415):

- Do some timed answers to past questions, see the *Tip: To Work Out How Much You Can Write, and To Keep On Target*.

- Ask someone, preferably a tutor, to comment on the plan of your answer and the content, and also on how you collected your ideas together during the time available.

- Randomise the past questions by putting several in a hat, or box or plastic bag, and doing the one you pick out first.

Tip: To Work Out How Much You Can Write, and To Keep On Target: p 420

Extra points for taking the exam:

- If you spend time preparing a skeleton outline, you write your answers more fluently and quickly.

- Use rough paper or a separate booklet for your plans, so that you can see them at the same time as you write your answers.

9   Maths and science exams

Some maths exams are set so that you answer as many questions as you can; in others you have to choose which ones to answer.

Read with:
Preparation: p 413
Taking Exams: p 428

Extra suggestions to 'practise the skills you need' (*STEP 6*, p 415):

- Maths and much of science include a lot of practical work, even in pen and paper exams.

- You are expected to know about processes as well as understand the concepts.

- You sometimes reproduce the processes, e.g. proofs, in a standard form; you will also have to apply them to unknown sets of data.

- There will be many skills that you need to demonstrate.

- Learning maths, and quite a bit of science, should be regarded as *DOING* and *TAKING-ACTION*.

- Developing and practising the necessary skills is often best achieved through doing past papers.

DOING: p 280
TAKING-ACTION: p 388

Both maths and science questions can contain a lot of information that you have to work with.

- Practise reading questions and deciding what concepts the question is about.

- Identify and mark the *PROCESS* words that tell you what you have been asked to do.

PROCESS AND CONTENT WORDS: p 189

- Recognise the maths processes that are relevant to the question.

- Identify the data.

- Work on strategies that help you move from one line of a proof or calculation to the next without making errors.

- Think how you will deal with turning over the page if you are someone who loses track of anything that goes out of sight.

Extra points for taking the exam:

For exams when you answer as many questions as you can:

- Don't spend too long on a question that you can't answer straight away.

- Mark the question as one to come back to; leave space in the answer book to go back; and carry on with the paper.

- As with essay questions, the answers may surface in your mind while you are working on a different question.

Problems and solutions

- The length of questions can be a considerable problem when data and question are on different sides of a sheet of paper; the short-term memory problems as discussed in *OUT OF SIGHT IS OUT OF MIND* mean information is not retained once the page is turned over. The best solution for this problem is to allow the candidate to have two copies of the exam paper.

OUT OF SIGHT IS OUT OF MIND: p 90

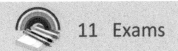

- The same problem can affect writing the answers and often the candidate needs to see both pages easily when an answer goes across two pages. Writing only on one side is one strategy that works; having loose paper might be suitable. The solutions will depend on the candidate.

- One student had found a particular spacing between lines allowed him to manage the flow of his equations. He was allowed to give the exams office a supply of the paper for his exams. This is a good example of a particular provision that enabled a student to demonstrate the knowledge and skills that are being examined.

- Recalling formulae can be a significant problem. If knowing the formulae is not part of the exam, formulae sheets are a good solution.

10 Multiple-choice questions (MCQ)

✶ indicates the points that are most relevant to ONLINE EXAMS which have a lot in common with MCQs.

Read with:
PREPARATION: p 413
TAKING EXAMS: p 428
ONLINE EXAMS: p 439

Extra suggestions to 'practise the skills you need' *(STEP 6, p 415)*:

- Find out the mechanics of answering the questions: straight into a computer or marking a sheet that will be fed into a computer.

- ✶Practise the mechanics of answering the questions as well as understanding and choosing the right answer.

- ✶You need to look for the most suitable methods of dealing with the format of MCQ that is being used for your exam.

Extra suggestions to 'practise in real conditions' *(STEP 7, p 415)*:

- ✶See if there is a mock, or past, paper that you can use for practice.

- ✶Practise using any provisions that have been set up for you.

Extra points for taking the exam:

- Don't spend too long on a question that you can't answer straight away; mark the question as one to come back to. As with essay questions, the answers may surface in your mind while you are working on a different question.

- Work on blocks of questions at a time, probably 5 at a time.
- Use a ruler to keep your place
- ✶You may need to re-write the question. Practise doing so under timed conditions.
- ✶You need to protect your confidence by knowing that the re-writing is better than puzzling over the wording.

Problems and solutions

For some dyslexic/ SpLD people, MCQ papers are the answer to taking exams; for others they can generate considerable problems with

- ✶reading the question
- ✶selecting the answer
- ✶keeping track of the lines
- marking the answer sheet on paper or online
- ✶switching thinking between subjects
- ✶switching thinking between tasks: reading, selecting answer, marking answer.

It can be difficult to spend so much time reading; it can be difficult to understand the questions if one cannot annotate the paper; it can be difficult to distinguish between closely worded versions of nearly the same ideas; it can be difficult to track across the answer sheets and fill in the correct box; if anything goes out of sight, it can be very difficult to retain the information. It can be difficult to switch thinking between different subjects as fast as is necessary to complete the exam or to switch thinking between the different tasks involved in dealing with MCQs.

✶Each person needs to understand his/her major problems and try to find solutions that are going to be robust enough to endure in the exam situation. It may be necessary to negotiate suitable provisions in order for your student to demonstrate his knowledge and skills, see *ACCOMMODATIONS*.

ACCOMMODATIONS: p 128

11 Practical exams

Read with:
PREPARATION: p 413
TAKING EXAMS: p 428

★ indicates the points that are most relevant to ONLINE EXAMS which have a lot in common with MCQs.

Extra suggestions to 'practise in real conditions' (STEP 7, p 415):

You need to find out the conditions of the exam in order to practise 'in *conditions* as near as possible to those of the exam'.

- In some practical exams you rotate through different stations and managing time is not solely in your control. The stations are areas set with different tasks that have to be dealt with by candidates in turn.

- In other exams, you are given an experiment to carry out.

- In a driving test you are expected to drive round a particular course as instructed by the examiner.

- In one geology exam, the practical element involved identifying samples of rock and moving from one group of rocks to another as the exam progressed.

★The examiners may not have had to think about provisions for dyslexia/ SpLD before. Appropriate provisions will depend quite significantly on the candidate taking the exam. Therefore a very early stage of preparation is to find out precisely what skills and strategies you will need in order to take the exam. It is no good practising the wrong set of strategies.

★In all of these examples you need to experience taking an exam in the place of the exam. That experience is the only reliable way of identifying the problems your dyslexia/ SpLD will cause and the possible solutions that you can develop to cope with them. Even for driving, if the conditions of the roads you practise on are quite different from the test course you may find your strategies are not robust enough. I suggest taking an exam rather than walking round the place because your actions during a pretend exam will reveal more to you than simply being in the place.

The possible problems are going to include:

- ✳not being able to work fast enough
- ✳not being able to read questions and information
- ✳not being able to annotate the questions and information as you read them
- ✳not being organised the right way for you, as you move from one station to another
- ✳not having time to set out equipment in a way that allows you to manage your dyslexia/ SpLD
- not responding to verbal instructions correctly (for example, not knowing left from right)
- ✳other; as exam practices alter there will be different problems.

Possible solutions:

- ✳Once you have inspected the exam site and the way the exam questions will be presented to you, you can work out what you need to do or what arrangements need to be made in order to demonstrate your knowledge and skills.

- ✳If it is a question of negotiating exam provisions see *ACCOMMODATIONS*.

ACCOMMODATIONS: p 128

REVISION: p 415

- ✳If it is a question of you developing and improving your knowledge and skills, make a *REVISION* programme, paying special attention to points flagged by the forklift truck. The programme should include practice of skills and knowledge in conditions as close to the exam conditions as possible.

12   Music exams

Extra points for taking the exam:

Music exams usually consist of pieces of music that have been learnt and are to be performed during the exam, technical work and supporting tests. The pieces and technical work come into the category of skills recalled and used directly, see *A MODEL OF LEARNING*. The supporting tests involve knowledge and skills recalled and used directly as learnt, as well as demonstrated by developed use.

Read with:
PREPARATION: p 413
TAKING EXAMS: p 428

A MODEL OF LEARNING: p 145

Choosing the right pieces to learn and learning them in a way that works for you is going to be fundamental to your success. You have no choice over the technical work: the material is set and the examiner tells you what to play out of a selection of possibilities. You can choose the supporting tests that you find easiest. You can choose when to sit the exam. You need to consider how to manage your preparation so that you reach the right level of competence without becoming bored by the practice.

There may well be dyslexic/ SpLD reasons why some parts of the tests will always be difficult for you and you may not be able to choose enough tests that you know you can practise to the level required. It is important to recognise the hazards and obstacles of your dyslexia/ SpLD and have a way of defusing any potential confidence knocks from lower than hoped for results. For your personal assessment, you could divide the pieces and tests that were not hampered by dyslexic/ SpLD issues from those that were. You can use the marks for the former to be a better assessment of your performance and preparation than the overall mark. It won't alter the mark that is officially registered, but it could allow you to maintain your self-esteem and to carry on enjoying the learning.

The object of such an approach is not to reduce the expectations, which remain high, but to allow exam-taking to be productive without low marks or failure having a devastating effect.

Having the full breakdown of marks for pieces and supporting tests can be important for continuing progress for the player. Music exam boards need to make them available, and keep doing so.

Extra suggestions to 'practise the skills you need' (*STEP 6*, p 415):

Preparation for performance often has to start from the very initial stages of learning, which is covered in *LEARNING A SKILL*. *PLANNING RELATED TO SKILLS* and *TAKING-ACTION* are also relevant to performance. It may be especially important to realise that playing pieces in a music exam is an example of a situation when there is *NO PAUSE BUTTON*. You need to know how you will deal with times when you play the wrong note in an exam.

LEARNING A SKILL: p 288

PLANNING RELATED TO SKILLS: p 208

TAKING-ACTION: p 388

NO PAUSE BUTTON: p 397

Extra suggestions to 'practise in real conditions' (*STEP 7*, p 415):

The environment may affect you as you play in many different ways. You need to get used to playing in different places; you need to observe what these differences are and decide how you will deal with them. Becoming confident in playing in different places to different listeners will increase your confidence in the exam itself.

Extra points for taking the exam:

Besides being very well prepared, the skills of being able to *THINK CLEARLY* should be practised so that they are as automatic as possible well before the exam. As you go into the exam, make sure you establish the technique that suits you best for *THINKING CLEARLY*.

THINK CLEARLY: p 79

13   Online exams

Newly qualified teachers (NQT) must pass some online tests. They very often run out of time to complete the exams; the only sensible solution is to practise until as many of the processes as possible are used automatically, including strategies to deal with the exams and techniques for *THINKING CLEARLY*.

THINKING CLEARLY: p 79

Online exams have much in common with *MULTIPLE-CHOICE QUESTIONS (MQC)* and *PRACTICAL EXAMS;* the relevant points in these two sections are marked with ✳.

MULTIPLE-CHOICE QUESTIONS (MQC): p 434

PRACTICAL EXAMS: p 436

The main themes are finding out:

- exactly what the exam will be like
- what the conditions will be like
- what preparation for the exam is needed and possible.

The possible problems are likely to include your student:

- not being able to see everything correctly together
- having information overload with too much in view
- not being able to go back and alter
- reading incorrectly because of the way items line up with each other
- not being able to track on screen as he reads
- not being able to mark his place or annotate the questions
- having a time limit for taking the paper.

One provision that might be suitable is a hard copy of the exam, or a computer format that can be edited or annotated with comments by the candidate.

14 Psychometric exams or tests

Comments about psychometric exams or tests:

Employers are increasingly using psychometric testing in job application processes before a candidate even gets interviewed. There are many websites which offer the opportunity to practise taking such a test and extra time is allowed in some cases. Psychometric tests have much in common with *MULTIPLE-CHOICE QUESTIONS* and with *ONLINE EXAMS*.

Psychometric tests are usually administered online or by computer in some way.

Psychometric tests are of three main types: intelligence, aptitude and personality. What makes them 'psychometric' is that they provide a direct comparison between the individual being tested and some kind of 'standard' group, which may be the general population or a specific group such as trainee nurses or engineers or call centre workers.

The scores on the test produced by the standard group are processed using psychological statistics, resulting in a 'standard' range of scores. When an individual is tested, his score can be placed within that range, and can be classified as, for example, average, above average, or below average. Generally a more precise form of numerical reporting is used.

Employers may then set the cut-off or threshold above which they are prepared to consider candidates.

Tests of intelligence or aptitude typically comprise a large number of questions that have to be attempted in a set time limit.

The total number of questions is usually more than even the most able candidate could be expected to attempt within the time limit.

Since all the questions are of equivalent difficulty, an individual's score is simply the number of correct answers they give.

Read with:
PREPARATION: p 413
TAKING EXAMS: p 428

MULTIPLE-CHOICE QUESTIONS: p 434

ONLINE EXAMS: p 439

Intelligence tests are designed to assess general ability and typically include items that measure verbal intelligence (such as vocabulary knowledge) and non-verbal intelligence (such as diagrammatic puzzles).

Intelligence tests are difficult to prepare for, but practice material is readily available both online and in booklets available from some bookshops.

The more practice intelligence tests that your student attempts the more confident he will be.

Aptitude tests cover acquired knowledge in a specific area, such as driving test theory, maths, electrical law and safety, etc.

As well as doing practice tests, your student can prepare for these by revising his knowledge in the subject.

Personality tests are different in that there is usually no time limit, and a smaller number of questions to which there are no correct answers.

Personality tests are designed to reveal what the person is like in terms of such traits as sociability, determination, persistence, team-working, honesty, helpfulness, adaptability, anxiety, etc.

It is risky to try to 'cheat' the test in order to pretend to be the sort of employee that the organisation might be seeking because the test producers are aware that this might happen and have built into the test subtle ways of detecting cheats.

One of the most critical factors in intelligence and aptitude tests is time management.

Since each question usually counts the same as every other question there is nothing to be gained (and much to be lost) by your student spending a lot of time trying to puzzle out an individual question that he finds tough.

It is better for him to skip questions he doesn't know the answer to, or choose an answer at random, than to waste precious time pondering. However, he should be aware that more sophisticated tests may present a selection of possible answers, which includes ones that are clearly wrong and choosing these could result in marks being deducted.

Psychometric exams or tests may be one type of test for which no suitable practice is possible and for which no accommodation will work. If your student finds he keeps failing these tests, he needs to observe objectively what problems he encounters, how he would usually deal with the problems and why it isn't possible to do so while taking a psychometric test. Your student should then request that his job application is considered without him taking the psychometric test. From your work with your student you are in a position to write a covering letter backing his case in terms of the impact of his dyslexia/ SpLD.

Useful sections:
BEHIND THE OBVIOUS:
p 64
ACCOMMODATIONS:
p 128
NEGOTIATING ACCOMMODATIONS:
p 550

Key point: Employers missing good employees

Employers should be aware that psychometric tests are ruling out some candidates who would have much to offer as employees.

For certain dyslexic/ SpLD people, asking them to succeed in psychometric tests is like asking a wheelchair user to go up a steep flight of stairs: practically impossible.

The following story illustrates lack of comprehension.

Story: The instructions don't make sense

One day, the post office introduced new procedures for paying in. I took the relevant leaflet home so that I would be able to use the new system.
I studied it hard and could not work out what to do, so I picked up everything I thought might be needed.
After the post-master had taken me through the system, I thought "That was easy, why weren't the instructions straightforward?"

When I re-read them, they were completely obvious. I couldn't improve them. I realised that one detail of the old system was sabotaging my attempts to understand the new.

Lack of comprehension like this is not an isolated experience. It was easily resolved when reality and words were matched. Accommodations need to be sorted out for psychometric testing so that similar problems do not result in capable people failing to get beyond the tests.

Possible problems:

Some of the problems likely to be encountered are listed below. It is not an exhaustive list. The problems encountered are likely to vary from one person to another depending on the effects of the dyslexia/ SpLD experienced by each individual.

Usual techniques can't be applied:

- Tests not specific to a topic: this rules out many techniques essential for reading and thinking e.g. chunking, mental set, preparation of long-term memory recall.

Reading:

- unfamiliar context
- complex wording makes meaning very obscure
- not able to annotate the text
- no time to re-write the questions or text
- no time, or insufficient text, to use scanning techniques to get the overall context
- mis-reading words, or sections
- short-term memory not carrying 1 or 2 words from one part of the question to another.

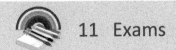

- Tracking with mouse to assist reading may result in distracting pop-ups: this disables one very important reading strategy.

- Pop-ups interfere with concentration.

- When a calculator is used it needs to be completely visible at the same time as the question to avoid short-term memory problems. Two linked screens should be available so that the full question is visible at the same time as the calculator.

- In numerical questions, one word or fact being mis-interpreted can lead to a wrong answer; without seeing the working, the capabilities of the candidate can be misjudged.

Extra suggestions to 'practise the skills you need' (*STEP 6,* p 415):

- Find out the type of psychometric paper you will be set.

- Practise doing this kind.

- Also practise doing some similar ones, but with slightly different format or range of questions.

- The reason for practising with other papers is to maintain a flexible approach and to avoid becoming set in one pattern.

- A level of flexibility will help you think effectively when taking the real test.

Extra suggestions to 'practise in real conditions' (*STEP 7,* p 415):

- Practise some papers without time constraints and check your answers with those given.

- Notice the kinds of difficulties you experience, and see what solutions you can find for them.

- Then, practise in as near test conditions as possible:
    - time
    - environment
    - computer settings
    - even including the clothes you wear.

Extra points for taking the exam:

- Taking the tests may be part of formal job applications and you may have to go to the prospective place of employment.

- You may be wearing more formal clothes than you are accustomed to.

- If you are someone who is strongly affected by your *ENVIRONMENT*, practising in formal clothes may reduce the impact of the whole set up.

ENVIRONMENT: p 70

15   Vivas and interviews

VIVAS AND INTERVIEWS: p 383

Vivas and interviews have been discussed in full in *VIVAS AND INTERVIEWS*. They are listed here for completeness only.

References

Stacey, Ginny, 2019, *Finding Your Voice with Dyslexia and other SpLDs*, Routledge, London

Website information

Series website: www.routledge.com/cw/stacey

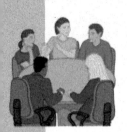

12 Group Work: Meetings, Seminars and Debates

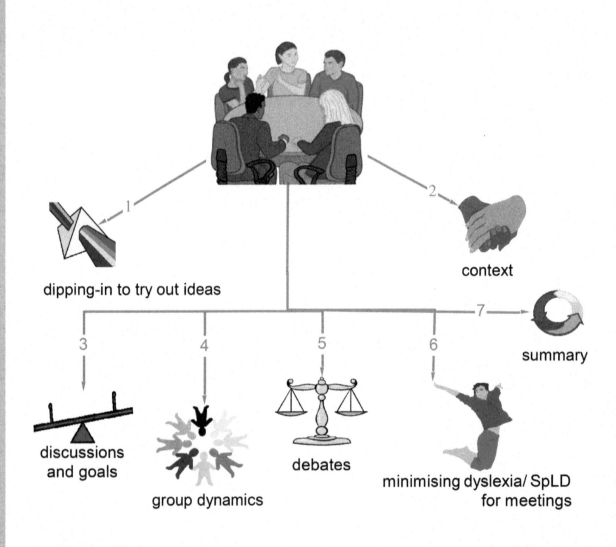

1 dipping-in to try out ideas

2 context

3 discussions and goals

4 group dynamics

5 debates

6 minimising dyslexia/ SpLD for meetings

7 summary

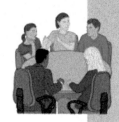

Contents

List of key points and summaries

K = key points
S = summaries

Information for non-linear readers

Before the context of the *Useful Preface* and *Chapters 1* and *2*, there is information that I hope will help non-linear readers as they approach the chapters. For chapters 4 – 14, this information would be identical except for which parts to scan and read. I have put all the information together into *Guidance for Non-Linear Readers, Chapter 3*. It is worth reading *Chapter 3* at some stage of working with this book.

Guidance for Non-Linear Readers: p 222

1 Dipping-in to try out ideas: reading and scanning lists

Start with *Dipping-in to Try Out Ideas: General Pattern*.

Dipping-in to Try Out Ideas: General Pattern: p 228

Read:

    Context, p 449

    Group Discussions and Useful, Relevant Sections, p 452

    Group Dynamics and Useful, Relevant Sections, p 456

    Group Leaders and Useful, Relevant Sections, p 459

    Enabling Dyslexic/ SpLD Group Members and Useful, Relevant Sections, p 461

    Debates and Useful, Relevant Sections, p 462

    What Could Happen and Useful, Relevant Sections, p 464

Scan:

    those sections that are relevant to students you work with or to your main interest.

1.1   Key points: for policy-makers and general readers

Key points: For policy-makers and general readers

Policy-makers:

- group work is difficult for some dyslexic/ SpLDs

- it can be the best way forward for others

- the policies for group work need to enable dyslexic/ SpLDs

Relevant discussion can be found in:
General Approaches: p 81
Dialogue: p 107
Indirect Communication: p 119

- important details include:
  - clarity in documents
  - paperwork well in advance
  - keeping all information about a meeting together; repeat all even if only one detail is changed
  - time given for people to collect their thoughts while contributing
  - clarity in summaries and about decisions.

General reader:

- focus on positive contributions

- understand the strategies dyslexic/ SpLD people use to deal with group work

- let each one explain her individual experience

- listen with curiosity

- be courteous and accepting of difficulties

- help when asked, if possible.

2 Context

To take part in *GROUP WORK: MEETINGS, SEMINARS AND DEBATES:*

- your student has to get to the right place at the right time
- with the right objects
- she needs to be prepared for the right discussion or debate
- she needs many strategies and skills to deal well with *GROUP WORK.*

She needs to deal with: paperwork; organisation; taking notes; talking; listening; recognising her own thoughts; remaining on good terms with others; etc.

Since dyslexic/ SpLD problems could affect any one of these stages of dealing with *GROUP WORK*, you could be drawing on many parts of the book in order to help her take part well.

Many other situations could similarly draw on applications of different parts of the book. *GROUP WORK* has been dealt with in this chapter in a way that could be adapted to other situations.

	Key point: Applying the ideas of this book

Analysis of skills tasks problems	The pattern used for Group Work:
	• group work has been divided into specific elements:
	  ○ communication with different aims: exchange of ideas (discussion) or to win an argument (debate)
	  ○ group dynamics: relationships within a group and what a group leader can contribute
	  ○ problems of dyslexia/ SpLD: how they might impact on group work

Resources for resolving problems	• references to other discussions in this book are given, where relevant and useful • a pattern for observing the problems your student encounters is set out, with an example

Observing, reflecting, monitoring	• the pattern can be used to monitor
	  ○ progress with any solution
	  ○ how well she is dealing with her dyslexia/ SpLD in general
	  ○ how good her confidence and self-esteem are.

'GROUP WORK: MEETINGS, SEMINARS AND DEBATES' is a long title. The chapter is about the discourse side of GROUP WORK. Teams doing physical work together still need to talk to each other. The practical side can be added by following the pattern set up in this chapter. For the rest of the chapter, 'GROUP WORK' is used as a shortened form of the full title and still does not include the practical side.

Meetings, seminars and group discussions are situations in which several people have come together to share ideas, to discuss them in some way and often to achieve some particular purpose.
Debates are situations in which different viewpoints are presented and defended. The aim of each set of presenters is to win the argument.

Key points: Elements of discussions in meetings, seminars and groups

• There is likely to be a goal.

• Your student will have to listen to others and understand what they are saying.

• She will have to form her own ideas.

• She will have to be able to speak clearly and in a way that contributes to the general discussion.

Meetings are likely to have agendas and minutes, with at least some people having roles of chairperson, secretary, treasurer, etc. The discussion and decisions will be minuted.

In seminars, often one person will be doing most of the talking, but others are expected to join in or ask questions at the end; there is probably a structure but it is unlikely that minutes will be taken. The goal is sharing knowledge and expertise.

Group discussions are less formal. If they are part of group work on an educational course, decisions may be taken during the discussion, but probably only those who have to take action will write down what they individually have to do.

Key point: The goal in debates

• There are several distinct parties in the debate.

• The parties have opposing points of view.

• The parties are trying to convince others of the rightness of their view.

• Maintaining the goal in mind is very important.

451

Debates are not about the exchange of views or information; they are competitive, with both, or several, teams aiming to win the argument. A lot of preparation is needed before a debate. It is very important to leave no gaps in the argument that can be exploited by the opponents.

Key point: Minimising dyslexia/ SpLD

Your student will need to minimise the effects of her dyslexia/ SpLD in all types of *Group Work*.

There are four sections in this chapter:

- *Discussions and Goals* is mostly about the discussion, *§3*.

§3: p 452

- *Group Dynamics* reflects on interpersonal issues, including those relating to leadership, *§4*.

§4: p 455

- *Debates* is about challenges that could increase your student's dyslexia/ SpLD and includes thinking skills, *§5*.

§5: p 561

- *Minimising Dyslexia/ SpLD for Meetings*, *§6*, is about strategies that allow your student to contribute well, including *Observing, Reflecting and Making Changes*, *§6.1*.

§6: p 464

§6.1: p 470

3   Discussions and goals

Group Discussions and Useful, Relevant Sections outlines the skills and strategies that will help your student to be able to take part in discussions and lists the relevant sections in the book.

Most of the skills and strategies are ones that can be developed in advance and then applied as necessary.

* marks those which will involve new work for each particular group discussion.

Group discussions and useful, relevant sections	
Your student needs to be able to understand the discussion; distinguish *Main Themes vs. Details*; and keep alert.	*Comprehension:* p 162 *Main Themes vs. Details:* p 178 *Being Alert:* p 91

	There is almost always some paperwork associated with group work; your student will need to have good reading strategies.	*READING:* p 230
*	The goals of a discussion provide the framework for it; if your student is clear about the goals, including her own, she will be able to take part in the discussion well.	Discussion of identifying goals is in: *GOALS FOR WRITING:* p 187
*	Doing some planning of ideas before the group work is a good idea.	*PLANNING RELATED TO KNOWLEDGE:* p 202
	Your student will need to listen to others; understand what they are saying and be able to remember what has been said.	*PREPARATION FOR LISTENING:* p 271 especially *EXERCISE FOR STUDENT: PREPARATION FOR A MEETING:* p 274 *STRATEGIES FOR LISTENING:* p 275
	She needs to be able to put her ideas across well. She needs to maintain her fluency as she talks.	*TALKING:* p 362 *TALKING FLUENTLY:* p 368
*	She may need to take notes so that she captures what was said and can use the notes later.	*TAKING AND MAKING NOTES:* p 300
*	She needs to be able to find her notes again, and any related paperwork.	*PAPERWORK, INCLUDING FILING:* p 71
*	She may well need to record and remember any decisions that are made.	*DECISION MAKING AND REMEMBERING:* p 71
	Contributing to discussions might seem daunting, so you need to teach your student how to maintain her confidence and self-esteem.	*BUILDING CONFIDENCE AND SELF-ESTEEM:* p 78

This table shows that contributing to discussions depends on a lot of skills which your student may have learnt in other circumstances, possibly working on her own. Working in groups has some specific challenges.

Key points: Challenges in meetings

The extra components in meetings are that:

- several people are contributing to the dialogue
- your student can't predict completely how the dialogue will progress
- there may be some distinct conclusion which she has to take note of
- the dialogue may wander too far from the topic under consideration and she won't keep the diversions clear.

Being clear about the goals of group discussions can make a significant difference to the way your student contributes. She may need to recognise where her own goals coincide with those put forward to the group and where they are different. For meetings that have no clearly defined goal, your student's experience of the discussion can be enhanced if she knows what she is contributing and what she would like to come away with.

Recognising the difference between the main idea and details will help your student to follow other people's points, see MAIN THEMES VS. DETAILS. She will also find it useful to be able to focus her mind and to be deliberately aware of many levels within the dialogue, see USEFUL ABILITIES OF THE MIND, especially METACOGNITION.

MAIN THEMES VS. DETAILS: p 178

USEFUL ABILITIES OF THE MIND: p 63

METACOGNITION: p 63

A further component in seminars is whether there is a single speaker or not, and whether questions or contributions from others are accepted throughout the seminar or just at the end. If ideas occur to her during a seminar, your student may need to capture them, see INSIGHT: CAPTURING THOUGHTS IN MEETINGS.

INSIGHT: CAPTURING THOUGHTS IN MEETINGS: p 473

For group discussions, taking notes and remembering decisions may or may not be important; your student needs to decide on the expectations of the group.

Summary: Discussion

Skills that are relevant:

- understanding the issues
- strategies for reading
- listening to and retaining what others say
- speaking fluently.

Good preparation for discussions:

- knowing the goal of a meeting
- knowing the topic of a seminar
- knowing one's own interests
- understanding any documents sent out in advance.

Paperwork (or e-work):

- collecting any papers together, in an organised way
- reading the papers
- taking and making notes
- recording decisions.

4 Group dynamics

Group dynamics can be one of the most important elements of group work. Comfortable relationships, even when there are differences of opinion, can produce the best results.

Many dyslexic/ SpLDs have good instincts for personal relationships, and can operate well in group situations; being in a group tends to diminish their dyslexic/ SpLD problems.

Others find working in groups quite a challenge. Sometimes, it is because their instincts for dealing with personal relationships are not so constructive; or sometimes, because the effects of their dyslexia/ SpLD interfere with engaging with the group. Whatever the reason, once dyslexia/ SpLD starts to get worse, more attention and energy is required to keep managing it.

Key points: Components of group dynamics:

- to remain on good terms with other people
- differing strength of feelings attached to topics
- differing levels of knowledge about the various topics
- the culture[1] of the group
- individual personality differences
- people not understanding your student's needs
- misunderstandings due to the way her mind works
- your student dealing with her dyslexia/ SpLD.

The last three components are covered in *WHAT COULD HAPPEN* along with other issues that can be affected by dyslexia/ SpLD.

WHAT COULD HAPPEN: p 464

In the following table, the other components are arranged in terms of:
A) strength of involvement and knowledge
B) culture
C) individual differences.

	Group dynamics and useful, relevant sections	
A	<ul><li>who cares about what?</li><li>who knows how much?</li><li>who's vulnerable?</li><li>where does your student fit in?</li></ul>	*GOALS FOR WRITING:* p 187 and *PLANNING RELATED TO KNOWLEDGE:* p 202 both have approaches that can be adapted to answer these questions.
A	<ul><li>different levels of knowledge and equal opportunity to ask questions</li><li>asking questions</li></ul>	see below and *QUESTIONS* in *ELEMENTS OF SKILLED THINKING:* p 171

[1] Culture: 'The distinctive ideas, customs, social behaviour, products, or way of life of a particular nation, society, people, or period. Hence: a society or group characterised by such customs, etc.' ('culture, n.7a' OED Online, 2020)

B	<ul><li>shared culture/ experience</li><li>unspoken code</li><li>shared basic assumptions</li><li>a single newcomer to a group can alter that culture</li><li>dyslexic/ SpLDs not picking up the culture</li></ul>	*DIALOGUE*, p 107, examines issues that may cause misunderstandings if a dyslexic/ SpLD person has a different culture to that of the group. Also see, *MINIMISING DYSLEXIA/ SPLD FOR MEETINGS:* p 464 entries under non-dyslexic/ SpLD in *INDEX:* p 589
C	<ul><li>the way dyslexic/ SpLD people think can lead to misunderstandings</li><li>different perspectives</li><li>personalities clashing</li></ul>	*DIFFERENCES IN THOUGHT PROCESSING:* p 114 *WHAT COULD HAPPEN:* p 464 entries under non-dyslexic/ SpLD in *INDEX:* p 589

A: Comments about strength of involvement

Your student needs to be aware that the depth of feelings expressed in the way people talk may mask the ideas being discussed. When working memory doesn't hold words very easily, it is difficult to run over a conversation in the mind and tone down any emotional context.

It can be important for your student to realise that others in a meeting will often know more than her; they will have good reason to do so and there may be no reason why she should be as knowledgeable as others. She needs to be comfortable with that and find a way to ask any questions that she has, to put her point of view and make her own decisions. Being clear about her ideas will often help your student in this kind of situation.

B: Comments about the culture within groups

Different groups of people will develop a culture of how they relate to each other. Your student could miss the unspoken communication and have a feeling of unease in the meeting.

She could try to find one of the group who will help her; someone who is able to listen well and not be judgemental; someone with whom she can work out anything she needs, whether that's in understanding the content and context of the meeting or in dealing with her dyslexia/ SpLD.

C: Comments about individual differences

It helps to remember that people with different personalities, or experience, will react differently. Personality systems, such as Myers-Briggs Personality Type (Stacey, 2019; Lawrence, 1993) can be a way of modelling the differences. Understanding the differences can lead to greater tolerance when the differences are manifest in discussion.

Stacey (2019)
Lawrence (1993)

4.1 Group leaders

Some groups have an official group leader; some have none; in some a person naturally acquires the role; in others there is a power struggle to be the group leader. Your student might be the group leader or a member within a group. The discussion in this section includes abilities of a group leader and what a group leader can do to enable a dyslexic/ SpLD member. The dynamics of power struggles are outside the remit of this book.

Key points: A good group leader

- knows the agenda
- is clear about timings
- can listen to members' ideas
- can direct the discussion and keep it close to the topic
- can defuse tensions
- can take decisions
- can summarise well

If your student is a group leader, she could use the following table to check how well she can provide these abilities to her group.

Group leaders and useful, relevant sections		
Task	*An able group leader:*	
direct the meeting	<ul><li>knows the agenda</li><li>can listen to members' ideas</li><li>can direct the discussion and keep it close to the topic</li><li>can take decisions</li><li>can summarise well.</li></ul>	KNOW THE GOAL OF ANY TASK: p 181 METACOGNITION: p 63 KEY WORDS: p 176 MAIN THEME VS. DETAILS: p 178 text 'MBPT characteristics', p 76
manage time	<ul><li>is clear about timings</li><li>can keep to time agreed</li></ul>	ORGANISATION: p 70
contain feelings	<ul><li>can defuse tensions</li><li>can remain calm.</li></ul>	STRESS: p 78 THINKING CLEARLY: p 79

There are some dyslexic/ SpLD people who are very good at interpersonal communication; they tend to have fluent spoken language.

Group leaders, often the chairperson, may be aware of someone in the group who's dyslexic/ SpLD. Even if no-one has said they are dyslexic/ SpLD, your student, as a group leader, could decide to use the good practice that enables dyslexic/ SpLD people to function well.

Key points: Group leaders and enabling dyslexic/ SpLDs

- Put practices in place that accommodate some key needs:
  - paperwork well in advance so that it can be read
  - clarity in documents
  - all information about a meeting kept together, even when only one detail is changed
  - timing set out clearly.
- Check for possible misunderstanding.
- Leave material and information visible as long as possible.
- Allow time for dyslexic/ SpLDs to collect their thoughts.
- Understand the problems that could arise.
- Observe what happens.
- Assist when asked, without patronising.
- Reduce stress or tension in any situation.

Most of these issues are discussed in other tables of this chapter:

GROUP DISCUSSIONS AND USEFUL, RELEVANT SECTIONS: p 452

GROUP DYNAMICS AND USEFUL, RELEVANT SECTIONS: p 456

DEBATES AND USEFUL, RELEVANT SECTIONS: p 462

WHAT COULD HAPPEN AND USEFUL, RELEVANT SECTIONS: p 464

A few are discussed in the following table.

Enabling dyslexic/ SpLD group members and useful, relevant sections		
date, time, place, papers	Make sure the date, time and place; minutes; agenda; and any other papers are sent out – this might be delegated, but the leader should know it will happen and with enough time for any dyslexic/ SpLD member to process.	*LECTURING AND TALKING:* p 124 in *INDIRECT COMMUNICATION:* p 119
clarity	Information clearly given and set out well can be understood more easily, so a dyslexic/ SpLD reader will be able to stay mentally switched on.	*UNIVERSALITY OF CLARITY:* p 121 *MENTAL ON/OFF SWITCH:* p 86
mis-understandings	*WHAT COULD HAPPEN* describes several possible causes of mis-understandings. Several sections in *INDIVIDUALS WITH DYSLEXIA/ SPLD* also enumerate other causes.	*WHAT COULD HAPPEN:* p 464 *INDIVIDUALS WITH DYSLEXIA/ SPLD:* p 57
assistance	Assist without patronising; looking for solutions is best done as a co-operative venture. You can use the *EXERCISE FOR STUDENT: OBSERVE WHAT HAPPENS IN GROUP WORK* and the ideas following the exercise.	*EXERCISE FOR STUDENT: OBSERVE WHAT HAPPENS IN GROUP WORK:* p 470

5   Debates

Debates have an adversarial element to them: two, or more, different teams are arguing and aiming to win support for their views and positions.

They usually have definite propositions and structures.

They take place within democratic, parliamentary systems.

They happen between barristers and solicitors in the courts of law.

They are practised at some universities and schools, often in debating societies.

Key points: Debates

The aim is to win the argument about a specific proposition.
Opposing teams are involved.
Important skills are:

- knowing the goal
- identifying key themes
- listening to the opposition
- talking fluently
- highly skilled thinking
- mental agility.

Debating is more intense than discussion because of the structure and the goal to win. Many of the points made under *Discussions and Goals* and *Group Dynamics* apply to *Debates* but there are some issues worth adding because of the increased intensity. Skilled thinking and mental agility are included here because they are so important in debating, but they can also be relevant to discussions. The issues in *Minimising Dyslexia/ SpLD for Meetings* also apply to *Debates*.

This section is not about debates, but the challenges debating presents to dyslexic/ SpLD people.

Discussions and Goals: p 452

Group Dynamics: p 455

Minimising Dyslexia/ SpLD for Meetings: p 464

Debates and useful, relevant sections		
roles and competition	- Learning anything new can be difficult: the roles and rules of debating can be quite tightly specified. - The tension caused by the competition has to be managed.	*Stress:* p 78 'anything new' in *What Could Happen:* p 468

multiple goals, identifying key themes	• Your team is aiming to win a particular argument. • There may be specific parts that are more important than others. • It is important to have no gaps in the argument that the opposition can attack. • Planning the way the argument is presented is likely to be important.	*KNOW THE GOAL OF ANY TASK:* p 181 *PLANNING RELATED TO KNOWLEDGE:* p 202
active listening	• You need to follow closely what the opposition are saying.	*LISTENING:* p 262
fluent talking	• You need to speak in a confident, convincing manner. • You have to think and speak on your feet. • You need to counter the opponents' points.	*TALKING FLUENTLY:* p 368
skilled thinking	• Very clear, analytic thinking is needed. • Critical analysis of what the opposition is saying allows you to expose logical flaws in its argument. • Two levels of thinking are required: ○ fast, instant response ○ identifying underlying argument.	*SKILLED THINKING:* p 167
mental agility	• Mental skills needed: ○ good working-memory strategies ○ rapid recall of knowledge ○ quick recognition of important themes vs. minor details.	*TECHNIQUES FOR USING THE MIND:* p 156 *MAIN THEMES VS. DETAILS:* p 178

6   Minimising dyslexia/ SpLD for meetings

Minimising your dyslexia/ SpLD for *GROUP WORK* will involve you in managing it:

- knowing the pitfalls that affect you
- knowing how to pause and recognise when you need to take steps to avoid a problem
- knowing your best strategies for avoiding pitfalls
- knowing when you need to ask for help.

The confidence and self-esteem you can gain from being proactive is worth the initial effort. You may find that the conditions that are VITAL for you are also GOOD PRACTICE for everyone else.

Ⓖ p 575 pitfall

WHAT COULD HAPPEN lists many sources of dyslexic/ SpLD problems and describes some of the ramifications. Your student may experience none of these problems, but they show how different sources of problems impact on *GROUP WORK* for dyslexic/ SpLDs.

What could happen and useful, relevant sections		
Source	*Details*	*SECTIONS*
reading	<ul><li>You take time to read and understand anything.</li><li>You don't notice underlying messages that are not explicitly stated.</li><li>Getting material too late means you don't understand the issues well enough for the meeting.</li></ul>	*READING:* p 230-241 *COMPREHENSION:* p 162-178 *GENERAL CONSIDERATIONS:* p 122 *WRITTEN COMMUNICATION:* p 123

Source	*Details*	SECTIONS
listening	• Listening to others and understanding might be a problem for you. • You may find you miss subtle, unspoken details. • You may find jokes cause problems.	STRATEGIES FOR LISTENING: p 275 LISTENING CHECK-LIST: p 265 MISUNDERSTANDINGS IN DIALOGUE: p 113-117
talking	• You have difficulty with speaking fluently. • You have problems finding the right words.	TALKING FLUENTLY: p 368-373 A WORD LOSING ITS CONTEXT: p 265
taking notes	• You have to take notes to keep engaged with the discussion. • Taking notes is a step too far in the context of meetings.	STRATEGIES FOR LISTENING: p 275 SEEING, LISTENING AND WRITING: p 309 TAKING AND MAKING NOTES: p 300-335
alternative THINKING PREFERENCES	• You interpret what you hear or read in a different way from what was intended. • Your ideas can be quite consistent and complete, or there can be gaps. ○ Either way, they don't match the ideas as others understand them. • One annoying result is that you do a lot of work on the wrong ideas. • Another result is that other people find you unpredictable; they can be unsettled as a result. • Also, other people don't understand your ideas.	THINKING PREFERENCES: p 72-78 DIFFERENCES IN THOUGHT PROCESSING: p 114 WAYS TO USE YOUR THINKING PREFERENCES: p 370 MISUNDERSTANDINGS IN DIALOGUE: p 113-117

Source	Details	SECTIONS
holistic thinking	• Holistic thinking holds many ideas in mind simultaneously; ideas from other people can set off many trains of thought. • Dyslexic/ SpLDs with this type of thinking can talk and write in incomplete sentences because their minds are jumping easily and fast between ideas. • They can also follow different trains of thought and easily go off 'at a tangent'. • Non-dyslexic/ SpLD people find it hard to follow the ideas.	HOLISTIC VS. LINEAR: p 75, 563 KNOW THE GOAL OF ANY TASK: p 181-182 DIFFERENCES IN THOUGHT PROCESSING: p 114 DIFFERENT EXPERIENCES: p 267

working memory	• The capacity of your working memory can be restricted
	
	  ○ by the slow processing of dyslexia/ SpLD
	
	  ○ unless you use deliberate techniques to enhance working memory.
	
	• You may miss significant information because you don't hold enough in working memory.
		MIND SET: p 158
		
		CHUNKING: p 158
		
		CAPACITY OF WORKING MEMORY: p 157

can't stop	• Sometimes, you may want to pause to deal with an immediate issue. • It can be difficult to stop in a meeting because other people are involved. • You need to work out what to do in such a situation, otherwise any tension could make your dyslexia/ SpLD more problematic.	THINKING CLEARLY (PAUSING): p 557-559 NO PAUSE BUTTON: p 397 CAPTURING THOUGHTS IN A MEETING: p 473 METHODS FOR EXPLORING BEHIND THE OBVIOUS: p 65

Source	Details	SECTIONS
static material constant content	• You may be helped if material stays in view during a discussion. • If you find text or pictures are being moved too fast, ask for them to stay in view as long as possible. • You will probably find this helps others too.	OUT OF SIGHT IS OUT OF MIND: p 90 STATIC MATERIAL AND CONSTANT CONTENT: p 91 CAPACITY OF WORKING MEMORY: p 157 MEANINGS OF WORDS: p 98

time and place	• If you are one of those who have difficulty with time and place,
	  ○ you can spend a lot of effort to get to the right place at the right time
	  ○ you still arrive very precisely at the wrong time or place.
	• These problems can be hard for non-dyslexics to understand.
		SUPPLEMENTARY ISSUES: p 68-70
		
		TIME MANAGEMENT: p 501
		
		DRIVING: p 485-489

environment	• Where you sit in a meeting can be important. • If you are uncomfortable, for any reason, your dyslexia/ SpLD may get worse. • You may need a flat surface to write on.	ENVIRONMENT: p 70, 377 CONCENTRATION: p 560 PREPARATION FOR READING: p 243-244
direction	• Following directions may be a problem. • Reading road signs could go wrong. • You may have no sense of where you are. • The problems can be the same for non-dyslexic/ SpLDs, but they can use words to ask for help more easily than dyslexic/ SpLDs can.	SPACE, PLACE AND DIRECTION: p 69 NAVIGATION: p 486 WHERE THE CAR IS PARKED: p 488

Source	Details	SECTIONS
organisation	<ul><li>Which end of the spectrum are you?</li><li>Dyslexic/ SpLDs are usually<ul><li>either completely organised because that is the only way they can function</li><li>or they are disorganised.</li></ul></li><li>There doesn't seem to be a middle way.</li><li>Some of the disorganised ones thoroughly enjoy it; others would have more enjoyment being organised.</li><li>Either extreme can prove difficult for non-dyslexic/ SpLDs; you need to be aware of their reactions.</li></ul>	ORGANISATION: p70-72 HIGHLY ORGANISED: p 501 MINIMALLY ORGANISED: p 502 CONSEQUENCES FROM MISINTERPRETATION: p 269
anything new	<ul><li>You may have a lot of strategies that mean your dyslexia/ SpLD is hardly a nuisance and then you are given a new task that sets you back to having no strategies.</li><li>You may feel your dyslexia/ SpLD has come back and got worse.</li><li>You just need to work out how to deal with the new task:<ul><li>you may develop new strategies</li><li>you may have to negotiate new accommodations for anything for which you can't find a solution.</li></ul></li></ul>	MAJOR PRECAUTION: p 10-11 FIRST LEARNING BECOMES FIXED: p 89 KEY POINT: USE INTERESTING BUT UNIMPORTANT TOPICS FOR NEW TECHNIQUES: p 316 ADAPTING A SKILL TO A NEW SITUATION: p 404

Source	Details	SECTIONS
your way of doing things	• Once each of us knows how we can do anything, we tend to stick to the way that works. • Since this may not be the way others do the same task, there can be conflict. • We can be regarded as stubborn and inflexible. • A lot of patience and good will may be needed on both sides to arrive at a workable solution.	STORY: TWO DYSLEXIC SAILORS: p 6 WHAT CAN GO WRONG, WHAT CAN GO RIGHT: p 54 CURIOUS BEHAVIOUR: p 116 TASKS DONE DIFFERENTLY: p 117

declaring your dyslexia/ SpLD	• You need to feel comfortable about telling anyone you are dyslexic/ SpLD.
	
	• Some people think too much is made of it
	  ○ some will think you are making excuses
	  ○ some won't think of the wide range of ways these syndromes affect your contribution to a meeting.
	
	• Once you've said it, you can't unsay it,
	  ○ but owning it can smooth out misunderstandings to the benefit of all.
		DECLARING DYSLEXIA/ SPLD OR NOT: p 84
		
		MISUNDERSTANDINGS IN DIALOGUE: p 113-117
		
		EMPLOYERS MISSING GOOD EMPLOYEES: p 442
		
		GENERAL LETTER TO EMPLOYERS: p 547
		
		DYSLEXIA/ SPLD AND INTERESTING JOBS: p 84

stress	• Stress and tension make you more vulnerable to your dyslexia/ SpLD.	STRESS: p 78 BUILDING CONFIDENCE AND SELF-ESTEEM: p 78-80 STORY: WORK FROM THE RIGHT PERSPECTIVE: p 402 USING EXTRA TIME: p 412 THINKING CLEARLY: p 557-559

Source	Details	Sections
accommodation	• There may be some tasks that it is not practical for you to do. • It is worth discussing any accommodation with the group leader who may be able to make suitable arrangements. • Accommodation for you is likely to be better for the whole group because you will be able to contribute more with it. • See how open you can be about it; o sometimes other members of a group can be unhappy unless they understand the reasons and benefits of accommodations.	ACCOMMODATIONS: p 128 MENTAL ENERGY TO MANAGE DYSLEXIA/ SPLD: p 541 CONTEXT (EXAMS): p 409 NEGOTIATING ACCOMMODATION: p 550-553 DECLARING DYSLEXIA/ SPLD OR NOT: p 84

6.1 Observing, reflecting and making changes

You can work with your student to sort out anything that is causing her dyslexia/ SpLD to hamper her contributions to GROUP WORK. She needs to objectively OBSERVE WHAT HAPPENS IN GROUP WORK so that you both can uncover the fundamental problem and work towards a solution.

Exercise for student: Observe what happens
in group work

• Collect your experiences together over several meetings.

• You could use one of the templates in COLLECTING INFORMATION TOGETHER.

• Find the solution most suited to you using the tables with USEFUL, RELEVANT SECTIONS in:
  o GROUP DISCUSSIONS: p 452
  o GROUP DYNAMICS: p 456
  o GROUP LEADERS: p 459

COLLECTING INFORMATION TOGETHER: p 526

- o   *ENABLING DYSLEXIC/ SPLD GROUP MEMBERS:* p 461
- o   *DEBATES:* p 462
- o   *WHAT COULD HAPPEN:* p 464.
- Gradually, build up knowledge of what makes a difference to the way you are able to understand and contribute to discussions.

If you need other resources to sort out problems, scan *INDIVIDUALS WITH DYSLEXIA/ SPLD.*

INDIVIDUALS WITH DYSLEXIA/ SPLD: p 57

Help your student to reflect on her observations and decide on any changes she can make. She can build the insights that she gains into her *INDIVIDUAL, PERSONAL PROFILE OF DYSLEXIA/ SPLD* and her *REGIME FOR MANAGING DYSLEXIA/ SPLD.*

INDIVIDUAL, PERSONAL PROFILE OF DYSLEXIA/ SPLD: p 540

REGIME FOR MANAGING DYSLEXIA/ SPLD: p 540

She can gradually accumulate a set of guiding notes for dealing with group work.

Tip: Guiding notes for group work

From the *EXERCISE FOR STUDENT: OBSERVE WHAT HAPPENS IN GROUP WORK,* above, your student may develop some guiding notes for dealing with group work.

It's a good idea to make sure that she will be able to see the notes at the right point in a meeting, see *TIP: REMEMBER THE SYSTEM.*

TIP: REMEMBER THE SYSTEM: p 474

For example:

- she could stick Post-it notes on pages with important ideas; and write a key word on the Post-it or highlight a key word on the page
- she could have a card with key words of the guiding notes; she could put this card with her note-pad or somewhere that she can always see it during the meeting.

12   Group Work: Meetings, Seminars and Debates

Observe What Happens in Group Work can also be used to monitor progress. She would be doing the exercise collecting information about any new strategies she is using. She would want to know whether the strategy is working as well as she hoped and whether any modifications were necessary.

Exercise: Observe What Happens in Group Work: p 470

Story: Too Many Ideas Sparked by Other People Talking has a list of observations from one student. *Insight: Capturing Thoughts in Meetings* is his solution with a few extra suggestions.

Story: Too many ideas sparked by other people talking

Members of one student's group objected to his many interruptions. Observing what happened showed the following:

- other people talking triggers ideas in his head
- remembering his ideas is difficult during a discussion
    - he doesn't remember his thoughts when he wants them
    - the thoughts come back at random times
    - he needs to catch them as they appear in his mind.
- he was interrupting because he spoke when an idea occurred which did not help the group dynamics
- often his ideas were rejected and mostly because the others were annoyed
- he needed to find the best way for him to record his thoughts.

Insight: Capturing thoughts in meetings

To capture his thoughts without interrupting in a rude way and be able to use them later:

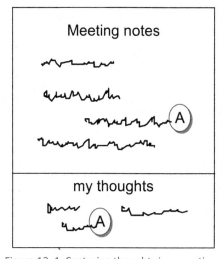

Figure 12. 1 Capturing thoughts in a meeting

- he took notes on paper, and reserved a space on one page for ideas that he wanted to mention; he labelled the space 'my thoughts', see *FIGURE 12.1*

- as he took notes about the meeting, he wrote in the main area of the page, under 'meeting notes'

- when an idea occurred that he wanted to capture he wrote it under 'my thoughts', then continued taking notes under 'meeting notes'

- when he wanted to connect one of his thoughts to a particular point in the meeting notes, he drew a link

  - you could use a symbol; in *FIGURE 12.1*, 'A' in a blue circle is demonstrated

- then when there was an opportunity, he said something like, "When we were talking about ... (he mentioned the topic at A in 'meeting notes') it occurred to me that ..." and he said the idea he had written at A in 'my thoughts'.

Further thoughts:
There will be several ways the same thing can be achieved electronically; how it is done will depend on the devices available to your student.

- She wants to keep the notes of the meeting separate from the ideas that she wants to raise.

- She wants to be able to go back to the ideas quickly and reliably.

- She wants to be able to link them to any relevant discussion during the meeting.

Tip: Remember the system

Once your student has developed a system that works for her,
she needs to remember it at the beginning of a meeting.
She could have an index card titled: 'My thoughts in a meeting',
with:

- purpose – to note my own thoughts and wait for the right
  moment to use them

- system – 'Meeting about....' area (in green ink) and 'My
  thoughts ...' area (in blue ink)

- to remember to use the system – she could use a
  paper-clip to fix the card to the top of her notes pad, or
  on the agenda.

Having worked out the system and how to remember it, your student
can monitor its use in future meetings by re-using OBSERVE WHAT
HAPPENS IN GROUP WORK. She might find that she is indifferent to the
ink colours in the instructions and not bother with that detail again.

OBSERVE WHAT HAPPENS IN GROUP WORK may also show her how well her
PROFILE and REGIME describe her best ways of working and her needs.
She could also use the same exercise to observe her levels of
confidence and self-esteem. The cycle of observation, reflection and
trying out changes can be repeated as many times as your student
finds useful.

EXERCISE: OBSERVE WHAT
HAPPENS IN GROUP
WORK: p 470

INDIVIDUAL, PERSONAL
PROFILE OF DYSLEXIA/
SPLD: p 540

REGIME FOR MANAGING
DYSLEXIA/SPLD: p 540

Key point: Operating from strengths

Operating from her optimum potential is powerful when it comes to minimising dyslexia/ SpLD. Your student can start by considering anything that is especially important for her, such as:

- being prepared

- knowing her own goals

- being comfortable, mentally and physically

- being able to use the strategies and techniques that allow her to function well

- other.

7 Summary: group work

- *GROUP WORK* covers group discourse and excludes practical team work.

- The discourse is divided into:
    - discussion, as exchange of ideas
    - debates, in which winning is the aim.

- Group dynamics is discussed in terms of relationships between members and leadership that can enable dyslexic/ SpLD people.

- Key elements of *GROUP WORK* are:
    1. skills relating to understanding
    2. mental techniques
    3. organisation
    4. enabling dyslexic/ SpLDs.

The following summary is an overview of the important issues.

Summary: Group work

Group Work presents a wide range of challenges for dyslexic/ SpLD people.
They may have strategies to deal with some of the challenges.
Anything new may require new strategies to be developed.

Other members of the group may not understand why dyslexic/ SpLD people work the way they do.
Group dynamics can be difficult to navigate.
Finding a friendly other member of the group can significantly help a dyslexic/ SpLD person deal with any problems.

Important issues are:

- clarity in documents
- documents and meeting details sent out with sufficient time for reading and processing
- clear goals and structures.

References

Lawrence, Gordon, 1993, *People Types and Tiger Stripes,* Centre for Applications of Psychological Types, Gainsville, FL, 3rd ed.
Stacey, Ginny, 2019, *Finding Your Voice with Dyslexia and other SpLDs,* Routledge, London

Website information

OED Online, September 2020, Oxford University Press Accessed 24 October 2020

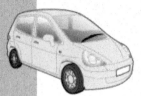

13   Driving

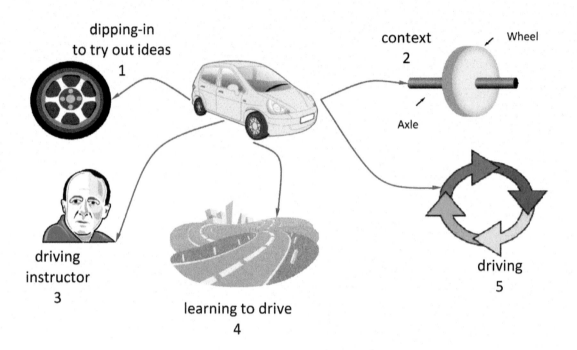

dipping-in
to try out ideas
1

context
2

Wheel

Axle

driving
instructor
3

learning to drive
4

driving
5

Contents

THINKING PREFERENCES, p 72, are highlighted in orange in this chapter.

Examples of their use are listed in the *INDEX:* p 589

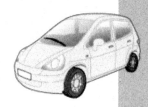

 ## List of key points and summaries

K = key points
S = summaries

Information for non-linear readers

Before the context of the USEFUL PREFACE and CHAPTERS 1 and 2, there is information that I hope will help non-linear readers as they approach the chapters. For chapters 4 – 14, this information would be identical except for which parts to scan and read. I have put all the information together into GUIDANCE FOR NON-LINEAR READERS, CHAPTER 3. It is worth reading CHAPTER 3 at some stage of working with this book.

GUIDANCE FOR
NON-LINEAR READERS:
p 222

1 Dipping-in to try out ideas: reading and scanning lists

Start with DIPPING-IN TO TRY OUT IDEAS: GENERAL PATTERN.

Read:

LEARNING TO DRIVE AND USEFUL, RELEVANT SECTIONS, p 483

SUMMARY: DYSLEXIC/ SPLD ISSUES AND DRIVING, p 490

TEACHING DYSLEXIC/ SPLD PEOPLE TO DRIVE, p 482

Scan:

the rest of the chapter.

DIPPING-IN TO TRY OUT
IDEAS: GENERAL PATTERN:
p 228

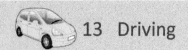

1.1 Key points: for policy-makers and general readers

Key points: For policy-makers and general readers

- Policies dealing with driving should incorporate awareness of dyslexia/ SpLD.
- Driving instructors and examiners need to be able to accommodate dyslexic/ SpLD people's needs.
- It needs to be recognised that *Stress*, anxiety and tension can increase the effects of dyslexia/ SpLD.
- Accommodation during the driving test should continue.
- The way the theory test is set out should avoid creating barriers; forms and instructions need to be clear and unambiguous.
- Clear, unambiguous signage[1] is very important.

Stress: p 78

2 Context

Most people drive and there is no reason why dyslexic/ SpLD people can't be as good as anyone else, but there are various problems to deal with.

- Learning to drive may be affected by dyslexia/ SpLD.
- Some dyspraxic people may find the effects of their dyspraxia mean they can't learn to drive safely.
- You have to navigate from one place to another.
- Often, you are trying to arrive at a particular time.
- Finding the car once it has been left may be challenging and frustrating.
- There is paperwork involved in owning a car.
- The car needs looking after.

For dealing with paperwork, see *Organisation*: p 70

---

[1] British road signs are used as an example of good signage in *Key points: Universality of Clarity*: p 121

Non-dyslexic/ SpLD people can also experience many of these problems. The added impact of dyslexia/ SpLD makes them worth mentioning.

To look at the way dyslexia/ SpLD affects driving, this chapter has thoughts about:

The chapter ends with a SUMMARY: DYSLEXIA/ SPLD ISSUES AND DRIVING, p 490

3 Driving instructor

For whatever reason, many dyslexic/ SpLDs find the first learning of anything new can become fixed in their minds so that it is very difficult to modify it or add to what they have learnt; examples are given in FIRST LEARNING BECOMES FIXED. Therefore, the early stages of learning to drive are very important. In MAJOR PRECAUTION, it is suggested that dyslexic/ SpLD students find out to what extent this is a factor for them.

FIRST LEARNING BECOMES FIXED: p 89

MAJOR PRECAUTION: p 10

It's a good idea for your student to find the right instructor who is able to teach in a way that suits his THINKING PREFERENCES.

THINKING PREFERENCES: p 72

The instructor and anyone helping him with driving practice (assisting experienced-driver) need to be aware of the particular difficulties your student has with his dyslexia/ SpLD.

It is important to sort out any problems as soon as possible, so as to enhance the correct learning and to avoid dyslexic/ SpLD confusion, see PARK PATHS AND PRUNING NEURONS.

PARK PATHS AND PRUNING NEURONS: p 7

13 Driving

Instructors and assisting experienced-drivers should bear in mind that a calm manner will help the learner more effectively than a tense one.

Instructors and assisting experienced-drivers are unlikely to be dyslexia/ SpLD support tutors. You may need to help your student to explain his dyslexic/ SpLD difficulties and how to deal with them.

The sections in the book that are likely to be helpful to instructors and assisting-experienced drivers are: *DIALOGUE* and *INDIRECT COMMUNICATION*.

DIALOGUE: p 107

INDIRECT COMMUNICATION: p 119

Key points: Teaching dyslexic/ SpLD people to drive

The initial stages of learning are very important for dyslexic/ SpLD people; it can be difficult to remove early mistakes, see *MAJOR PRECAUTION*.

MAJOR PRECAUTION: p 10

- What is the best way to give instructions? See *INPUT, OUTPUT AND MOTIVATION*.

INPUT, OUTPUT AND MOTIVATION: p 73

- How good is your student's knowledge of left and right? Is it:
  - o as words with consistent meaning
  - o as directions without reliable words
  - o not good?

ROTE LEARNING: p 89

- You need to find out whether *ROTE LEARNING* and *SUBLIMINAL LEARNING* work for the learner.

ⓖ p 575 subliminal
SUBLIMINAL LEARNING: p 88

- *EPISODIC MEMORY* can cause problems when sections of sequences need to be used as individual units.

EXPERIENCE AND EPISODIC MEMORY: p 156

4 Learning to drive

Encourage your student to be careful about his learning from the beginning; these are skills he will want to use for a long time, so he wants them to be reliable.

Some of the most important or common issues that affect learning to drive are listed below, together with the sections that have more information.

* indicates aspects that may continue after your student has learnt to drive.

Learning to drive and useful, relevant sections	
The instructions need to be given in a way that your student finds easy to understand.	*THINKING PREFERENCES:* p 72 *MODEL OF LEARNING:* p 145 especially *INPUT, OUTPUT AND MOTIVATION:* p 73
Driving is a practical skill with some factual knowledge that has to be learnt. His interests might be a way of helping him to remember all the rules and regulations.	*DOING:* p 280 *THINKING PREFERENCES:* p 72
* Being able to think clearly and keep focused on the task in hand are good skills while driving.	*THINKING CLEARLY:* p 79 *METACOGNITION:* p 63
* Learning problems that may hinder his progress are that: • rote learning doesn't work for him • he can't learn subliminally • episodic memory may stop him breaking skills into useful components.	*ROTE LEARNING:* p 89 *SUBLIMINAL LEARNING:* p 88 *EXPERIENCE AND EPISODIC MEMORY:* p 156
* His sense of space and of time may be issues for him in driving.	*SPACE, PLACE AND DIRECTION:* p 69 *TIME:* p 69

There is a lot to process when learning to drive. It may be useful to establish the necessary thought patterns away from the roads. *Mental Rehearsal of Movements* could be used to good effect; or even a slightly different situation which is already known.

Mental Rehearsal of Movements: p 292

Insight: Practising to learn a skill

Your student could practise without driving.

- Just before the test, I used to mentally rehearse the sequences for turning right and left while cycling to work every morning; I used to manoeuvre the bike while doing it. (kinaesthetic)

- Your student could sit on a chair and do the same. (kinaesthetic)

- He could have recordings of the instructor taking him through all the driving sequences. (verbal)

Help your student to reflect on any part that is proving more difficult to learn than most of the driving processes.

Is there some point of confusion in his thinking that is blocking progress?

Is there any way his mind goes blank at that point?

He can pull his reflections together by:

- using the resources in *Collecting Information Together*

- adapting the *Figure 1.2: The Root of a Problem*.

Collecting Information Together: p 526

Figure 1.2: The Root of a Problem: p 66

The insights for *Practical Exams* will be useful in preparation for taking the driving test.

Practical Exams: p 436

Don't forget that good *Breathing* will help with driving just as much as with any other action.

Breathing: p 557

5 Driving

Once your student has learnt to drive and he is driving on his own, his dyslexia/ SpLD may still impact on his use of cars. Many of the pitfalls of dyslexia/ SpLD can cause problems when driving or giving instructions to other drivers. He won't have anyone else to help him manage any difficulties. In all situations, including taking the driving test, your student needs to stay safe.

Driving was mentioned in *No Pause Button* as one of those situations when once you've started, you have to keep going. You can't always suddenly stop to sort out any difficulty that has arisen. For example, if you have been told to turn left and you move to turn right, you may find the traffic conditions are such that you have to go right. It could be a long time before you can stop and try to find the best way back to where you should be going. A sensible approach to dealing with times when he can't stop is to prepare himself, as suggested in *No Pause Button*.

No Pause Button: p 397

Car maintenance is important when you own the car you drive and there is paperwork to be dealt with. Finding out what you have to do is similar to the *Thinking Processes for Plumbing Job* or *Householder Decision*. Good *Organisation* will save effort and tension.

Thinking Processes for Plumbing Job: p 167

Thinking Processes for Householder Decision: p 168

Organisation: p 70

You can't drive without fuel. Have enough fuel in the car so that you don't have to worry about running out. If you find getting fuel is a problem, have a fuel notice permanently in the car. When you see you are going to run out in the next couple of days, you put the notice where you can see it and where you won't ignore it. Leave it there until you fill the car up again. I have an envelope with 'fuel' on and I clip it round the steering wheel with a clothes peg.

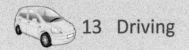

5.1 Navigation

Many people have difficulty with directions and spatial awareness, with or without dyslexia/ SpLD. There is the added dimension that your student's dyslexia/ SpLD will cause further confusion.

Key points: A few of the dyslexic/ SpLD difficulties while driving

- You know the directions spatially, but don't reliably say left and right correctly.

- You can't concentrate long enough to take in the directions.

- You don't remember to organise the route in advance.

- You don't hear the words correctly when given directions.

- You transpose the road numbers; you transpose letters or words.

- You don't mentally process the sequence of different directions.

- You don't process what you see on the road signs quickly enough to take the appropriate action.

There are benefits. The following story is worth relating to your student because it is such a good example of a positive perspective.

Story: The benefits of getting lost

"Do you often get lost in a new place?" is a standard question in a dyslexia screening test.

One person said, "No" and when I probed a bit further, "I enjoy getting lost. I have seen more of Paris getting lost in one weekend, than most people see in years."

Using a good Sat Nav (Satellite Navigation) system can help with directions.

For some people, reading road signs is a major difficulty:

- numbers and letters can be transposed and wrong directions taken
- converting vertical diagrams of road layout to the horizontal reality can be difficult
- dealing with road works and diversion signs can disrupt previous planning
- other: there are many ways road signs can prove difficult.

Your student needs to recognise which ones he finds difficult.

- There may be specific solutions.
- He may have to leave extra time for journeys.
- He may have to manage other people's expectations.
- He should certainly find out how to remain calm and to be tolerant of himself and others.

5.2   Time constraints

Key points: Driving and time issues

Timings can present problems.

Your student may not be good at remembering how long a particular journey takes, even if it is one he does very frequently.

He may have difficulty setting off in time to arrive when he is expected.

He may be reluctant to arrive early because he doesn't like having nothing to do.

As with the other problems, your student needs to decide exactly what the source of the problem is and then work out his solution from his strengths. Use ideas from METHODS OF EXPLORING BEHIND THE OBVIOUS to help him.

METHODS OF EXPLORING BEHIND THE OBVIOUS: p 65

It may be that he always has to set out early and take something to do so that when he does arrive early he isn't bored.

He may need to tell the people expecting him that he is apt to go wrong or get lost[2] and therefore needs to arrange a flexible arrival time.

It is usually better to keep the other people informed of his progress than to travel in the hope that everything will go smoothly and he won't be late, when underneath he knows he will be late.

5.3   Where the car is parked

Remembering where you have parked is a problem for many with and without dyslexia/ SpLD.

If your student has a recording device, he could record where he is; either by taking photos or by recording the location as text. Record the day, date and time as well, so that he knows which data he needs to use to find the car again.

---

[2] Going wrong and getting lost are not the same thing, though both can cause a person to be late. You can go wrong because your knowledge of the words 'left' and 'right' is not secure and at the same time you can know exactly where you are, so you are not lost.

If the car has remote central locking, once your student is fairly near the car, pressing the lock button will activate the car lights, which he should be able to see.

Insight: One way to find the car

I rarely have this problem, but I would use the envelope + clothes peg system, with a dedicated note book that fitted in a back pocket.

- The envelope would go on the driver's inside door handle and it would be a reminder to write down where I have parked; I would discipline myself to take-action before doing anything else.

- Once I had written in the note book and put that in my pocket, I would leave the envelope on the driver's seat to remind me to put the note book back in the car rather than leave it in my pocket.

Versions of these techniques are a major part of solving the dyslexic memory problems that could cause chaos in my life.

Key point: Finding the parked car

- Work with your student to identify exactly what happens when he can't find the car.

- What sort of strategies work for him in other situations?

- What could he do to record the place?

- What could he do to record the route from the car, and therefore back to the car?

- What can he do to make sure he is systematic about knowing where the car is, what is around it, and the route back?

5.4 Summary: dyslexic/ SpLD issues and driving

Summary: Dyslexic/ SpLD issues and driving

Learning to drive

- Recognise the ways your dyslexia/ SpLD will cause difficulties while you learn to drive. Be as open as you can.

- Make sure you can easily understand your driving instructor and avoid generating dyslexic/ SpLD problems in your driving.

- Remember that it can be difficult to remove early mistakes, see *MAJOR PRECAUTION*.

MAJOR PRECAUTION:
p 10

Driving practice

- 'Little and often' is good advice for practising skills.

- Before the test, make sure you drive around roads very similar to the ones that are used for tests.

Driving and time issues

- If time is an issue for you, keep a record of how long journeys take you until you have built up a good sense of time for journeys.

- Leave with extra time to complete a journey.

Navigation and finding the parked car

- Recognise your strengths and difficulties with navigation.

- Develop secure systems to deal with any difficulties with:
  o finding your way about
  o finding your parked car.

Owning a car

- Be organised with the paperwork.

- Make sure you have enough funds for all the extras related to driving.

- Have a schedule for maintenance.

- Have a reliable system to make sure you don't run out of fuel.

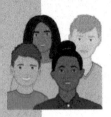

14 Social Examples

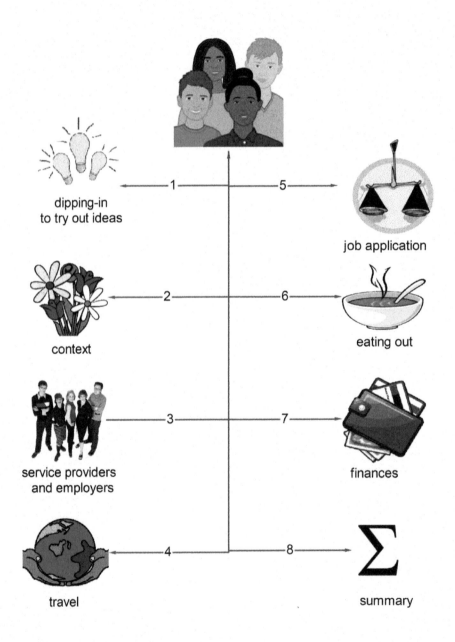

dipping-in
to try out ideas — 1

5 — job application

context — 2

6 — eating out

service providers
and employers — 3

7 — finances

travel — 4

8 — summary

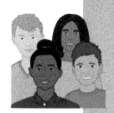

Contents

List of key points and summaries

K = key points
S = summaries

Templates on the website

TEMPLATES

COMPANION @ WEBSITE

Templates useful for systematically comparing information from different sources are:

B5-8   RECORDING TEMPLATES - 1-4

Templates useful for observing what is happening in a particular situation and monitoring possible solutions are:

B3   COMPARE EXPECTATIONS AND REALITY

B4   ACTIONS, RESULTS, NEXT STEP

A template useful for dealing with deadlines is:

B9   A CALENDAR MONTH FOR PRIORITISING – 5 WEEKS

Use these templates as appropriate while working with your student on any social situation, including the SOCIAL EXAMPLES discussed in this chapter.

Information for non-linear readers

Before the context of the USEFUL PREFACE and CHAPTERS 1 and 2, there is information that I hope will help non-linear readers as they approach the chapters. For chapters 4 – 14, this information would be identical except for which parts to scan and read. I have put all the information together into GUIDANCE FOR NON-LINEAR READERS, CHAPTER 3. It is worth reading CHAPTER 3 at some stage of working with this book.

GUIDANCE FOR
NON-LINEAR READERS:
p 222

1 Dipping-in to try out ideas: reading and scanning lists

Start with DIPPING-IN TO TRY OUT IDEAS: GENERAL PATTERN.
Read:

DIPPING-IN TO TRY OUT
IDEAS: GENERAL PATTERN:
p 228

    CONTEXT, p 495
    SUMMARY: SOCIAL SITUATIONS, p 522
    SERVICE PROVIDERS AND EMPLOYERS, p 496
    TRAVEL, p 498
    SUMMARY: JOB APPLICATION, p 504
    The opening paragraph of EATING OUT, p 514
    The Box: ISSUES TO THINK ABOUT (finances), p 519

Scan:
    other KEY POINT boxes, the stories and tips
    the rest of the chapter.

1.1 Key points: for policy-makers and general readers

Key points: For policy-makers and general readers

- Policies need to incorporate the good practices that are VITAL for dyslexic/ SpLD people.

Key general principles are:

- an openness that accepts differences easily
- clarity of expression
- a basic understanding of the difficulties from dyslexia/ SpLD and the solutions
- accommodations to meet the needs of dyslexic/ SpLD people when their own strategies can't provide solutions.

2 Context

Four different social situations have been chosen for a discussion of managing dyslexia/ SpLD by applying knowledge and skills. The areas of life chosen are:

- *TRAVEL* because it allows your student to work far afield and to widen her perspective on life
- *JOB APPLICATION* which is usually a necessary stage for getting a job
- *EATING OUT* which is an activity that can allow good relationships to develop and grow
- *FINANCES* because we need money to engage with others in so many ways.

TRAVEL: p 498

JOB APPLICATION: p 504

EATING OUT: p 514

FINANCES: p 518

They are all fairly important situations in many people's lives. Three involve service providers and one involves employers.

SERVICE PROVIDERS AND EMPLOYERS outlines ways the other people involved in these situations can enable dyslexic/ SpLD people to function well in the various situations.

SERVICE PROVIDERS AND EMPLOYERS: p 496

The four areas are discussed in slightly different ways:

- *TRAVEL* is used to highlight two extreme levels of organisation and shows how it can be important for your student to be aware of her characteristic approaches
- *JOB APPLICATION* is divided into different stages which are discussed and the discussion is annotated in terms of the skills and issues covered elsewhere in this book
- *EATING OUT* is discussed in terms of possible problems and how your student can find her solution
- *FINANCES* are discussed in terms of what might be involved, what your student needs to think about and where she might find useful ideas in this book.

The chapter ends with an overview in the *SUMMARY: SOCIAL EXAMPLES*.

SUMMARY: SOCIAL EXAMPLES: p 496

3   Service providers and employers

In all four examples, other people are engaging with your student. In three, your student is a customer receiving a service. In the fourth, your student is trying to match what she wants with the needs of an employer and the relationship is slightly different.

In a best case scenario, the other people want:

- to give your student information in a way that is easy for her to understand and use
- to have connection with her in a mutually beneficial way
- to enable her to use their services or systems with the least possible hassle – for her or themselves.

Service providers and employers connecting with dyslexic/ SpLD people and useful, relevant sections	
Service providers and employers should realise that it is to their benefit to communicate well with dyslexic/ SpLD people. They need to remember that dyslexic/ SpLDs may well process information in alternative, unexpected ways which could lead to quite a different understanding. Approaches that are VITAL for them are GOOD PRACTICE in relation to everyone else.	CONTEXT of IMPARTING KNOWLEDGE AND SKILLS: p 53 WHAT COULD HAPPEN AND USEFUL, RELEVANT SECTIONS: p 464 DIALOGUE: p 107
An open attitude, that enables dyslexic/ SpLDs to voice their difficulties, will get to the heart of any problems more quickly.	ATTITUDES: p 82 BEHIND THE OBVIOUS: p 64
Clear, unambiguous speech, texts and signs will be important.	INDIRECT COMMUNICATION: p 119
Understanding the difficulties arising from dyslexia/ SpLD should help you to be more patient.	INDIVIDUALS WITH DYSLEXIA/ SPLD: p 57 STATIC MATERIAL AND CONSTANT CONTENT: p 91

Service providers and employers can:

- scan through the rest of this chapter and notice the problems dyslexic/ SpLD people encounter and the possible solutions
- think about their communications with dyslexic/ SpLD people to consider what could be done to make anything more straight forward.

It could be useful for you to talk through these ideas with your student, so that she has insights about other people's side of communication.

4 Travel

People travel for work, for hobbies, to see friends and family, for relaxation, and for many other reasons. Sometimes your student will be asked to travel by other people, sometimes she will travel from her own choice. Some people don't travel because they are afraid of certain consequences. For dyslexic/ SpLD people, some of the major problems are:

- getting lost
- not being able to find out where they are going
- high levels of stress while maintaining any kind of organisation
- difficulties with time.

If your student can't travel easily, she may either restrict the opportunities in her life or she may have to live with high levels of STRESS.

STRESS: p 78

To indentify your most comfortable approach to travel you could:

- objectively assess what your worries and difficulties might be
- imagine yourself as a traveller and work out what you need
- assess how your own characteristics and THINKING PREFERENCES can be used to help you.

THINKING PREFERENCES: p 72

You can test out possible solutions by going on short, unimportant journeys to find out how they work. These journeys will also help you to expand your knowledge of how you want to be as a traveller. Make sure you have a backup plan that will ensure that you arrive at your final destination safely.

If a journey is likely to be repeated, make notes so that you don't have to re-invent it each time.

The STORY: BENEFITS OF GETTING LOST shows a creative approach to situations that could otherwise be regarded undesirable.

STORY: BENEFITS OF GETTING LOST: p 487

In this section, I am going to look at some objects and information that need organising, some of the issues of travel and then describe two different approaches; one highly organised and one with minimal organisation.

4.1 Important objects and information

There are some things that your student probably can't travel without.

A passport if she is going abroad; she needs to find a way of making sure it doesn't go out of date.

Tickets if she's using public transport; some tickets are much cheaper if she buys them early. She then needs to be careful about her organisation so that she has them to hand when she needs them. If she uses electronic devices to buy tickets, she needs to be systematic about where she stores them on her device because she will need to find them fairly quickly while travelling. She also needs to make sure to charge the batteries of any electronic devices with tickets on them.

Money is probably important however she is travelling; she may need to get foreign currency; she may need to tell the bank she is going abroad so that she can use her bank card; she may simply need to get cash. She may need to assess how much money she wants; it may be useful to keep records from one trip to another. Again, organising the money so that it is to hand when wanted will be useful.

Information about her route or about her destination may be something that she needs to get in advance. She could get the information from the Internet or the public library or people she knows. She needs to give herself enough time to get the information and then she needs to maintain good organisation so that it is also to hand.

There could well be changes at short notice or no notice at all; she needs to be mentally prepared for these in such a way that she keeps the adventure alive.

At an early stage it can be worth thinking about the language if she's going to a foreign country. She may need to think about how she will deal with communicating with people who don't speak her language or any of those that she knows.

Also, she should think about anything that will make a difference to the way she travels. She might like always to have a book with her; she might be artistic and want art materials with her. She should ask herself what she wants to do in the long stretches of time during travel.

Useful sections of the book:
BEHIND THE OBVIOUS:
p 64

SUPPLEMENTARY ISSUES:
p 68

ORGANISATION: p 70

4.2   Dyslexic/ SpLD problems

Your student needs to be aware which of her dyslexic/ SpLD problems
are likely to affect her while travelling:

- she might experience difficulty reading notices

- she might have difficulty with directions

- her organisation might be vulnerable

- keeping together with others or with her luggage might be difficult

- or something else that is particular to her may affect her
  travelling.

If your student assesses any problem as accurately as possible before
she travels and she works out possible solutions, she is more likely to
be able to deal with it. She needs to minimise the effects of STRESS
because of the way it makes the dyslexic/ SpLD problems worse, see
BUILDING CONFIDENCE AND SELF-ESTEEM.

STRESS: p 78

BUILDING CONFIDENCE
AND SELF-ESTEEM: p 78

Listening to unintelligible announcements is difficult for everyone and
particularly so for some dyslexic/ SpLDs who already find
listening difficult as part of the pitfalls they experience. Again
your student needs to minimise the effects by reducing the
level of her stress.

Difficulties may also arise because the information she is expecting to
see is not the information being used. For example if she is
changing trains at a major city, say Birmingham, she could be
looking for 'Lancaster', the town where she will get off, but the
station uses 'Glasgow', the final destination of her train.

There may be nothing your student can do the first time she
experiences a particular travel problem but, if she keeps a log
of the type of problems that happen to her, she will gradually
know how to deal with them and know what precautions to
take.

Your student can use any travel difficulties as a creative way of
investigating her THINKING PREFERENCES and the pitfalls of her
dyslexia/ SpLD. This is all part of her REGIME FOR MANAGING
DYSLEXIA/ SPLD and living confidently with it. I would only
suggest that she is as adventurous as possible while remaining
just slightly out of her comfort zone.

THINKING PREFERENCES:
p 72

REGIME FOR MANAGING
DYSLEXIA/ SPLD: p 540

4.3 Time management

TIME: p 69

It's a good idea for your student to expect preparation tasks to take longer than she thinks they should. Any time she saves because they are quicker is a bonus and can be used for something else. If she runs out of time or is pressured for time, she is likely to have more problems than otherwise. Preparation may include interacting with officialdom. On the whole, your student cannot hurry official systems.

Journey deadlines at both ends may need managing. Getting to the start of the journey needs to be organised. Details about the end of the journey should be thought about in advance.

Journey times can also be unpredictable and it is worth having something to occupy herself (unless she finds twiddling her thumbs satisfying).

If she finds telling the time and reading clocks problematic, again it is worth allowing herself sufficient time to take care.

4.4 Highly organised

MATERIALS AND METHOD: p 565

ADAPTING DIPPING-IN TO TRY OUT IDEAS: GENERAL PATTERN: p 400

Your student may prefer to be highly organised. She can choose her best *MATERIALS AND METHOD* for organisation and gradually build up a body of knowledge from many different journeys. She can use *ADAPTING DIPPING-IN TO TRY OUT IDEAS: GENERAL PATTERN* to build a system that works for her, with the following adjustments:

The purpose of the project: why she is travelling.

Keeping in contact with people: other people might be:

- service providers
- fellow travellers
- people involved with any stage of the travel.

Dividing the preparation into sections:

what to take
timetable for preparation
journey details
official documents.

For each one of the sections, your student can have a master list that is her accumulated wisdom for travel. Then for each journey, she uses the relevant ideas from the master list.

These master lists might include how your student goes about:

- planning the journey
- getting the necessary documents together
- any equipment she might need for work or her hobbies
- keeping everything together as she collects:
    - the clothes that she will need for different temperatures and seasons
    - materials she might need for different activities.

Your student will have her journey planned from beginning to end. She will probably have contingency plans in case anything goes wrong. She will think about food that she needs on the journey. She will generally have covered all the possibilities that she can think of and be confident that the journey will go as smoothly as possible, even when it is not going to plan.

4.5   Minimally organised

At the other end of the organisation spectrum, your student may thoroughly enjoy travelling with much less planning; the best way to describe such travelling is with a story.

Story: Travelling with no time constraints

A colleague was joining friends and travelling from Wales to a town in Normandy. She didn't bother with cheap tickets bought in advance because of the time constraints. She looked forward to stress-free travelling. She had her passport, medical insurance and money, and knew that the train from Wales left for Birmingham every two hours. She left home when she was ready.

On the first train there was a map showing the routes from Birmingham and the places you could get to. She knew she would try to get the next train to Southampton, but as she couldn't do anything about time, she didn't worry, she just enjoyed the journey. She changed with no rush onto the Southampton train.

In Southampton, she had no idea where the St Malo ferry would go from, but she knew the signs saying 'for car drivers arrive at ferry' would get her to the right place, so she set off.

When she arrived at the dock, she found that the next ferry was going in 4 hours; it was the overnight one. She decided to have a cabin. She had a peaceful evening and a restful night. Her French is good enough to find a train, so next morning she found and took the train going to her destination.

As luck would have it, one of her friends was buying baguettes just outside the station when she arrived; that's not a guaranteed end result of minimal organisation, but the relaxed state of mind and of being is.

4.6 Summary: travel check-list

Summary: Travel check-list

What is the purpose of your journey?

How organised do you need to be?
How organised do you like to be?
What do you need to organise?

What problems might happen because of your dyslexia/ SpLD?

Are there people you need to contact?

5 Job application

Job applications are one of the major tasks that most people encounter at some stage during their working life, so this section is a full discussion of the processes involved. There are examples in boxes.

Themes from elsewhere in the book are indicated in the right-hand margin; you can find the relevant sections through the *INDEX*. Issues arising in employment have been discussed in *Organisation and Everyday Life with Dyslexia and other SpLDs* (Stacey 2020a). CVs and job applications are used as types of written work in *GOALS FOR WRITTEN WORK*.

Job applications are often done online and your student may have difficulty. See whether *FORMS ONLINE* has any useful suggestions and whether any recommendations in *INDIRECT COMMUNICATIONS* would help.

Some people find their jobs through chance encounters and never have to engage with the application process.

Themes in the book.

INDEX: p 589

Ⓖ p 574: CV

Stacey (2020a)

GOALS FOR WRITTEN WORK: p 187

FORMS ONLINE: p 354

INDIRECT COMMUNICATIONS: p 119

Summary: Job application

- Deciding on priorities for a job.
- Master CV (Curriculum Vitae) and application letter.
- Job searching.
- Deadlines.
- Application forms.
- Covering letter.
- Disclosure of dyslexia/ SpLD.

5.1 Clear idea of the job your student wants

Your student can brainstorm about the job she wants, including:

- the skills she has
- her interests and anything else that might be relevant, such as:
    - pay/salary
    - working hours
    - flexibility
    - the structure of the job
    - inclusion, or not, of initiative.

Work with your student to check whether her dyslexia/ SpLD is affecting her employment choices.

- Use one of the *METHODS OF EXPLORING BEHIND THE OBVIOUS*.
- Reflect with your student about her dyslexia/ SpLD using *RESPECTING THE LEARNING NEEDS OF THE FOUR SPLDS*.
- Use *THINKING PREFERENCES*, *THINKING CLEARLY* and *TECHNIQUES FOR USING THE MIND*.

Key point: Choice of job and avoiding dyslexia/ SpLD

- The effects of dyslexia/ SpLD could well be magnified, if your student chooses a job that she is uninterested in but which she hopes will not challenge her dyslexia/ SpLD.
- A job that interests her is likely to help her manage her dyslexia/ SpLD, see *DYSLEXIA/ SPLD AND INTERESTING JOBS*.

Group the ideas. Suitable categories are likely to be your student's:

- skills
- interests
- qualifications
- conditions of employment.

There may be other categories, but they will emerge from the brainstorming.

Ⓖ p 575: brainstorm

> recall;
> metacognition

METHODS OF EXPLORING BEHIND THE OBVIOUS: p 65

RESPECTING THE LEARNING NEEDS OF THE FOUR SPLDS: p 60

THINKING PREFERENCES: p 72

THINKING CLEARLY: p 79

TECHNIQUES FOR USING THE MIND: p 156

DYSLEXIA/ SPLD AND INTERESTING JOBS: p 84

> chunking

In each category, help your student to arrange the items from the one most important to her to the one least important to her.

Then she can decide across the categories which are her first, second and third priorities; include as many of the priorities as she needs, but three are probably enough to work with, see *EXAMPLE: JOB PRIORITIES FOR OBOIST,* below.

>
>
> ### Example: Job priorities for oboist
>
> The oboist had completed a music degree.
>
> | | |
> |---|---|
> | primary importance: | music |
> | secondary importance: | teaching |
> | third in importance: | flexibility |

5.2 Curriculum Vitae (CV) and letter of application

The CV contains factual information about your student's education and qualifications, and it will contain certain standard information that is required in job applications. She can put her name (represented by *'name'* below) in the heading.

The letter of application is a separate document and contains further information that could be relevant to any job your student might apply for. The purpose of the letter is to show prospective employers how her experience makes her particularly suitable for the job she is applying for.

Writing these two documents before she even starts searching for a job will help your student to be really clear about the type of jobs she would like to do. Many careers centres in universities or colleges or schools will help students write these documents. Your student can get templates for them so she doesn't have to design them completely herself.

CV (see *EXAMPLE: CURRICULUM VITAE (CV) FOR 'NAME'* below)

- It is useful to colour code anything that needs to be filled in later, such as the date the CV is prepared for a particular application.

- Your student can put her name and the page numbers in the footer.

prioritising

knowing the goal

be prepared

knowing the goal

be organised

- She can use a master CV to keep other information that she may need; it is useful to collect it in one place for use whenever necessary.

Education: include dates and start with the most recent.
List of your student's places of education

facts

Qualifications:
education: degree/certificates
               A levels
               GCSE
qualifications in any specialism
publications

facts

Other information likely to be asked for
date of birth, address, age, sex,

facts

Example: Curriculum vitae (CV) for *'name'*

Date dd/mmm/yyyy
Application for the job of XXX

Education
    last place, beginning and end dates
    second to last place, beg-end dates
    backwards through all other places, beg-end dates
    first school, beg-end dates

facts

Qualifications
    Degree, from whom, date, class
    certificates, from whom, date
    A-levels, date
    GCSEs, date
    other qualifications with similar details

facts

Other information likely to be requested
    date of birth
    address
    age, gender
    etc.

facts

Letter of application

This is a separate document from the CV; as in her CV, your student can put her name and page numbers in the footer. She should have one master letter of application that has absolutely everything in it and for which she has spent time creating a good layout. When making an application and using her letter of application, she can make a copy of her master and then edit the copy to suit the job she is applying for, see *EXAMPLE: PRESERVING THE MASTER DOCUMENTS*.

time management; be prepared

time management

Example: Preserving the master documents

Even if your student has just edited a master document, it is a good idea to close it first; otherwise, the most recent edits may not be saved in the master.

For example, if she has just edited her letter of application which has the file name: *letter_applic_master.docx*:

close:	the file, which will save it
find:	*letter_applic_master.docx*
open:	the file
save as:	*letter_applic_JOB_ONE.docx*
edit:	the file to suit the particular job application.

Tip: Complete copies of CV and job application letter

Make sure that you always have a complete copy of your master letter of application and of your CV.

The letter of application includes everything that your student has done from 11 years old onwards: part-time jobs and work experiences while at school, any voluntary experiences, driving experiences, all hobbies, sports, see *EXAMPLE: EXPERIENCES OF AN OBOIST*.

Writing about each one, your student can include: her interest, what she gained from the experience and why it is relevant to her as an employee.

If this last instruction is difficult, your student can think of an interested person to whom she could be writing and write as if they will be reading her letter of application as part of a job application process.

facts; arguments

writing techniques;
know the goal of any task

chunking

Example: Experiences of an oboist, as above

- jobs in music
- summer schools
- playing in bands
- sports activities
- horse riding
- driving experience
- school work experience
- voluntary work

Your student will edit this letter when making an application, so her master copy is not the final document that is sent. It is just very helpful to have it all in one place before she starts looking for a job, and she may gain important insights about the type of job she really wants to do.

Your student can group her experiences in categories with the most recent first; in the oboist example above, the categories are: music, sport, driving and work.

5.3 Job searching

At the beginning of any period of job searching, help your student to use mind set to bring to mind her priorities for a job, her skills and anything else she can remember from the work she did on her CV and letter of application.

mind set

She can scan likely sources of job opportunities; as these will change with time, this book is not the right place to give a definitive list. She is likely to be looking on the web, at newspapers on the web or in hard copy, and in local information sources. She can bookmark or highlight anything that looks attractive or suitable; when she has found half a dozen or so, then she can look at them in more detail.

reading skills

time management

She can make notes about the various jobs she is interested in, see TAKING AND MAKING NOTES. Using the same template, or list order, for collecting the information for the different jobs will allow her to compare the different jobs relatively easily; TABULAR NOTES is a particularly useful format for comparisons.

taking notes

TAKING AND MAKING NOTES: p 300

TABULAR NOTES: p 321

As far as possible, she should identify the culture of her prospective employers. If she keeps the notes for each job separate, they will probably be helpful when she prepares for an interview, see SUBJECT MATTER FOR JOB INTERVIEWS.

SUBJECT MATTER FOR JOB INTERVIEWS: p 385

It is worth identifying at this stage what your student thinks the most difficult task will be for her in the rest of the job application process. Use the appropriate parts of this book to make sure she makes the application process as easy and as smooth as possible.

dyslexia/ SpLD management

She needs to:

- keep any paperwork organised
- make sure she's handling time well
- think what she will need to have to hand when she telephones a potential employer
- practise job application interviews with a friend or with a professional.

organisation; time management

It is better to identify the stages that worry her, and put the strategies in place, rather than to hope it will all go well.

talking

However, this excellent advice doesn't suit everyone and there are some who do better with very little preparation. Look at your student's experience to decide which category she comes in.

5.4   Deadline for application

As part of the job-seeking process, your student must notice the deadlines for application, and any dates that relate to part of the application process, for example interview dates, or aptitude test dates. Make sure that she allows time for making her application well in advance of the deadline. If possible, include time for someone else to proof-read her application.

time
management

5.5   Application forms

Help your student to look at the criteria for any job that she is interested in, especially checking which ones are essential and which are desirable. Your student should make sure that she can satisfy all the essential criteria for the job; they are what the employer is looking for. If she doesn't meet the essential criteria, it is not worth applying for that job.

metacognition;
reading skills;
time
management;
self-esteem

She can print off the advert, the job description, and the application form if they are on a website, or else ring up and ask for them to be sent to her. She can make copies so that she can work on the hard copy and still have the original.

strategy to help
your student
work well

metacognition;
knowing the goal

Key points: Criteria for a job

- Help her to look at the desirable criteria and the section that says "Your duties will be ...".

- Make sure that your student feels she can fulfil 80% of these criteria and duties; these will give the guidelines for editing her letter of application, as set out below.

Guide her through filling in the application form using the information she has accumulated in her master CV. If it requires information that she hasn't already included under 'other information' on her master CV, then she can add the extra information to her master CV so that it is to hand if it's needed for another application form. In this way her master CV contains as much information as possible to help her.

> reading skills;
>
> strategy to help your student work well;
>
> copying skills[1]

She can make a copy of her CV, fill in any missing information as already highlighted, edit out the 'other information' that is either included in their form, or not relevant to this application.

> copying skills;
>
> time management

She can make a copy of her letter of application. Looking at the desirable criteria for the job and "Your duties will be...", your student should alter her letter so that it tells her prospective employer how well she can satisfy these criteria and how well she can do the job. She should delete anything in her letter that the employer is not interested in. She should expand or edit her application letter so that it addresses the desirable criteria and what her duties would be. "This is what I did; this is how it will be valuable to the job; these are my reasons for saying my experiences will be valuable."

> metacognition; knowing the goal
>
> know what your correspondent wants
>
> prioritising; facts, arguments, evaluation

Sometimes the application form will have sections where your student is invited to give further information; many dyslexic/ SpLD people find these sections very hard to fill in. They may ask for details that are very similar to the information that your student has put in her letter of application and the employers may not want a separate letter of application.

> metacognition; knowing the goal

Your student needs to decide:

- whether to use a brief summary of the information and refer to a more detailed version in her letter

- or to include in these sections as much as she can from her letter of application and to abandon the letter.

> know what your correspondent wants
>
> prioritising; facts, arguments, evaluation

Encourage your student to plan to finish her application well before the deadline for submitting the application. If she can give herself a break of 24 hours her final proof-reading will be more effective.

> time management

---

[1] 'Copying skills' are not in the Index. Treat them as a combination of comprehension, reading and practical skills. Find out exactly what is causing any problem.

5.6 Covering letter

If your student sends the application form, her CV and her letter of application by post she needs a covering letter.

She needs to include:

- the employer's name and address on the left-hand side
- her name and address, phone number and email address on right-hand side
- the date on right-hand side.

Starting at the left-hand margin:

- Dear Sir/ Madam (or name of person),
- Re: Application for XX (all in bold)   where XX is the name of the job
- I enclose (list what she encloses)
- I look forward to hearing from you.
- Yours truly/ sincerely,
- (Your student's signature)
- Your student's name printed
- Enc. then a list of the names of the documents.

Space the sections and paragraphs out well. If your student doesn't know the name of the person she is writing to she should end with 'Yours truly'. If she has put the name of a person, she should end with 'Yours sincerely'[2].

If she is emailing her application, she could also email a covering letter, set out as if it were going to be posted. Alternatively, she needs to make sure that the email is basically the same as a covering letter.

---

[2] 'Yours faithfully' is another phrase used to end letters. It is used when writing on behalf of a firm or company.

5.7   Interviews

Preparing for interviews is discussed in *Vivas and Interviews*, including visiting the place in advance and arriving in good time.

dyslexia/ SpLD management; self-esteem; talking well

Vivas and Interviews: p 383

Much of *Talking* is relevant to interviews:
- §2, *Context*
- §3, *Talking Fluently*, though probably not the ideas in that section about taking notes
- §4, *The Listeners*
- §6, *Environment*, it is important for your student to know how she reacts to the environment although she will not be in control of it during an interview;
- §8, *Equipment*, will be important if your student has to do a presentation as part of the interview or if, as a teacher, she usually has to deliver a lesson.

sections of *Talking*:
§2: p 364
§3: p 368
§4: p 374
§6: p 377

§8: p 379

Strategies for Listening will be relevant to your student's understanding of the questions asked.

Strategies for Listening: p 275

5.8   Special provisions

To disclose one's dyslexia/ SpLD is a hard decision to make, see *Declaring Dyslexia/ SpLD or Not*. If there are aptitude tests as part of the job application process, it may be necessary for your student to disclose that she is dyslexic/ SpLD in order to have a chance of performing well. Many careers service departments in universities or colleges can give help with aptitude tests and with obtaining appropriate accommodation.

dyslexia/ SpLD management

Declaring Dyslexia/ SpLD or Not: p 84

6   Eating out

Eating out can be an emotionally highly charged event with the potential for small incidents to trigger uncomfortable levels of *Stress*. When your student feels confident in herself and socially at ease, it is possible to relax and be comfortable about any problems she experiences and then she can ask others for help or she can ask them questions as necessary. Observing objectively what she experiences when eating out will help her find the solutions that suit her.

Stress: p 78

6.1   Difficulties when eating out

Some of the difficulties listed here stem from the basic problems of dyslexia/ SpLD; others are derived from more adult, advanced problems (Stacey, 2020b) of dyslexia/ SpLD.

Stacey (2020b)

Initial organisation:
>   remembering to take your bank card or money
>   getting to the right place, at the right time, in the right
>   clothes.

Menu difficulties – all reading problems, including:
>   unusual fonts
>   the layout of the menu
>   unfamiliar terminology or words or language
>   not understanding the answer when you have asked the
>   waiter a question.

Group dynamics:
>   wanting to fit in with the group in choice of food
>   keeping an eye on what the rest of the group is doing about
>   food and drink
>   where to sit so that you can listen and talk comfortably
>   knowing when and how to use the cutlery
>   trying not to be out of step with the group in many subtle
>   ways.

Decisions can be made difficult in various ways:
>   too much choice
>   whether to select on type of food
>   whether to select according to cost of food
>   whether to deselect rather than select
>   wanting to feel neither hungry nor bloated at the end of the
>   meal
>   needing to achieve a good balance of food; therefore it
>   matters whether the group decides to have starters
>   or puddings or both.

Paying:
>   calculating any tip
>   dividing the cost between members of the group
>   dealing with change.

Other:
>   This is definitely an area of life where the category 'other' is
>   useful. The difficulties you experience may be quite
>   different from those given in the list above.

6.2 Eating out with confidence

FIGURE 14.1 is one way of working out how to eat with confidence.
Your student may have different issues depending on the
circumstances of eating out, so she may need to work separately on
different situations.

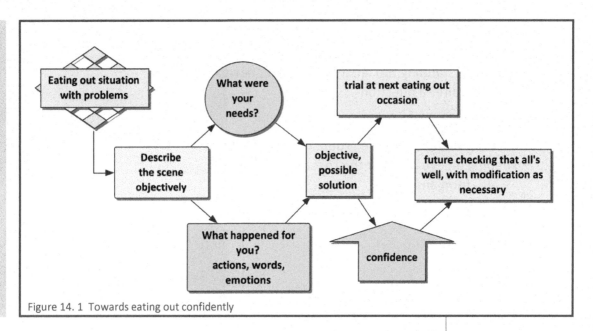

Figure 14. 1 Towards eating out confidently

The first step is to observe as accurately and as objectively as
possible what happens in a typical situation that you would like to
improve.

Observe the general situation, what you are saying and doing
and feeling.

Can you identify an underlying need that influences how you are
feeling?

In response to that need, is there something that you could do,
or think, differently to satisfy that need?

Is there a way you could express your need to other people in
the group and so find a satisfactory solution?

It might be useful to record the possible solutions you have
thought of.

If you are reflecting on a situation in the past, you should be using
your imagination as vividly as possible, which is why I have used
the present tense in the questions.

It might be better to decide to work with a future situation than a previous one because it hasn't yet been uncomfortable for you. So imagine a likely eating out event and use the questions above.

Organise a time to eat out with friends so that you can try out your solution in a safe situation. It is a good idea to build confidence securely rather than risk undermining new processes by using them in challenging circumstances. Again, observe the situation and monitor how well your proposed solutions worked. You can repeat the process until you find your way of eating out comfortably and pleasurably.

Story: Deciding what to eat

One dyslexic person is never comfortable eating out with others until orders have been placed, unless he is paying the bill in which case he can order exactly what he likes.

There are many ways he feels the need to fit in with the group, for instance:

- he would not like to be the only one ordering a starter and then have everyone else waiting while he ate it
- he finds reading the menu difficult
- he finds making choices difficult.

By talking through the issues to see what was at the heart of them, he decided:

- he needed a mental check-list for making his choice of what to eat
- he could put the list on a card the size of a bank card
- he can quickly check the card before or during choosing food.

With this easy-to-remember strategy, he has more confidence about the initial stages of eating out.

6.3 Summary: eating out

Summary: Eating out

Dyslexia/ SpLD might affect:

- organisation: time, place, money or debit card, clothes
- choice of food: reading menu, making a choice, using cutlery, fitting in with others
- paying: calculating how much tip or change
- other: what specific problems does your student face?

Being able to relax will help your student to maintain her self-esteem and confidence.

7   Finances

Money enables many different exchanges to happen within society, so it is difficult to opt out of dealing with finances. Many of the ideas in COMPREHENSION will be relevant to dealing with finances. Your student needs to get an overview of what's involved and then decide which areas affect her directly. She will need detailed and reliable information of those areas that are relevant to her. She can modify the process described above in EATING OUT WITH CONFIDENCE to identify any problems in situations dealing with finances and possible ways to maintain her confidence.

COMPREHENSION: p 162

EATING OUT WITH CONFIDENCE: p 516

Theories of finance and models of good practice will change. They may be dependent on many different factors, including the economic climate of the time, the country and the work or life situation of the people involved. There will be many different sources of information. Your student needs to identify and find those that will help her.

Tip: Good sources of information

- It is good to find at least one source that is applicable to the finances you are dealing with.
- You also need one that you find easy to work with.
- You may need to find a basic source of information to start with to give you the overview and after that it will be easier to work with more advanced sources.

The following comments are some suggestions to help your student process the information and make decisions about the way she will handle finances.

Issues to think about	Strategies and ideas in this book
Organisation	
Finances are an area of life where it is probably better to be more organised than less; it can be very time- and energy-consuming for your student to get her money sorted out again once it has got in a muddle. She is likely to be dealing with: information, correspondence, details about money, budgeting, and paying taxes on time, amongst other things.	ORGANISATION, p 70, especially PAPERWORK, INCLUDING FILING, p 71, will help your student keep everything under control.

Issues to think about	Strategies and ideas in this book
Criteria for decisions and attitudes	
If it is your student's own finances that she is dealing with then it will be her own criteria that matter; if she is dealing with finances as part of her work or for other people then it will be their criteria that apply. Knowing the criteria will help her to assess the information and processes that she will use.	The right MATERIALS AND METHODS, p 565, for organisation will make the work easier for your student. Useful techniques to sort out the criteria could include: MIND SET, p 158, METACOGNITION, p 63, and KNOWING THE GOAL OF ANY TASK, p 181.
Gathering information	
Your student is likely to be using many different sources. Help her to start by finding an overview of the information that she needs. Then she can search for the details of topics she has identified as relevant; comparing different sources of information is often useful.	As appropriate, use ADAPTING DIPPING-IN TO TRY OUT IDEAS: GENERAL PATTERN: p 400. COLLECTING INFORMATION TOGETHER, p 526, has some useful strategies.
Decision-making, including budgeting	
Decision-making is made easier for your student when she understands the information she has gathered, and she knows her criteria. One possible decision is that she hasn't got all the information and she needs to find more. She may need to decide how she will deal with budgeting. Remembering her decisions may be an important issue.	Any of the ideas above in this column could be useful as well as DECISION-MAKING AND REMEMBERING: p 71

Issues to think about	Strategies and ideas in this book
Knowing when something is important	
Your student will probably gain more knowledge of what is important the longer she deals with finances; alternatively, she could seek advice. Once she understands which aspects are important, she should deliberately look for them and attend to them; she should look for deadlines in correspondence and paperwork.	*MAIN THEMES VS. DETAILS:* p 178
Deadlines	
Knowing when the deadlines are, what they are about and what your student needs to do are all important aspects of dealing with deadlines.	*TIME:* p 69, and *KNOW THE GOAL OF ANY TASK:* p 181

Summary: Finances

Your student should:

- develop and use a reliable organisation
- find a reliable source of information
- know how to prioritise, and make sure she does it
- make sure she doesn't miss deadlines.

8   Summary: social situations

Summary: Social situations

You only have one physical brain; you might:

- be managing it well and not experience any effects from your dyslexia/ SpLD

- be vulnerable to being triggered into dyslexic/ SpLD functioning

- know a particular situation always presents problems because of your dyslexia/ SpLD.

In any situation knowing how you manage your dyslexia/ SpLD is likely to be important.

Describing situations objectively, knowing your characteristic strengths and your vulnerabilities will allow you to work out solutions for many of the situations.

When you've done all you can to maximise your potential and minimise your dyslexia/ SpLD, find the right person to help you with anything that is presenting a problem.

Other people involved can make a significant difference when they:

- easily accept differences

- adopt the good practices that are VITAL for dyslexic/ SpLD people

- are willing to accommodate your needs.

References

Stacey, Ginny, 2020a, *Organisation and Everyday Life with Dyslexia and other SpLDs*, Routledge, London

Stacey, Ginny, 2020b, *Development of Dyslexia and other SpLDs*, Routledge, London

Website information

Series website: www.routledge.com/cw/stacey

Appendix 1: Resources

Contents

Series: *Living Confidently with Specific Learning Difficulties (SpLDs)*

Book 1: *Finding Your Voice with Dyslexia and other SpLDs*
Book 2: *Organisation and Everyday Life with Dyslexia and other SpLDs*
Book 3: *Gaining Knowledge and Skills with Dyslexia and other SpLDs*
Book 4: *Development of Dyslexia and other SpLDs*

Stacey (2019, 2020a, 2021, 2020b)

To Readers of Books 3 and 4

The appendices are written for dyslexic/ SpLD people.

Dyslexic/ SpLD people are the readership of books 1 and 2. They are the learners for books 3 and 4, so the appendices are written for them, even when they are not the direct readership.

Many people supporting dyslexic/ SpLD people are themselves dyslexic/ SpLD; therefore, many of the readers of books 3 and 4 may benefit by using the material in the appendices for themselves.

Templates on the website

1   General resources

This is a collection of resources and ideas that will help you to capture any ideas that seem important to you. Ideas that are captured will then be available to you for use later on.

Notice anything that doesn't work for you, and use it to design your own way to capture and use information that seems relevant to you.

Tip: Margin

You can use the right-hand margin to jot down your ideas as you scan or read the book.

I have used it for cross-referencing and for references to help you find these when you want them.

---

2   Collecting information together

- Create a mind map of the information; there are examples in the book. Experiment with different styles to find which work well for you. (Don't use mind maps if you don't like them.)

- Use a digital recording device; make sure you label the files so that you can remember what they are about.

- Create tables of information; this section has several suggestions for using tables.

- Use electronic note-collecting devices.

B1 - *COLLECTING IDEAS THAT RELATE TO YOU*

TEMPLATES

This *TEMPLATE* will help with building your *INDIVIDUAL, PERSONAL PROFILE OF DYSLEXIA/ SPLD* and your *REGIME FOR MANAGING DYSLEXIA/ SPLD*.

G p 575: profile, regime

Column 4 allows you to reflect whether you are learning more about
1   your profile
2   your regime for managing dyslexia/ SpLD.

Column 5 allows you to note which elements are involved:
      thinking preferences
      pausing
      pitfalls
      accommodations
      goals.

B3 - *COMPARE EXPECTATIONS AND REALITY*

TEMPLATES

If you are going to observe objectively you need to keep a record of your expectations and what actually happens. The *TEMPLATE: COMPARE EXPECTATIONS AND REALITY* is one way of doing this. It can be easier to rule horizontal lines after writing in the template than forcing yourself to keep within lines already printed.

The template suggests you record the *situation* and *date*. It has 4 columns headed: *Events, Expected, Actual, Comments*.

For example:

Situation: to have everything ready for football on Saturday morning (include the date), in order to arrive on time.

Events	Expected	Actual	Comments
wash kit	Tuesday		
assemble kit	Friday		
put boots with kit	Friday		
get up	8.30 am Saturday		
breakfast	9.00		
leave house	9.45		
arrive at *venue*	10.15		

THE ACTUAL COLUMN WOULD BE FILLED IN AS CLOSE TO THE EVENT AS POSSIBLE. THE COMMENTS COULD THEN REFLECT PLEASURE AT SUCCESS OR ANY ADJUSTMENTS NEEDED TO ACHIEVE THE DESIRED RESULT.

B4 - ACTION, RESULTS, NEXT STEP

TEMPLATES

This *TEMPLATE* is very similar to *COMPARE EXPECTATIONS AND REALITY*. In *COMPARE EXPECTATIONS AND REALITY* you are planning ahead and monitoring how well the plan was executed. In *ACTION, RESULTS, NEXT STEP*, you are observing the results of actions, whether planned or not, and considering any implications for the *Next Step*, whenever that might be.

For example

Event	Action	Results	Next Step
conversation with friend	I created pictures in my mind as we talked	I remembered the details next day	try putting pictures on my lists
shopping	I drew some of the items on the list and left the list at home!	I remembered the drawings and some connected items; forgot others	see what other line drawing I can use

B5, B6 - *RECORDING TEMPLATES - 1 AND - 2*

These templates can be used for a number of different purposes. In *B5 - RECORDING TEMPLATE - 1* the columns are uneven, which is suitable for those times when you want to use one column for a lot of detail while the others are only needed for brief information. *B6 - RECORDING TEMPLATE - 2* has 4 equal columns.

B7, B8 - *RECORDING TEMPLATES - 3 AND - 4*

These templates are similar to *B5, B6 - RECORDING TEMPLATES - 1* and *- 2*, but with a 5th column. Often the fifth column is very useful for a brief key word or symbol. It allows you to code the information you are collecting so that you can find sections that belong together. For instance, if you are exploring how you use different senses, you can put visual/ hearing/ smell/ taste/ kinaesthetic or V/ H/ S/ T / K in the fifth column. Then you only have to look for the V/ visual to find all the notes about the way you use your vision.

Useful headings for linear lists or text notes

Any of the column headings suggested for tabular forms of collecting information could be used as headings for lists or a sentence-based way of collecting information.

You might divide a page into spaces for different categories of information and label the spaces.

You might write down the information you are gathering and leave space to add in the headings later.

TEMPLATES

MARGIN NOTE: when these 4 templates are recommended, headings are usually suggested.

3   Prioritising

Given a collection of tasks, situations or topics (not an exhaustive list), what are the priorities for you?

1   You might have to prioritise bearing in mind limited time and resources.
2   You might be trying to decide the relative importance of each of a set of topics.
3   You might be deciding the order in which to do a series of tasks.

You can use any style for taking notes to collect the information together. The suggestions here use a calendar, a mind map and a tabular form.

Step 1   With limited time or resources

First you have to establish the constraints:

- Do you have enough time or resources to do everything?
- Does anything depend on another thing being done first?

Assessing the constraints first stops you trying to do more than you possibly can.

The *TEMPLATE: B9 - A CALENDAR MONTH FOR PRIORITISING* allows you to mark deadlines and block out sections of time. You can often then decide the priority of the various tasks and the order in which to do them.

Put everything that is happening in your life onto the calendar. In particular, include time for the ordinary, everyday tasks.

It can be helpful to highlight the beginning and end of the month, whether using paper or an electronic device.

You then continue with the second stage below.

Step 2   What is involved?

A second stage is simply to brainstorm about the tasks, situations or topics under consideration. You can use any of the shapes of mind map used in the book. You could make lists of ideas.

In terms of reading a book, a useful set of questions might be:

What do I know already?
Why have I picked up this book?
What do I think it might give me?
What am I interested in? or Who am I interested in knowing more about?
What aspect would it be interesting to know more about?
What do I really want to know?

If you are prioritising actions, a set of useful questions might be:

What do I want to achieve?
What equipment do I need?
Who else is involved? How? Why?
What individual tasks are there?
What do I need to find out?

TEMPLATES
COMPANION @ WEBSITE

See the *INDEX:* p 589, for a list of mind maps

MARGIN NOTE:
GENERATING USEFUL QUESTIONS, p 530 could help you find the right questions.

Step 3   Deciding relative priorities

When you have decided what is involved, you can put the information together in a table and then decide the relative priorities of the tasks.

B5, B6 - RECORDING TEMPLATES - 1 AND - 2 can be adapted to gather the information.

TEMPLATES

Title = the reason for sorting out a set of priorities.

A = the priority assigned to each task once you've assessed them all

B = name of a task

C = details of the task

D = resources or time requirements.

B7, B8 - RECORDING TEMPLATES - 3 AND - 4 could be used if a 5th column is useful.

TEMPLATES

E = Vital/ important/ non-essential.

This information would help in assigning the priorities that are written in column A.

Step 4   Plan of action

Use the priorities list in column A and the calendar to make a plan of action. Keep monitoring your progress. Adapt your plan as necessary.

4 Generating useful questions

Making a list of questions can be a very useful way to guide yourself through many different situations or tasks. The purpose of the list is to clarify what you are attempting to do, to help you be realistic and to help you achieve the end goal. Discussion around these ideas has come under: useful questions, ultimate goal, know your goal, research questions and probably a few other terms too.   It is hard to pick out any common themes that lead to a direct set of principles. However, the idea of useful questions is sufficiently important that there is an *INDEX* entry: *QUESTIONS, USEFUL, EXAMPLES*.

INDEX: p 589

TEMPLATE: B10 - QUESTIONS TO ASK ONESELF TO HELP OBSERVATION is an example of a good set of questions.

The style and wording of the questions will be slightly different depending on the circumstances, for example:

When you're organising something, you might think about how you're going to organise it and why you're organising it in a particular way.

When you are reading something or listening, having some questions you want answered gives a structure to the material. You then understand it faster.

When you're writing an essay, doing a presentation, or communicating by some means, the purposes for your work need to be defined clearly. This approach usually gives a coherence to the work.

When you are making major decisions for your life, you can be helped by a set of questions about what you want to do, what you are most interested in, how your decisions will affect others. The list is not exhaustive.

When you need to keep your attention focused on a specific task and stop yourself getting diverted, you can use a set of questions to:

a) define the specific task

b) relate what you are doing at any moment to the specific task.

Pulling yourself back from distractions can make a task more enjoyable, or it can shorten a task you don't really want to do.

TEMPLATES

The Basic Set of
USEFUL QUESTIONS:
Why?
Who?
When?
Where?
How?
What for?

Exercise: To practise generating useful questions 1

You are going to use *USEFUL QUESTIONS* to search the book in order to find any discussion on a specific topic:

- Think of a topic that interests you.
- What questions need answering to help you find out about the topic?
- List your questions.
- Use them as you scan the *INDEX ENTRY: QUESTIONS, USEFUL, EXAMPLES*. Then scan the rest of the *INDEX,* the *CONTENTS* and the book to find topics that are similar to the one you have in mind.
- How good were your questions? Did they help you to find the sections that deal with the topic you had in mind?
- What changes would you make to the questions for the next time?

MARGIN NOTE: this exercise could be applied to all 4 books in the series (Stacey, 2019, 2020a, 2021, 2020b)

INDEX: p 589
CONTENTS: p xv

Exercise: To practise generating useful questions 2

You are going to use *USEFUL QUESTIONS* to search the book in order to find the nearest match to a specific task:

- Think of a task that needs doing.
- What questions need answering to help you find the best match, in the book, to your task?
- List your questions.
- Use them as you scan the *INDEX ENTRY: QUESTIONS, USEFUL, EXAMPLES*. Then scan the rest of the *INDEX* the *CONTENTS* and the book to find tasks that are similar to the one you have in mind.
- How good were your questions? Did they help you to find a good match to the task you had in mind?
- What changes would you make to the questions for the next time?

MARGIN NOTE: this exercise will work best with Organisation and Everyday Life with Dyslexia and other SpLDs (Stacey, 2020a) and Gaining Knowledge and Skills with Dyslexia and other SpLDs (Stacey, 2020b)

INDEX: p 589
CONTENTS: p xv

Tip: The skill of generating useful questions

This skill is worth developing until it becomes natural. You could add the *Exercise: To Practise Generating Useful Questions 1 & 2*, above, to the card index for *Systematic Review*. It is a skill that could be usefully practised once a week until it is easy to use.

Systematic Review in *Finding Your Voice with Dyslexia and other SpLDs* (Stacey, 2019)

5 Surveying

In surveying you are looking over material to find out, in broad terms, what the material contains and where certain ideas are. As part of the process you will probably decide your priorities for exploring the ideas. 'Material' could be instruction manuals for household goods, books, articles, web pages.

Step 1 Key ideas

You need to establish a set of key ideas that you want to find out about. These will be your focus of attention as you survey any material.

Margin Note: Exercise: Initial Purpose for Reading, p 17 is a good example of surveying.

You can use one of the *Exercises: To Practise Generating Useful Questions*.
You can brainstorm around the associated topics to see if key ideas emerge.
You can look at other examples using *Questions, Useful, Examples* in the *Index*, and see if any of them help you to recognise the key ideas you want to read about.

Exercises: To Practise Generating Useful Questions: p 532

Ⓖ p 575: brainstorm

Index: p 589

You can discuss your interest with someone else and use ideas that come out of the conversation.

It doesn't matter how you do it, but find a set of key ideas.

The set of key ideas will still be helpful, even when they are not quite right. They will help you to focus your mind as you survey. You will be more attentive to the material than if trying to read with a wide open mind that is not looking for anything specific.

Step 2   Recording your survey

TEMPLATES

Use *B5 - RECORDING TEMPLATE - 1.*

Headings   A = key topic   B = where in the book

C = main ideas   D = order to read.

(Complete D at the end of Step 3)

Step 3   Survey (as applicable to this book)

INDEX: p 589
CONTENTS: p xv

- Use the *INDEX* and *CONTENTS* of the book to find sections of the book that cover the topics you want to find out about.
- Scan the book for useful indications of important material, such as headings, words in bold or italic; scan graphs and other visual material.
- Cover all the topics you have identified in the key ideas list.
- Have a quick look at each section to gather its main ideas.
- Write in column D the order in which you would like to read the various sections.

Surveying other books

Some books don't have an index or contents list. You can use chapter headings. You may have to use introductions and conclusions to chapters. You may have to scan the beginnings of paragraphs every few pages.

Surveying can be used with any source of information. It can be extended to work with several sources at the same time. Column B would then be headed: Source, and where in the source. Or you could use the *B7 - RECORDING TEMPLATE - 3.*

TEMPLATES

6 Recording as you scan

Scanning a section: you can randomly move through a section deciding roughly what it is about. You don't try to understand the ideas.

Several times in this book you are recommended to scan several
        sections to find material and ideas that are relevant to you.
It is frustrating to see something interesting or useful and not be able
        to find it again.

TEMPLATE: A1 - JOTTING DOWN AS YOU SCAN allows you to make brief comments as you scan.

If you want to write more, and a landscape page would suit you better, use *B5 - RECORDING TEMPLATE - 1*.

The headings would be:

A = Source and page   B = Section/ Keywords

C = What is interesting   D = Priority.

Drawing a line after each entry can help to separate the ideas that you want to record.

7 Monitoring progress

It's really useful and encouraging to see how well you are doing. It's useful to see anything that isn't working so well, because then you can do something about it.
You might want to see:

> your progress with a skill
>
> knowledge you are gaining
>
> how a situation is developing
>
> how you are managing a task
>
> other ... the list is not exhaustive.

You can collect the information by any means that suits you:

> notes   on paper or electronic device
>
> voice recordings   art work.

Use the ideas below, in *USING TEMPLATES ON THE WEBSITE*, to help you decide what to record and how to label or annotate your information. You want to remember the key ideas and your reflections so that you can use them again later.

You can gather the information together by category, e.g. keep all the information about situations together.

Appendix 1   Resources

Using the templates on the website

If you collect information using the TEMPLATES: *B3 - COMPARE EXPECTATIONS AND REALITY* and *B4 - ACTION, RESULT AND NEXT STEP,* you can use the last columns, *Comment* and *Next Step* respectively, to reflect on your progress and anything you want to change.

Templates

The TEMPLATE: *B11 - MONITORING PROGRESS* has 5 columns.

1   = date
2   = focus of interest
3   = current state of play
4   = last application
5   = reflection.

Templates

Comments about the columns:

1   It is almost always useful to have the date recorded.
2   A few words that capture what you want to monitor.
3   Record your summary of how far you have progressed.
4   Describe what happened when you tried out your progress to date.
5   Reflect on your progress; maybe think about the next step; anyone you could usefully consult; anything that will bring further progress or satisfaction.

References

Series: *Living Confidently with Specific Learning Difficulties (SpLDs)*
Stacey, Ginny, 2019, *Finding Your Voice with Dyslexia and other SpLDs,* Routledge, London
Stacey, Ginny, 2020a, *Organisation and Everyday Life with Dyslexia and other SpLDs,* Routledge, London
Stacey, Ginny, 2020b, *Development of Dyslexia and other SpLDs,* Routledge, London
Stacey, Ginny, 2021, *Gaining Knowledge and Skills with Dyslexia and other SpLDs*, Routledge, London

Website information

Series website: www.routledge.com/cw/stacey

Appendix 2:

Individual, Personal Profile of Dyslexia/ SpLD
and
Regime for Managing Dyslexia/ SpLD

Contents

Series: *Living Confidently with Specific Learning Difficulties (SpLDs)*

Book 1: *Finding Your Voice with Dyslexia and other SpLDs*

Book 2: *Organisation and Everyday Life with Dyslexia and other SpLDs*

Book 3: *Gaining Knowledge and Skills with Dyslexia and other SpLDs*

Book 4: *Development of Dyslexia and other SpLDs*

Stacey (2019, 2020a, 2021, 2020b)

Templates on the website

TEMPLATES

1   Living confidently

The aim of the whole series LIVING CONFIDENTLY WITH SPECIFIC LEARNING DIFFICULTIES (SPLDS) is that dyslexic/ SpLD people have ownership of their dyslexia/ SpLD; therefore this appendix is addressed to dyslexic/ SpLD people. It is essentially the same throughout the series, with the addition of the sub-sections in this section. These sub-sections are summaries of key elements about the PROFILE and REGIME covered in *Finding Your Voice with Dyslexia and other SpLDs* (Stacey, 2019).

Stacey (2019)

1.1   Individual, personal profile of dyslexia/ SpLD

A profile is a summary of information. This profile is about your dyslexia/ SpLD. It contains:

how you think best	THINKING PREFERENCES
how you pause well	THINKING CLEARLY
the pitfalls of your dyslexia/ SpLD	PITFALLS
any accommodations you need	ACCOMMODATIONS

THINKING PREFERENCES: p 562

THINKING CLEARLY: p 557

PITFALLS: p 569

ACCOMMODATIONS: p 128

Thinking well and pausing at the right times allow you to deal with any pitfalls that come your way. When you know what they are likely to be, you can recognise your pitfalls in advance. You are in a better position to arrange necessary accommodations when you are clear about your pitfalls and the strategies you have tried to use in order to deal with them.

1.2   Regime for managing dyslexia/ SpLD

Your regime is about the day to day management of dyslexia/ SpLD in the light of life's unpredictable moments. It has 3 elements in common with your profile; it has goals instead of accommodations.

In day-to-day life, you carry on assuming all's OK, then a pitfall looms. You may be able to notice it before it has become a problem. You may be into a dyslexic/ SpLD way of functioning before you notice what is happening to you. Either way, having a regime allows you options for managing the situation.

Noticing the pitfall as early as possible is the first step. The second is pausing, being able to step back and take a moment to reflect on what is happening. Your thinking preferences are valuable tools for rescuing you. If you are not clear as to what you are aiming to achieve (*YOUR GOAL*), you are likely to fall back into the pitfall even after pausing well and deciding to use your best thinking.

KNOW THE GOAL OF ANY TASK:
p 181

1.3   Testing and developing your profile and regime

You test your profile and regime by using them and assessing how well each section works for you. Your profile and regime are unlikely to be fixed for all time; they will develop as you use them and as you gain more insights into the way your mind best works.

1.4   Mental energy to manage dyslexia/ SpLD

(Copied from *Finding Your Voice with Dyslexia and other SpLDs*, Stacey 2019)

Stacey (2019)

Insight: Mental energy to manage dyslexia/ SpLD

By using thinking preferences and various strategies, it is possible to function at a level that is comparable to your best intelligence.

If you are a dyslexic person that means using language at a level that is much better than the dyslexic language, see *FIGURE APPENDIX 2.1.*

However, the dyslexia/ SpLD doesn't get removed. It is still there in the mind and you can be triggered into using those thought processes.

Mental energy often has to be reserved to monitor progress in order to stay out of your dyslexic/ SpLD processing.

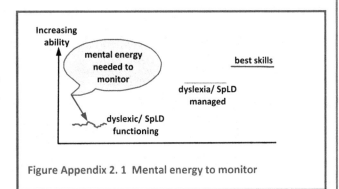

Figure Appendix 2. 1 Mental energy to monitor

2 Building up insights

The table shows the overlap between the elements of your individual profile and your regime for managing dyslexia/ SpLD. It also shows the key way for developing and testing each element.

Element	Individual, personal profile	Regime for managing dyslexia/ SpLD	For developing and testing processes	Covered in Book (or see Appendix 3 for summaries)	Page
Thinking preferences	1	3	recall & check	1	562
Pausing	2	2	practise & reflect	1	557
Pitfalls	3	1	observe & reflect	2 & 4 partly in 1	569
Accommodation	4		negotiate, use and reflect	2, 3 & 4 partly in 1	128
Goals		4	via applications	3 partly in 1	181

The aim is to build up the insights into a *Tool Box for Living Confidently*. The tool box will develop and expand over time, see *Updating the Tool box*.

If you keep your records in a way that you can easily review, you will build on your insights in an effective way. You will be able to use them and discuss them with others.

B1 - *Collecting Ideas That Relate to You - Template*

Collect the stories, insights, examples, etc. from the book that relate to you. Collect what happens when you try any of the exercises.

To fill in the 4th column, write 'profile' or 'regime/ managing'.
Use the elements in the table above to fill in the 5th column.
It is then easy to scan these two columns to bring your insights together.

Tool Box for Living Confidently: p 545

Updating the Tool box: p 548

Templates

Look at the layout for the summary templates:

TEMPLATES
COMPANION
@
WEBSITE

> D3 - REGIME FOR MANAGING DYSLEXIA/ SPLD (SPATIAL)
> C1 - INDIVIDUAL, PERSONAL PROFILE OF DYSLEXIA/ SPLD (SPATIAL)
>
> E2 - TABLE OF THINKING PREFERENCES
>
> D5 - REGIME FOR MANAGING DYSLEXIA/ SPLD (LINEAR EXAMPLE)
> C3 - INDIVIDUAL, PERSONAL PROFILE OF DYSLEXIA/ SPLD (LINEAR)

Which do you think will suit you best?

Which do you think would be worth trying out?

You can use them as soon as you start gathering insights. They may well change as further insights are gained.

Observe and reflect

Templates that can be used for gathering insights are:

TEMPLATES
COMPANION
@
WEBSITE

> B2 - KNOW YOUR OWN MIND
>
> B7, B8 - RECORDING TEMPLATES - 3 OR - 4
>
> D1 - MANAGING DYSLEXIA/ SPLD (MIND MAP)
>
> D2 - MANAGING DYSLEXIA/ SPLD (LINEAR)

Suggestions for headings for the RECORDING TEMPLATES - 3 OR - 4 are:

A = date   B = situation   C = what I was trying to do

D = details, including strategies being used

E = notes on success or otherwise.

Column E could either be narrow for a single word that rated your success or it could be wider for more detailed notes. Choose the template depending on whether you want column E to be narrow or wide.

E4, E5 - THINKING PREFERENCES, one spatial, one linear, are two useful TEMPLATES for recording brief notes as you build your profile.

TEMPLATES
COMPANION
@
WEBSITE

Examples from a log book

A log book is another way of recording incidents and reflections. You can pull the insights together by using key words in columns down the edges of the pages. You gradually have confidence in your insights because you have experience and evidence, which you are recording in a systematic way.

These notes were taken over several weeks while observing behaviour patterns:

MARGIN NOTE:
I usually shorten my headings to fit the columns
e.g. Th-Pref for Thinking Preferences

Date	Details	Other	Pitfall	Th-Pref (Thinking Preference)
DD/ MM/ YY	Total absorption in what's current in my mind – nothing rings any bells to warn me that something else needs attention. (Example) Focusing on writing reports before a deadline meant I missed an evening class		frequent problem	
DD/ MM/ YY	Can't remember from top of stairs to bottom that I need to add something to the shopping list. Crossing my fingers at top of stairs will remind me at the bottom that I have to remember something (that's enough to remember what to add).		poor short-term memory	kinaesthetic
DD/ MM/ YY	A friend explained the mechanism of blood circulation and capillary healing; now I know how to look after my ankle injury. I had forgotten the list of instructions. When there is no logic behind information, I forget what I'm told; or I modify half-remembered instructions by trying to make sense of incomplete information.		poor short-term memory	logic needed

Date	Details	Other	Pitfall	Th-Pref (Thinking Preference)
DD/ MM/ YY	Total confusion in my paperwork. If it isn't organised and doesn't stay organised, I've had it. I won't remember where any relevant other pieces of information are; I won't remember if it exists. Not having a printer in this room is causing major problems. I can't multi-task when paper is involved.		reading problem & recall	
DD/ MM/ YY	After I've been reading black-on-white intently for a while, my vision has the black print lines across it. Bright images also leave a strong imprint.	eyes: after images		

3   The tool box for living confidently

If you consistently work through the ideas in this book and build a picture of how you think well, how you take-action well and how you manage your dyslexia/ SpLD well, you will accumulate a body of knowledge and skills. You can summarise what you learn in three templates:

Ⓖ p 575: taking-action

  D3 - *REGIME FOR MANAGING DYSLEXIA/ SPLD (SPATIAL)*

  C1 - *INDIVIDUAL, PERSONAL PROFILE OF DYSLEXIA/ SPLD (SPATIAL)*

  E2 - *TABLE OF THINKING PREFERENCES*

or use the linear alternative templates:

  D4 - *REGIME FOR MANAGING DYSLEXIA/ SPLD (LINEAR)*

  C3 - *INDIVIDUAL, PERSONAL PROFILE OF DYSLEXIA/ SPLD (LINEAR)*

If some of the insights are more important than others, add this information to the summaries.

TEMPLATES

Make cross-references to any notes you have about the insights you put on the summaries. For example, you could have a log book entry which gives a good example of you using your kinaesthetic strength. You list 'kinaesthetic' in your thinking preferences table with cross-reference '(log book, date)'.

You could also have:

> a collection of stories that reflect your experiences
>
> a log book or other systematic collection of evidence that you can easily access.

What you know about yourself will change and develop over time, which is the same for everyone. Any summary should be dated so that you know when it was the current one.

Even when nothing is causing you to update your tool box, it is worth reflecting on the whole tool box from time to time, to see whether any element needs to be developed further.

This accumulated knowledge and skills is your tool box for living confidently with your dyslexia/ SpLD.

You can use the *A3 - BOOKMARK – PROFILE AND TECHNIQUES* to record your profile and the techniques that help you. Then use the bookmark when you are reading to make sure you are doing everything possible to ease your reading.

TEMPLATES

Examples of insights of some other people are in *TEMPLATES*:

TEMPLATES

> *D5 - EXPERIENCES FOR MANAGING DYSLEXIA/ SPLD (LINEAR EXAMPLE)*
>
> *C2 - EXAMPLE: INDIVIDUAL, PERSONAL PROFILE OF DYSLEXIA/ SPLD (SPATIAL)*
>
> *C4 - 2 EXAMPLES OF INDIVIDUAL, PERSONAL PROFILES OF DYSLEXIA/ SPLD (LINEAR)*
>
> *E3 - EXAMPLE: TABLE OF THINKING PREFERENCES (SPATIAL)*

It can be useful to see what insights other people have gained.

General letter to employers

It might be possible and useful to have a general letter in your tool box from someone who has given you dyslexia/ SpLD support. These are extracts taken from a single page for a student (PG) with dyslexia. He had decided that he wanted any future employer to know he was dyslexic.

Example: Extracts from a letter to employers

To Whom it May Concern (with qualifications of author somewhere)

Re: PG and dyslexia in the workplace

Dyslexia
Short paragraph about dyslexia and giving a reference to a book that shows a positive approach to dyslexia.

Dyslexia in the workplace
Short paragraph about management rather than cure of dyslexia and that suitable environment allows dyslexic people to be as effective as any others.

PG's choice of career
PG wants to work in pharmaceutical and medical marketing. PG has done a biology and chemistry degree at Y University. He has also discovered that he likes dealing with people and that he has appropriate, interpersonal skills. He has chosen pharmaceutical and medical marketing as a career because he will be able to use both his degree and his interpersonal skills.

Most of the time in this job, PG does not expect his dyslexia to hinder him. He may find certain electronic devices extremely useful, such as a voice recorder and an electronic organiser. The one task he may need to take extra care with is report-writing. He has found at university that he can deal with coursework assignments providing he leaves adequate time, does not work right up to the deadline and gets someone else to read his work before the final stage. He will need to use the same strategies for any report-writing at work.

Conclusion
A couple of sentences about dyslexics in general having intellectual strengths.
PG should be able to contribute his knowledge and thinking strengths to any employer provided his different ways of working are accommodated so that he can effectively manage his dyslexia.

4 Updating the tool box

Any time the tool box seems to be unhelpful:

- look after your confidence
- check you are pausing in ways that help you
- read (re-read) about fluctuations between the *4 LEVELS OF COMPENSATION*.

4 LEVELS OF COMPENSATION: p 568

Observe and reflect

Use any of the formats that have worked for you in building your tool box to find out what is undermining the management of your dyslexia/ SpLD and to develop any necessary new skills and knowledge.

In particular, the following could be table headings or arms of mind maps:

Date, situation	*Insights as to why the strategy didn't work
What I want to do	*What was going well
Strategy I thought would work	*Insights as to why the strategy worked
*What was going wrong	What to try next.

*In a table, I would combine these headings into one column, 'Details'. It would be wide enough to write quite a bit. I'd have a narrow column beside it which would categorise the details:

✓	or	OK
✓ ?		OK/ why?
x		not OK
x ?		not OK/ why?

Working in this way, you can find new insights about the contents of your tool box. You may simply be adding to it. You may find some of the insights you had were not as robust as you thought they were. You may be replacing them or developing them. You may find the source of your decreased management had nothing to do with the dyslexia/ SpLD. The processes set out here should help you to identify the root of the problem.

Tip: Adding new significant insights to the tool box

Whenever something significant comes to light:

- add it to the summaries

- date it.

Keep the stories that led to the new insight.
Make sure you can connect the summary to the stories.

Progress report

Progress reports can be useful.

- They can show you what you have achieved so far; they can demonstrate how those achievements have come about and what skills or capability you have.

- They can state the problems that remain.

- They can make the case for accommodations and continued support. They can contribute to updating the tool box.

- They should have a declared benefit, especially for you. The issues addressed need to be pertinent to you.

Example: Extracts from a progress report

Name XX - Progress report on dyslexia support tuition

This report outlines the progress that XX has made in study skills, and the support she is likely to need to complete her course successfully.

549

Five areas relevant to XX have been covered recently:

1) time management

2) organisation

3) reading and taking notes

4) essay-writing

5) exams stress control.

For example: Reading and taking notes

XX has learnt to read more effectively. She now scans contents lists and headings to get an overview and to find the sections of immediate relevance; she no longer works her way slowly through every word. She continues to have difficulty understanding some texts, and benefits from translating them with the help of pictures. For taking notes, she now uses mind maps. She still needs support to group notes by topic. She has developed various personal 'shorthand' symbols and also uses colour very effectively.

[Any significant comments about the other areas.]

General conclusion

XX has made considerable strides towards becoming a confident student, able to use appropriate strategies to overcome the range of difficulties caused by her dyslexia. She has become much more willing to try new approaches.   Her results in a number of modules show that she has the potential to achieve a good degree.

5 Negotiating accommodation

It is fairly hard to negotiate accommodation for yourself. You may need to get someone, your advocate, who has been working with you or who knows you well, to put your case.

Ⓖ p 575: accommodation

These are suggestions as to how to make the case for accommodation. The request might be in a formal letter or in an email from your advocate.

The role and expertise of the advocate need to be stated, and the contact they have with you in relation to the case being made. If these details are already known, they could be excluded.

The advocate should:

Propose the requested accommodation directly and simply.

Explain the situation that prompts the request. Include any information about dyslexia/ SpLD that may be relevant.

Give any comparisons with the experiences of other people (if possible and useful).

Explain any solutions that you have tried in order to deal with the situation and why nothing has worked.

Give evidence of your capabilities (if not known to the person who would agree to the accommodation).

Re-state the request, possibly in greater detail.

End as fits the document being written.

Example request for accommodation

Situation: dyslexic mathematician receiving support at university, including:
notes taken by a fellow student at lectures;
a university department organising support;
a support tutor;
a system of feedback between support tutors and the university department.

It was necessary for the student to attend the lectures in order to be eligible to receive the notes from the note-taker.

⌃

Dear [name of person, or person's job title],

Can XX opt out of lectures and still receive the notes from the note-taker?

I had email contact with XX before the beginning of term and then didn't hear from him. Last week I contacted him, asking whether the silence meant everything was OK or whether he was drowning. It was the latter.

He came to see me this morning. Last week he got so demoralised that he was considering giving up the course.

He has 9 lectures a week and is getting nothing from them. He has compared experiences with a couple of other students. One doesn't understand the lectures either, but she gets enough so that she is able to use the relevant sections to help her complete the problem sheets. The other finds that in the end everything falls into place, and that the maths doesn't all have to make sense immediately.

XX doesn't work like this; as I mentioned in the feedback sheet last term, he needs to understand everything as he goes, to build up the whole subject, and he cannot make progress when there are gaps in his knowledge. He has tried to use the on-line handouts before lectures so that he has some framework to listen with, but the lecturers don't follow the handouts and XX can't work out quickly enough how the lecture relates to the printed pages. Also, the handouts are very wordy so trying to understand them takes XX a long time. He records the lectures and finds that a bit useful. At the moment XX is spending 9 hours at lectures without understanding them, and is getting nowhere.

On Sunday he decided to go back to his preferred way of working and he solidly worked through all the maths relating to his problem sheets, making sure he understands everything. He managed to get the problem sheets done, albeit one was late.

⌄

He used the notes made by the note-taker. They are bullet points, succinct and clear. Just occasionally he has had to find extra information from the on-line lecture handouts. They are a very good resource for him.

We have worked on trying to find a solution to the problem of the lectures, but I am not very hopeful within the current situation; the lectures are really 9 hours that take time and destroy his motivation and morale.

Can XX receive the lecture notes if he doesn't go to the lectures? Is an understanding of the way he needs to work and of the problems he is having with the lectures sufficient evidence? Can receiving the notes without going to the lectures be accepted as suitable accommodation for his dyslexia?
Best wishes
Support Tutor

Result of this request

XX was allowed to have the notes from the official note-taker even though he didn't go to the lectures. He had a conversation with the subject tutor, which resulted in a radical change to the way he worked on his course. He finished his degree.

References

Stacey, Ginny, 2019, *Finding Your Voice with Dyslexia and other SpLDs*, Routledge, London

Stacey, Ginny, 2020a, *Organisation and Everyday Life with Dyslexia and other SpLDs*, Routledge, London

Stacey, Ginny, 2020b, *Development of Dyslexia and other SpLDs,* Routledge, London

Stacey, Ginny, 2021, *Gaining Knowledge and Skills with Dyslexia and other SpLDs*, Routledge, London

Website information

Series website: www.routledge.com/cw/Stacey

Appendix 3:   Key Concepts

Contents

Series:
Living Confidently with Specific Learning Difficulties (SpLDs)

Book 1	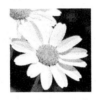	*Finding Your Voice with Dyslexia and other SpLDs* (Stacey 2019)

Book 2	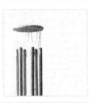	*Organisation and Everyday Life with Dyslexia and other SpLDs* (Stacey 2020a)

Book 3	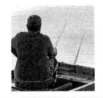	*Gaining Knowledge and Skills with Dyslexia and other SpLDs* (Stacey 2021)

Book 4		*Development of Dyslexia and other SpLDs* (Stacey 2020b)

Useful template on the website:

B1 *COLLECTING IDEAS THAT RELATE TO YOU*

TEMPLATES

To Readers of Books 3 and 4

The appendices are written for dyslexic/ SpLD people.

Dyslexic/ SpLD people are the readership of books 1 and 2. They are the learners for books 3 and 4, so the appendices are written for them, even when they are not the direct readership.

Many people supporting dyslexic/ SpLD people are themselves dyslexic/ SpLD; therefore, many of the readers of books 3 and 4 may benefit by using the material in the appendices for themselves.

Templates on the website

B1   COLLECTING IDEAS THAT RELATE TO YOU
E1   LIST OF OPTIONS FOR THINKING PREFERENCES

Context

The books in this series are written to be used individually, but people's lives can't be separated quite so neatly. In any situation, you may need information from more than one book.

THINKING PREFERENCES are highlighted in orange in this appendix.

This appendix has summaries of many of the skills and knowledge that I cover when going over all that is useful in managing dyslexia/ SpLD. It has been included to allow the books to be used individually.

The book that covers each key concept is indicated by the icons and the coloured lines in the CONTENTS, and the coloured lines on the left hand side of the text.

1   Thinking clearly (pausing)

Pausing is the second element in both your *INDIVIDUAL, PERSONAL PROFILE OF DYSLEXIA/ SPLD* and your *REGIME FOR MANAGING DYSLEXIA/ SPLD. Finding Your Voice with Dyslexia and other SpLDs* (Stacey, 2019) discusses the benefits of thinking clearly and gives you several different methods for doing so.

INDIVIDUAL, PERSONAL PROFILE OF DYSLEXIA/ SPLD: p 540

REGIME FOR MANAGING DYSLEXIA/ SPLD: p 540

Stacey (2019)

Thinking Clearly in *Finding Your Voice with Dyslexia and other SpLDs* also discusses confidence and self-esteem. Maintaining good levels in these two states of being is important.

You need to practise some of the methods for pausing in order to experience the benefits. As you work with the ideas in this series of books, you will be able to reflect on what is happening for you. You can add your insights to your *PROFILE* and *REGIME.*

This section repeats 2 of the exercises from *Finding Your Voice with Dyslexia and other SpLDs.*

1.1   Breathing

If you switch on good breathing, you switch off panic, anxiety and many other unhelpful emotional states.   Focusing on your breathing allows you mental space to stop and step back from the immediate situation.

Tip: CAUTION

If you feel dizzy, get up and walk about, or hold your breath for a count of 10. Dizziness, from poor breathing, is caused by too much oxygen and you need to use it up by walking about or to retain CO_2 by holding your breath for a while.

If you carry a lot of tension in your body, you may find it more useful to work through the relaxation *EXERCISE: PHYSICAL RELAXATION* before attempting the following exercise.

EXERCISE: PHYSICAL RELAXATION: p 559

Exercise: Breathing

First, see the *TIP: CAUTION* above.

During the exercise, as you breathe in you feel the sensations in different parts of your body; as you breathe out you let go of the sensations. You can imagine the out-breath flowing easily into each part of the body.

Sit comfortably and close your eyes.
    Breathe naturally while doing the exercise.
As you breathe in[1],

  feel the sensations in your:

face	and let go
neck and shoulders	and let go
arms and chest	and let go
stomach	and let go
buttocks and legs	and let go
whole body	and let it relax further

Repeat the cycle several times.

1.2   Relaxation

Being able to deliberately stop and relax is another way to give yourself the opportunity to pause well. Relaxation, however you do it, allows you to focus on the here and now and to step back from any situation that requires you to manage your dyslexia/ SpLD.

---

[1] When I lead this exercise, I usually say "As you breathe in" just once.
I say "feel the sensations in your (*name the part of the body*)" for at least the first cycle.
When it feels right, I just say the part of the body and "and let go".

Exercise: Physical relaxation

Sit comfortably and close your eyes.

Tighten
the muscles   of your face   and let go
   "   of your neck and shoulders   "
   "   of your arms, clench your hands   "
   "   of your chest   "
   "   of your stomach   "
   "   of your buttocks and legs   "

Tighten your whole body and let go.

Repeat this cycle several times.

2   Using the mind well

Using the Mind Well is a chapter in *Finding Your Voice with Dyslexia and other SpLDs* (Stacey, 2019) which discusses many techniques and skills for thinking. A selection of the techniques is summarised here.

Stacey (2019)

2.1   Mind set

If your mind is expecting a particular subject, it is able to handle relevant information more effectively.
Take about 5 minutes to switch your brain onto the subject you are about to deal with. Recall to mind what you already know or what your most pressing questions are.

2.2   Chunking

Working-memory stores information more effectively when it is linked together in some way that makes sense to you. The packages of linked information are known as 'chunks'.
Deliberately notice the links between pieces of information, or create your own links if necessary, or if you prefer. The process of making links is known as 'chunking'.

Ⓖ p 575: chunking, working memory

559

2.3 Recall and check

You strengthen your memory of information, knowledge or skills by recalling what you know and then checking against a reliable source. Re-reading material is not nearly as effective.

2.4 Memory consolidation

Your memories of knowledge are made much more permanent by having a pattern of repeated recall and check. You start by recalling your knowledge the next day, then after a week, then after a month, then after 6 months.

Done efficiently, memory consolidation is an extremely effective strategy.

The same memory consolidation is required for memories of skills. 'Little and often' is a better time scale for skills.

2.5 Concentration

Concentration is often a problem for dyslexic/ SpLD people. As you observe the way you do things more precisely, you should look out for those places, times and conditions when you can concentrate easily. Gradually build up your knowledge of the things that help you and see how you can use them when you find concentration difficult.

2.6 Metacognition

Metacognition is the awareness of the fact that you are doing or thinking something; it is not awareness of how or why. Just by noticing what is happening as you manage your dyslexia/ SpLD you will be developing the skill of metacognition. Be positive about the things you notice: enjoy those things you do well; find ways that enable you to be positive about anything you don't do so well.

2.7 Objective observation

Ⓖ p 575: objective

Observation is most effective when it is objective. If you keep factual records and reduce any emotional aspect to a minimum, the way forward with anything you want to change will be clearer.

2.8   Reflection

Once you have collected some observations on a common theme, you can look at them all together and see what sense to make of the whole group together. This is the skill of reflection, which is helpful in making decisions.

2.9   Prioritising

PRIORITISING: p 528

PRIORITISING is also a skill for using the mind well. It is a section in *APPENDIX 1*.

2.10   A model of learning

There are various stages in learning when you need to pay attention to how you are processing information, these are:

Input: any time new information is given.

Immediate use: very shortly after input.

Feedback loop: when what is being learnt is checked against what is intended to be learnt.

Recall: information is brought back from memory some time after input.

Direct use: information and skills are used exactly as they were given.

Developed use: knowledge and skills are modified in some way.

Long-term memory: knowledge and skills are established in long-term memory, and can be recalled.

Understanding: an appreciation of significant concepts has taken place.

You might use different ways of thinking:

- for each stage of a task
- for different tasks
- at different times for any particular task.

You need to experiment to find out what works for you. You will often have to be quite determined about what's right for you, and not let others persuade you to adopt ways that you know don't suit you so well.

3   Thinking preferences

THINKING PREFERENCES are part of both the *PROFILE* and *REGIME* (Stacey, 2019). They are often key to a dyslexic/ SpLD person being able to function well. Often in this series there is a section on *THINKING PREFERENCES.*

Stacey (2019)

INDIVIDUAL, PERSONAL PROFILE OF DYSLEXIA/ SPLD: p 540

REGIME FOR MANAGING DYSLEXIA/ SPLD: p 540

It is unusual for people to pay attention to how they think, so the usual – orthodox – approach is to ignore how anyone is thinking. These thinking preferences can be seen as unorthodox simply because they are outside the orthodox approach.

The *TEMPLATE: E1 - LIST OF OPTIONS FOR THINKING PREFERENCES* has suggestions for using the different preferences.

TEMPLATES

One way to find out about your *THINKING PREFERENCES* is to use *RECALL AND CHECK*, together with *MEMORY CONSOLIDATION*; then to reflect on your ways of thinking.

RECALL AND CHECK: p 560

MEMORY CONSOLIDATION: p 560

Make sure you know what your preferences are and that you have the confidence to use them.

Attention is often given to visual and verbal aspects of communication and education. The same attention should be given to kinaesthetic processing and to the *RATIONALE OR FRAMEWORK*. If kinaesthetic processing and the need for a framework are part of your thinking preferences, do find ways to make sure these needs are met.

RATIONALE OR FRAMEWORK: p 563

3.1   Sense-based: visual, verbal and kinaesthetic

The five physical senses are vision, hearing, taste, smell and kinaesthesia. The use of taste and smell to help use information is not covered in this series, although they are important for some people.

Ⓖ p 575: kinaesthesia

Kinaesthesia is used as an umbrella term for the physical senses, touch, position and movement. The term also includes experiences that are primarily remembered through a connection with the physical part of the experience.

The visual thinking preference uses spatial awareness and other visual patterns to process thinking.

See *INDEX* for examples in this book.

The **verbal** thinking preference uses language and words to process
thinking.

The **kinaesthetic** thinking preference uses the kinaesthetic sense as
the basis for thinking processes.

See *INDEX* for
examples in this book.

To facilitate discussion of kinaesthetic thinking processes, 'doing' and
'taking-action' are used for acquiring and applying knowledge and
skills, in parallel with reading, writing, listening and talking:

Acquiring	*Applying*
Reading	Writing
Listening	Talking
Doing	Taking-action

3.2   Rationale or framework

Some dyslexic/ SpLD people do not keep hold of information or
understanding if they don't know what the overall rationale or
framework is. Their minds don't retain the seemingly random
information long enough for the framework to emerge; it has to be
given in advance.

Ⓖ p 575: rationale,
framework

3.3   Holistic vs. linear

'Holistic thinking is happening when a large area of a topic is held in
the mind and processed simultaneously. An example is when you
look at a scene in front of you, you see that scene as a whole. This
type of thinking doesn't involve words, but you are definitely
thinking.' (Stacey, 2019)

Stacey (2019)

'Linear thinking involves analysing and breaking topics into their
component parts. Linear thinking is thought to be localised to definite
areas for specific tasks, whereas holistic thinking is diffused over
larger areas.' (Stacey, 2019)

3.4   Motivation

Two schemes for looking at individual differences between people are
used in *Finding Your Voice with Dyslexia and other SpLDs* (Stacey,
2019):

Stacey (2019)

> Myers-Briggs Personality Type
>
> Multiple Intelligences.

In the context of this appendix, the most interesting characteristics from both schemes are the motivations that people have, and which some dyslexic/ SpLD people can use to help themselves think well.

3.4.1   Myers-Briggs Personality Type (MBPT)

The Myers-Briggs scheme is based on 4 mental functions and 4 attitudes. The scheme characterises people as:

4 mental functions:	4 attitudes:
sensing	extroverted
intuiting	introverted
thinking	perceiving
feeling	judging (deciding).

MARGIN NOTE:
Judging is used in the sense of being able to make decisions, not in judging right or wrong.

The motivations of the different types come from their approach to the world around them.

Mental functions

- Sensing people are practical, pay attention to the here-and-now, like practical skills and learning with their hands.

- Intuiting people focus on concepts, ideas and plans.

- Thinking people tend to be logical, to like structures and organisation.

- Feeling people engage with people dynamics and feelings.

Attitudes

- Extroverted people sort out their ideas with the people and environment around them.

- Introverted people sort out most of their ideas on their own, before engaging with anyone else.

- Perceiving people like to carry on gathering information.

- Judging people like to come to a decision.

3.4.2   Multiple Intelligences (MI)

The Multiple Intelligences scheme includes 8 different, independent intelligences. Most of the intelligences have overlap with the Myers-Briggs system, as far as motivation is concerned, so I don't use them. However there is one intelligence that is distinct and worth noting.

The Naturalist Intelligence involves accurate observation of the world around. People skilled with this intelligence are able to see parallels between topics or within a group of objects. They are able to classify ideas or objects and they instinctively sort information into categories.

3.5 'Other'

The list of thinking preferences has grown as I have worked with dyslexic/ SpLD people and tried to make sense of what happens to or for them. There was no point in trying to make them fit already known patterns, so I have always worked with a category titled 'Other'.

'Other' is a holding category that allows you to keep hold of experiences that don't fit any category you already know.

4   Useful approaches

You will be managing your dyslexia/ SpLD during everyday events and while you tackle tasks. *Organisation and Everyday Life with Dyslexia and other SpLDs* and *Gaining Knowledge and Skills with Dyslexia and other SpLDs* deal with the practical application of using your *PROFILE* and *REGIME*. The approaches summarised here are those that help you make a good start with most tasks.

Stacey (2020a, 2019)

4.1 Materials and methods

For many situations or tasks, you will want to collect information together. You should find out your best way of doing it. The options depend on how you think best.

Materials include: paper, recording device, computer; using colour; using pen or pencil with a suitable grip. You need to think how you manage your materials, e.g. being able to spread out can make a significant difference.

Methods include: making lists (**linear** thinkers); mind maps (**holistic** thinkers); doing for yourself (**kinaesthetic** learners); bouncing ideas off other people (Myers-Briggs **feeling**, **extroverted** people).

When something is working well for you, notice what you are using and how you are doing it.

4.2   Model for developing organisation

The model puts forward 5 steps that need attention in organisation:

Step 1   gather strengths

Step 2   assess hazards

Step 3   describe what needs organising

Step 4   recognise insuperable obstacles

Step 5   develop constructive ways forward.

Ⓖ p 575:
hazard, obstacle

By changing the text at step 3, this model can be adapted to work with different situations or tasks when no organisation is required.

As you work with the tasks and situations, record what happens for you. Have a system so that you can see what is working for you and you can deliberately make the progress you want.

4.3   Comprehension

To comprehend something is to have a mental grasp of it.

You need your mind to hold information together and for long enough so that you can understand, comprehend, what it is all about.

All the skills in this appendix will help with comprehension. Observe how you comprehend anything. Keep records so that you can reflect on your experience over time. Explore different approaches until you find the ones that work best for you.

4.4   Key words

Key words are the words that hold the essence of
          an idea, a paragraph, a subject ...

Take something that you are very familiar with. Jot down some words that are most important for describing it. Cut the number of words down and find the fewest words that you feel comfortable with. These words should be the keywords of your chosen topic. Repeat the exercise over time, until you are good at producing a minimum collection of words to hold the essence of a subject.

When you can work well with key words, you can use them to give an overview of something or to help you sort out a main theme from minor details.

4.5   Know your goal

Knowing your goal is the 4th element of your *REGIME FOR MANAGING DYSLEXIA/ SPLD*. Quite often, when you are using *MENTAL ENERGY TO MANAGE DYSLEXIA/ SPLD*, you can do all the right things:

- observing what is happening
- pausing well
- deciding how to use your thinking preferences

but you still can't get matters under control and you still find yourself struggling in a circle.

Knowing what you want to achieve can help you to see the way out, or the way to resolve the situation.

Key words can help with knowing your goal. Learning how to hold your goal in a few keywords means it is much easier to stay focused and not get lost in a maze of ideas.

4.6   Planning

Planning is when you consider all the steps necessary to achieve a given outcome.

Almost all dyslexic/ SpLD people need to plan their work in order to minimise problems; for example, dyslexic people often write well when they have a good plan, but without a plan their writing will rarely reflect their ideas.

You need to find the level of detail that yields the result you want.

A big project can be broken down into smaller sections and separate plans constructed to achieve each section. This process makes the big plan less daunting and allows you to tackle it more readily.

REGIME FOR MANAGING DYSLEXIA/ SPLD: p 540

MENTAL ENERGY TO MANAGE DYSLEXIA/ SPLD: p 541

5   Aspects of dyslexia/ SpLD

You need to stay confident and positive in order to manage dyslexia/ SpLD. The aspects summarised here help you to know more about the characteristics of dyslexia/ SpLD so you are prepared for the inevitable fluctuations; the full discussions are in *Development of Dyslexia/ SpLD* (Stacey, 2020b).

Stacey (2020b)

5.1   Learned confusion

As a dyslexic/ SpLD person develops, certain patterns of confusion tend to become established in your brain, see *USEFUL PREFACE CONTEXT*. When you are older, you probably learn in better ways but you don't erase the original confused ways; they remain in your brain. They are there for your brain to activate.

USEFUL PREFACE CONTEXT: p 5

5.2   Oldest memory trace

When you unexpectedly need to think of something it is often the oldest memory trace that is used, not a later one. For example, you have learnt correct spellings, but when you use the words the older incorrect versions spring to mind.

5.3   Attention to learning

Most dyslexic/ SpLD people have to pay attention to all levels of a task; they do not learn subliminally. Reading a large number of books does not teach spelling.

Ⓖ p 575: subliminal learning

5.4   Average level of language skills a disadvantage

Intelligent students are often first recognised as being dyslexic/ SpLD at college or university, when they can no longer find ways round underlying problems. They have language skills that lift them above the group who are recognised as being in need of extra help at school, but those skills are not at the level of overall intelligence and the difference makes its mark in Higher Education.

5.5   4 levels of compensation

As you work on managing dyslexia/ SpLD, you gain skills and you become a 'compensated' dyslexic/ SpLD (McLoughlin et al., 2001).

McLoughlin et al. (2001)

There are different levels of compensation:

1   'People at level 1 are not aware of their weaknesses and have developed no strategies to overcome them.

2   'Those at level 2 are aware of their weaknesses but have not developed strategies to overcome them.

3   'People at level 3 are aware of their weaknesses and have developed compensatory strategies, but have developed them unconsciously.

4   'Finally, people at level 4 are aware of their weaknesses and they have consciously developed strategies to overcome them.'

The most important aspect is to realise that you do not remain consistently on any particular level. Even when you mostly operate as a 'compensated' dyslexic/ SpLD, i.e. on level 4, you may find you have dropped back into one of the less compensated ways of managing.

5.6   Pitfalls

Gradually as you learn to manage your dyslexia/ SpLD, you will recognise certain things that often tip you into dyslexic/ SpLD functioning: these things are called pitfalls in the context of these books.

('pitfall, n.', OED Online, 2020)

A pitfall is defined as 'a hidden or unsuspected danger, drawback, difficulty or opportunity for error' ('pitfall, n.4' OED Online, 2020).

I've divided pitfalls into 'hazards' and 'obstacles'. I've used the term 'glitch' for those moments when you notice a potential pitfall and deal with it immediately.

Ⓖ p 575: hazard, obstacle, glitch

5.7   Accommodation

Accommodations are adaptations put in place to address or reduce the problems caused by dyslexia/ SpLD; sometimes called 'reasonable adjustments' or 'provisions'.

There are certain situations in which a PITFALL of your dyslexia/ SpLD is very likely to be a significant issue, and it is known in advance. For some of these situations, e.g. exams and tests, accommodations are well established. Other situations may be specific to your circumstances.

5.8   Degrees of severity

Dyslexia/ SpLD is not like short- or long-sightedness: there is no equivalent pair of glasses that you can put on and find that the problems are reliably sorted. Learning 'coping strategies' gives you ways of dealing with issues, but you will constantly have to be putting effort into doing so.

I argue that 'degrees of severity' is not a useful concept. The statements usually used are that someone is 'mildly dyslexic/ SpLD' or 'severely dyslexic/ SpLD' as if this describes a static level of being dyslexic/ SpLD. The lived experience of dyslexia/ SpLD is that how you will be is variable and unpredictable.

It would be more useful to talk in terms of McLoughlin's 4 compensation levels (McLoughlin et al., 2001). For each person:

> What does level 4 consist of?
>
> How well can the person maintain level 4?
>
> How often does the person get triggered out of level 4?
>
> How much time and effort are required to get back to level 4?

4 LEVELS OF COMPENSATION: p 568

McLoughlin et al. (2001)

5.9   Stress

Stress usually makes the problems of dyslexia/ SpLD worse. You and those around you need to recognise this.

5.10   Benefits of recognising the problems

It is very difficult to do anything about problems that are not being recognised. When you know what your strengths are, and you realise you can make useful contributions, it is easier to acknowledge the problems and discuss them fruitfully with those around you.

References

McLoughlin, David, et al., 2001, *Adult Dyslexia: Assessment, Counselling and Training*, Whurr, London, 6th re-print
Series: *Living Confidently with Specific Learning Difficulties (SpLDs)*
Stacey, Ginny, 2019, *Finding Your Voice with Dyslexia and other SpLDs*, Routledge, London

Stacey, Ginny, 2020a, *Organisation and Everyday Life with Dyslexia and other SpLDs*, Routledge, London

Stacey, Ginny, 2020b, *Development of Dyslexia and other SpLDs*, Routledge, London

Stacey, Ginny, 2021, *Gaining Knowledge and Skills with Dyslexia and other SpLDs*, Routledge, London

Website information

OED Online, September 2020, Oxford University Press Accessed 24 October 2020

Series website: www.routledge.com/cw/Stacey

Glossary

Contents

1 Table: Symbols

Symbol	Explanation
§	Symbol used to denote a section.
Ⓖ	Symbol used to indicate an entry in the *GLOSSARY*. The page number is to the beginning of the appropriate section of the glossary.
@ COMPANION WEBSITE	The symbol signifies material on the companion website, www.routledge.com/cw/stacey. The section of the website is indicated.
text	Thinking preferences are highlighted in orange.
Book icon and blue line	Used in *USEFUL PREFACE* to show text that is significantly different from one book to another.
Green line on the margin	Sections of the book to teach to your student, as appropriate. In Appendix 3, the green line represents this book, as opposed to the other books.
Green strip inside the margin	Sections of the book in which 'you' specifically addresses a dyslexic/ SpLD person.
The two together.	Sections of the book in which 'you' specifically addresses a dyslexic/ SpLD person and ones to teach your student.

572

2 Table: Specific Learning Difficulties (SpLDs) descriptions

Dyslexia/ SpLD is used in most of this book because dyslexia is the most researched and recognised form of SpLD and because the dual term keeps the variations in mind.

SpLD	Definitions from DfES Report (2005)
Dyslexia	'Dyslexia is a combination of abilities and difficulties; the difficulties affect the learning process in aspects of literacy and sometimes numeracy. Coping with required reading is generally seen as the biggest challenge at Higher Education level due in part to difficulty in skimming and scanning written material. A student may also have an inability to express his/her ideas clearly in written form and in a style appropriate to the level of study. Marked and persistent weaknesses may be identified in working memory, speed of processing, sequencing skills, auditory and/or visual perception, spoken language and motor skills. Visuo-spatial skills, creative thinking and intuitive understanding are less likely to be impaired and indeed may be outstanding. Enabling or assistive technology is often found to be very beneficial.'
Dyspraxia / Developmental Co-ordination Disorder (DCD)	'A student with dyspraxia/DCD may have an impairment or immaturity in the organisation of movement, often appearing clumsy. Gross motor skills (related to balance and co-ordination) and fine motor skills (relating to manipulation of objects) are hard to learn and difficult to retain and generalise. Writing is particularly laborious and keyboard skills difficult to acquire. Individuals may have difficulty organising ideas and concepts. Pronunciation may also be affected and people with dyspraxia/DCD may be over/under sensitive to noise, light and touch. They may have poor awareness of body position and misread social cues in addition to those shared characteristics common to many SpLDs.'
Dyscalculia	'Dyscalculia is a learning difficulty involving the most basic aspect of arithmetical skills. The difficulty lies in the reception, comprehension, or production of quantitative and spatial information. Students with dyscalculia may have difficulty in understanding simple number concepts, lack an intuitive grasp of numbers and have problems learning number facts and procedures. These can relate to basic concepts such as telling the time, calculating prices, handling change.'

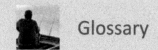

SpLD	Definitions from DfES Report (2005)
Attention Deficit Disorder ADD AD(H)D reflects the first sentence in the description	'Attention Deficit Disorder (ADD) exists with or without hyperactivity. In most cases people with this disorder are often 'off task', have particular difficulty commencing and switching tasks, together with a very short attention span and high levels of distractibility. They may fail to make effective use of the feedback they receive and have weak listening skills. Those with hyperactivity may act impulsively and erratically, have difficulty foreseeing outcomes, fail to plan ahead and be noticeably restless and fidgety. Those without the hyperactive trait tend to daydream excessively, lose track of what they are doing and fail to engage in their studies unless they are highly motivated. The behaviour of people with ADD can be inappropriate and unpredictable; this, together with the characteristics common to many SpLDs, can present a further barrier to learning.'

3 Table: Acronyms

Acronym	Explanation
ADD, ADHD, AD(H)D	Attention Deficit Disorder with or without Hyperactivity
DCD	Developmental Co-ordination Disorder
CV	Curriculum Vitae (plural Curricula Vitae)
DfES	Department for Education and Skills
MBPT	Myers-Briggs Personality Type
MCQ	Multiple-choice Question
MI	Multiple Intelligences
NLP	Neuro-Linguistic Programming
OED	Oxford English Dictionary
SENCO	Special Educational Needs Co-ordinator
SpLD	Specific Learning Difficulty

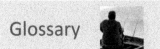

4 Table: Words and phrases, alphabetical list

Entry	Explanation
Accommodation	Accommodation refers to adaptations put in place to address or reduce the problems caused by dyslexia/ SpLD; sometimes called 'reasonable adjustments' or 'provisions'.
Argument	Statement of the reasons for and against a proposition; discussion of a question; debate. ('argument, n.5a', OED Online, 2020)
Autonomy autonomous	Control over your life by self-determination: acting and thinking for yourself; independent; free; self-governing. An autonomous person has autonomy.
Brainstorm	Collect all your ideas or thoughts about something; collect them in a concrete way, either on paper or on a white board, etc., straight into a computer or using a recording device; the collection of ideas is then available for further processing. The initial stages of brainstorming are often not selective; all ideas are captured even if they don't seem very relevant.
Blueprint	Used in this book to refer to a set of notes against which you check your knowledge. More usually, it is the working instructions for a project.
Chaotic chaos theory	Chaos theory is a field of mathematics. 'Behaviour of a system which is governed by deterministic laws but is so unpredictable as to appear random owing to its extreme sensitivity to initial conditions' ('chaos, n.6' OED Online, 2020).
Chunk	A chunk is 'a package of information bound by strong associative links within a chunk, and relatively weak links between chunks' (Baddeley, 2007). The capacity of working-memory is discussed in terms of chunks that can be stored.
Chunking	The process of making strong links between pieces of information so that more can be stored in chunks in working-memory (Baddeley, 2007).

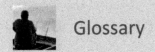

Entry	Explanation
Concrete	Concrete in contrast to abstract: anything that has a physical reality. Abstract ideas are always in the mind; they do not have a physical presence. Concrete includes: people, animals, buildings, water, air. Abstract includes: happiness, self-confidence, theories, expectations.
Doing See also KINAESTHETIC and TAKING-ACTION	In this series of books, 'doing' is used to refer to acquiring knowledge and skills using kinaesthetic processing.
Episodic memory	Episodic memory retains a whole event from start to finish; the memory of reciting the alphabet is a good example of episodic memory.
Framework	A structure made of parts joined to form a frame; especially one designed to enclose or support; a frame; a skeleton ('framework, n.1a' OED Online, 2020).
Goal	The end result of a task or activity. Knowing the goal of anything is often an important element in managing dyslexia/ SpLD.
Glitch	A sudden short-lived irregularity in behaviour ('glitch, n.a' OED Online, 2016). A glitch is a time when dyslexia/ SpLD has an effect on your behaviour, but you see it immediately and correct it. Any error is short-lived and there is no impact to prolong dyslexic/ SpLD functioning.
Hazard	A hazard is a danger or a risk which you can take steps to deal with. 'Hazard' is used to describe one category of the pitfalls of dyslexia/ SpLD.
Kinaesthesia kinaesthetic See also PROPRIOCEPTION and TAKING-ACTION.	Used as an umbrella term for the physical senses (touch, body-sense, movement), by comparison with the visual sense or the hearing sense. The term also includes experiences that are primarily remembered through a connection with the physical part of the experience.

576

Entry	Explanation
Mnemonics	Memorable phrases, words or sounds that help you to remember something. For example: Naughty Elephants Squirt Water gives the directions north, east, south and west round a compass or map; HONC gives the four most common elements in organic chemistry, hydrogen, oxygen, nitrogen and carbon.
Mind set	A process of switching your mind on to the topic you are about to work on: for study, for a meeting, for planning a project, etc. It is the equivalent of warm-up exercises before vigorous exercise. (Mindset as one word is something quite different.)
Neural networks	Neural networks are established when neurons repeatedly fire in set patterns. These set patterns are related to learning.
Neuro-Linguistic Programming (NLP)	NLP is about the mind and how we organise our mental life; about language, how we use it and how it affects us; about repetitive sequences of behaviour and how to act with intention. Some of the ideas from NLP are used in *THINKING CLEARLY* (Stacey, 2019). For further information, see O'Connor and McDermott (1996).
Neuron	A basic cell of the nervous system.
Neuron firing	A neuron fires a signal along its axon when the conditions in the neuron rise above a certain threshold; the conditions depend on all the many other neurons that input to that neuron.
Objective vs. subjective	Objective: existing as an object of consciousness, as opposed to being part of the conscious [person]. (OED, 1993) Subjective: of or belonging to the thinking [person]; proceeding from or taking place within the individual's consciousness.
Obstacle	An obstacle is something that blocks your way or prevents progress; you have to go round it, or avoid it. 'Obstacle' is used to describe one category of the pitfalls of dyslexia/ SpLD.

Entry	Explanation
Other	Other is a useful category. Whenever I'm sorting something out, for myself or a student, I keep the category 'other' in mind or give it space on the sheet of paper I'm working on. I use it for anything that I don't want to forget and that doesn't fit into the categories I already have.
Paradigm	A conceptual or methodological model underlying the theories and practices of a science or discipline at a particular time; (hence) a generally accepted world view ('paradigm, n.' OED Online, 2016).
Pitfall	A hidden or unsuspected danger, drawback, difficulty or opportunity for error ('pitfall, n.4' OED Online, 2020). Used as part of an individual's profile with respect to dyslexia/ SpLD.
Profile: Individual or personal	A representation of a structured set of characteristics of someone or something. A description of a person, organisation, product, etc. ('profile, n.II.10' OED Online, 2020). The dyslexia/ SpLD profile used in this book is an outline of: 1 the thinking preferences 2 the dyslexia/ SpLD pitfalls 3 strategies for pausing 4 accommodations that need to be made. The profile is highly personalised and is the foundation for managing the dyslexia/ SpLD.
Proprioception	The reception of information by sensors which receive signals relating to position and movement ('proprioception, n.' OED Online, 2020); part of the kinaesthetic senses.
Pruning	Has been proposed as an idea to account for the reduction in synaptic connections that occurs during normal development (Kolb, 1995, p154).

Entry	Explanation
Rationale	1 A reasoned exposition of principles; an explanation or statement of reasons 2 The fundamental or underlying reason for or basis of a thing; a justification ('rationale, n.2.1 and 2' OED Online, 2020).
Regime	A way of doing things, esp. one having widespread influence or prevalence ('regime, n.2a' OED Online, 2020). The regime for managing dyslexia/ SpLD profile used in this book includes: recognising the pitfalls pausing using best thinking preferences knowing the relevant goal. The regime is highly personalised.
Schema	An (unconscious) organised mental model of something in terms of which new information can be interpreted or an appropriate response made (OED, 1993).
Self-esteem	Esteem: value, worth, favourable opinion (OED, 1993); hence self-esteem is valuing oneself.
Senses	The five physical senses are vision, hearing, taste, smell and kinaesthetic, which is made up of touch, position and movement. The use of taste and smell to help use information is not covered in this book, although they are important for some people.
Subliminal Subliminal learning	Subliminal: below the level of consciousness. Subliminal learning is learning which happens without conscious effort or attention; it simply happens alongside other learning or through everyday life.

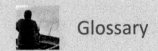

Entry	Explanation
Taking-action	Used in this book to mean: 'applying knowledge and skills in a practical way through kinaesthetic processing. The hyphen is deliberate.
	Taking-action is used in conjunction with 'doing' to facilitate discussing kinaesthetic processing and learning. It is used in parallel with reading, writing, listening and talking to give the following table for acquiring and applying knowledge and skills:

Acquiring	Applying
Reading	Writing
Listening	Speaking
Doing	Taking-action

Entry	Explanation
Thinking preferences	A major component of dealing with your dyslexia/ SpLD is to know how you think best (Stacey, 2019).
Working memory	Part of the mind/ brain which has the capacity for complex thought; it has temporary storage and its workings can be monitored and directed by conscious attention.

References

Baddeley, Alan, 2007, *Working Memory, Thought, and Action,* Oxford University Press, Oxford

Kolb, Bryan, 1995, *Brain Plasticity and Behaviour,* Lawrence Erlbaum Associates, Mahwah, NJ

OED[1], Brown, Lesley, Ed in Chief, 1993, *The New Shorter Oxford English Dictionary on Historical Principles*, Clarendon Press, Oxford

O'Connor, Joseph and McDermott, Ian, 1996, *Principles of NLP,* Thorsons, London

Stacey, Ginny, 2019, *Finding Your Voice with Dyslexia and other SpLDs,* Routledge, London

Website information

DfES Report, 2005, https://www.patoss-dyslexia.org/Resources/DSA-Working-Guidelines Accessed 10 June 2020

OED Online, September 2020, Oxford University Press Accessed 24 October 2020

---

[1] The online OED has been consulted every time, and the meanings are consistent. Sometimes the words used in the hard copy of OED (1993) are clearer, or more to the point in the context of this book; in which case the reference is to the hard copy edition that I have consulted.

List of Templates
on the Website

This table lists the *TEMPLATES* on the companion *WEBSITE* that are recommended in each chapter.

		Table	page
The sections on the *WEBSITE* are:			
A: Aids for Reading		2A-B:	p 584-585
B: Gathering Insights		2A-B:	p 584-585
C: Individual, Personal Profile of Dyslexia/ SpLD		3B:	p 587
D: Regime for Managing Dyslexia/ SpLD		3B:	p 587
E: Thinking Preferences		3A-B:	p 587-588
G: Developing skills		3A:	p 587
H: Check-lists		1:	p 583

There is no significant difference between ✓ and ◊; having 2 symbols just makes tracking easier.

Table 1 lists the check-lists that can be used with this book.

Chapter 3 acts as the opening for chapters 4 – 14, so the templates listed for chapter 3 will be useful for chapters 4 – 14.

For chapters 9, 12 and 13, no extra templates are listed in these tables.

Table 2 lists the templates from sections A and B as recommended in the Useful Preface, chapters and appendices.

Table 3 lists the templates from sections C, D, E, and G recommended for chapters 1, 4, 6. Appendix 2 and Appendix 3.

Website information

Series website: www.routledge.com/cw/stacey

Table 1

These check-lists are described in *CHECK-LISTS FOR READERS*, p 21.
The most relevant sections of the book are also listed in *CHECK-LISTS FOR READERS*.
Several of the check-lists cover ideas from the whole book.

		Name of template
H	1	Check-list for researchers and assessors
H	2	Check-list about the general background
H	3	Audit of understanding and skills – for an individual dyslexic/ SpLD person
H	4	Check-list for direct support
H	5	Check-list for general teaching
H	6	Check-list for professional people exercising responsibility or authority
H	7	Check-list for policy-makers, campaigners and media personnel
H	8	Check-list for indirect communication

Table 2 A

Name of Template U-P is Useful Preface			✓ U-P	◊ 1	✓ 2	◊ 3	✓ 4	◊ 5	✓ 6	◊ 7
Jotting down as you scan	A	1	✓	◊	✓	◊				
Bookmark – purpose	A	2	✓	◊	✓	◊				
Bookmark – profile and techniques	A	3					✓			
Jotting down as you read, with a few guiding questions	A	4	✓	◊	✓	◊				
Collecting ideas that interest you	A	5	✓	◊	✓	◊				
Collecting ideas that relate to you	B	1	✓	◊	✓	◊				
Know your own mind	B	2		◊						
Compare expectations and reality	B	3		◊				◊		
Action, results, next step	B	4		◊				◊	✓	
Recording template - 1 (4th column narrower for coding)	B	5		◊			✓	◊		◊
Recording template - 2 (4 equal columns)	B	6		◊			✓	◊		◊
Recording template - 3 (5th column narrower for coding)	B	7		◊		◊	✓	◊		◊
Recording template - 4 (5 equal columns)	B	8		◊			✓	◊		◊
A calendar month for prioritising – 5 weeks	B	9								
Questions to ask oneself to help observation	B	10								
Monitoring progress	B	11		◊						

Table 2 B

Name of Template / A1 – A3 are Appendices 1 – 3			◊ 8	✓ 10	◊ 11	✓ 14	◊ A1	✓ A2	◊ A3
Jotting down as you scan	A	1					◊		
Bookmark – purpose	A	2							
Bookmark – profile and techniques	A	3						✓	
Jotting down as you read, with a few guiding questions	A	4							
Collecting ideas that interest you	A	5							
Collecting ideas that relate to you	B	1					◊	✓	◊
Know your own mind	B	2						✓	
Compare expectations and reality	B	3				✓	◊		
Action, results, next step	B	4				✓	◊		
Recording template - 1 (4th column narrower for coding)	B	5				✓	◊		
Recording template - 2 (4 equal columns)	B	6	◊			✓	◊		
Recording template - 3 (5th column narrower for coding)	B	7		✓		✓	◊	✓	
Recording template - 4 (5 equal columns)	B	8				✓	◊	✓	
A calendar month for prioritising – 5 weeks	B	9			◊	✓	◊		
Questions to ask oneself to help observation	B	10					◊		
Monitoring progress	B	11					◊		

Table 3 A

Templates from sections E and G recommended for chapters 1, 4, 6.

Chapter 1

		Name of template
E	1	List of options for thinking preference
E	7	The box 'other'
G	1	The function of 'round' and other words
G	2	The functions of words
G	3	Constant content to demonstrate language function
G	4	Basic sentence pattern
G	5	Basic sentences from a complex one

Chapter 4

		Name of template
G	6	Eye-span exercises 1&2
G	7	Eye-span exercises 3
G	8	The story Paper split to show word groups
G	9	The short story: Paper

Chapter 6

		Name of template
E	1	List of options for thinking preference
E	7	The box 'other'

Table 3 B

Templates from sections C, D and E recommended for Appendix 2 and Appendix 3.

Appendix 2

		Name of template
C	1	Individual, personal profile of dyslexia/ SpLD (spatial)
C	2	Example individual, personal profile of dyslexia/ SpLD (spatial)
C	3	Individual, personal profile of dyslexia/ SpLD (linear)
C	4	2 Examples of individual, personal profiles of dyslexia/ SpLD (linear)
D	1	Managing dyslexia/ SpLD (mind map)
D	2	Managing dyslexia/ SpLD (linear)
D	3	Regime for managing dyslexia/ SpLD (spatial)
D	4	Regime for managing dyslexia/ SpLD (linear)
D	5	Experiences for managing dyslexia/ SpLD (linear example)
E	2	Table of thinking preferences (spatial)
E	3	Example: Table of thinking preferences (spatial)
E	4	Thinking preferences (spatial)
E	5	Thinking preferences (linear)

Appendix 3

		Name of template
E	1	List of options for thinking preference

Index

*in front of an entry marks a word or phrase that is in the GLOSSARY, ⓖ, p 572

The following may be useful INDEX entries:

Interest	Entries	
Everyday life	SpLD experience words, comments about pitfalls time management confidence motivation	preparation listening communication, indirect practical work employment
Using the mind	mind, using the mind set thinking preferences memory recall	metacognition thinking skills techniques key words comprehension
Teaching	teaching learning education SpLD support SpLD exploring	reading entries writing spelling exams
Managing SpLD	SpLD exploring questions, generating useful, confidence prioritising	exercises goals accommodation pitfalls stress
Reader groups	SpLD vital for SpLD, good practice for all communication, indirect dialogue misinterpretation	policy-makers professional people key points, list of summaries, list of assumptions

Tip: To find a word in the text

If the word you are looking for doesn't show quickly, try running a ruler or envelope or other straight edge down the page. Doing this makes your eyes look at each line and you are more likely to find the word.

Occasionally, the entry refers to the context and not a specific word; so sometimes you need to read the text.

BBC SOUNDS

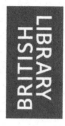

The BBC Listening Project records conversations between different people about many different kinds of experiences between people with a wide range of relationships.

Ginny and Sally — A Dyslexic Brain

Sally and I have enjoyed our journey working together on these four books and we recorded our thoughts about the experience for The Listening Project in April 2018. Though we are both dyslexic, our experience of dyslexia is quite different; we have different processing strengths and different ranges of problems. We are both positive about dealing with any problems and we both enjoy our various strengths. It has been huge fun working together, as we hope you can hear from our conversation.

An extract from our conversation is available on the BBC website at
https://www.bbc.co.uk/sounds/play/b0b1tmbl

The whole conversation is archived at the British Library and will be made available later this year (2020) at https://sounds.bl.uk

Full details of the recording can be found on the British Library's Sound and Moving Image catalogue at http://sami.bl.uk (search for C1500/1554).

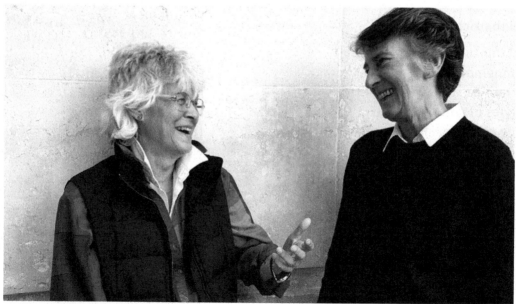

Ginny Stacey and Sally Fowler
Photo by Louise Pepper for the BBC Listening Project